Core Curriculum *for*
OCCUPATIONAL*&*
ENVIRONMENTAL
HEALTH NURSING

Core Curriculum *for* OCCUPATIONAL& ENVIRONMENTAL HEALTH NURSING

American Association of Occupational Health Nurses, Inc.

Edited by

Mary K. Salazar, EdD, RN, COHN-S, FAAOHN

Associate Professor
Director, Occupational Health Nursing Program
University of Washington School of Nursing
Department of Psychosocial and Community Health
Seattle, Washington

Second Edition

W. B. SAUNDERS COMPANY
A Harcourt Health Sciences Company
Philadelphia   London   Montreal   Sydney   Tokyo   Toronto

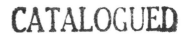

W.B. SAUNDERS COMPANY
A Harcourt Health Sciences Company

The Curtis Center
Independence Square West
Philadelphia, Pennsylvania 19106-3399

Library of Congress Cataloging-in-Publication Data

Core curriculum for occupational and environmental health nursing /
American Association of Occupational Health Nurses, Inc. ; edited by
Mary K. Salazar.—2nd ed.
   p. ; cm.
  Rev. ed. of: AAOHN core curriculum for occupational health nursing /
American Association of Occupational Health Nurses ; edited by Mary K.
Salazar. c1997.
  Includes bibliographical references and index.
  ISBN 0–7216–9207–9
  1. Industrial nursing. I. Salazar, Mary K. II. American Association of
Occupational Health Nurses. III. Title: AAOHN core curriculum for
occupational health nursing.
  [DNLM: 1. Occupational Health Nursing—education. 2. Education,
Nursing. 3. Environmental Health. WY 18 C79677 2001]
RC966 .A26 2001
610.73′46′0711—dc21   2001017014

Vice President and Publishing Director, Nursing: *Sally Schrefer*
Executive Editor: *N. Darlene Como*
Associate Developmental Editor: *Laura Selkirk*
Project Manager: *Catherine Jackson*
Production Editor: *Jodi Everding*
Designer: *Amy Buxton*

CORE CURRICULUM FOR OCCUPATIONAL AND ENVIRONMENTAL HEALTH
NURSING   ISBN: 0-7216-9207-9

Second Edition

Printed in the United States of America

Last digit is the print number: 01 02 03 04 05 GW/MV 9 8 7 6 5 4 3 2 1

NOTICE

Pharmacology is an ever-changing field. Standard safety precautions must be followed, but as new research and clinical experience broaden our knowledge, changes in treatment and drug therapy may become necessary or appropriate. Readers are advised to check the most current product information provided by the manufacturer of each drug to be administered to verify the recommended dose, the method and duration of administration, and contraindications. It is the responsibility of the licensed prescriber, relying on experience and knowledge of the patient, to determine dosages and the best treatment for each individual patient. Neither the publisher nor the editor assumes any liability for any injury and/or damage to persons or property arising from this publication.

CONTRIBUTORS

Jacqueline Agnew, PhD, MPH, COHN-S, FAAN
Associate Professor, Director of Occupational Health Nursing Program, and Director of Education and Research Center in Occupational Health and Safety
Johns Hopkins School of Hygiene and Public Health
Baltimore, Maryland

Mary Amann, MS, RN, COHN-S
Faculty Member
University of Illinois College of Nursing
Department of Public Health, Mental Health and Administrative Nursing
Division of Occupational Health Nursing
Independent Consultant
Occupational Health Information and Management Systems
Chicago, Illinois

Randal D. Beaton, PhD, EMT
Research Professor, Clinical Psychologist
Occuaptional Health Nursing Program
University of Washington School of Nursing
Department of Psychosocial and Community Health
Seattle, Washington

Barbara J. Burgel, MS, RN, COHN-S, FAAN
Clinical Professor and Adult Nurse Practitioner
University of California San Francisco School of Nursing
Occupational Health Nursing Graduate Program
San Francisco, California

Kay N. Campbell, EdD, RN-C, COHN-S
Manager, Health and Wellness Resources
GlaxoSmithKline, Inc.
Research Triangle Park, North Carolina

Eleanor McCarthy Chamberlin, RN, COHN-S, CCM
Disability Account Manager
Kemper National Services
Plantation, Florida

Frances Childre, MS, RNC, ANP, COHN-S
Director, Employee Health/Workers' Compensation
Emory Hospitals & University
Atlanta, Georgia

Catherine Connon, PhD, RN
Public Health Advisor
Washington State
Department of Labor and Industries
Olympia, Washington

Janet deCarteret, MN, RN, COHN-S
Consultant
Self-employed
Bellevue, Washington

Deborah V. DiBenedetto, MBA, BSN, RN, COHN-S/CM, ABDA
President
DVDiBenedetto & Associates Ltd.
Yonkers, New York

Mary E. Dirksen, MN, RN, COHN-S
Occupational Health Nurse Consultant
Seattle, Washington

Michelle Kom Gochnour, MN, RN, COHN-S
Lecturer and Assistant Director
Occupational Health Nursing Program
University of Washington School of Nursing
Department of Psychosocial and Community Health
Seattle, Washington

Marilyn Hau, MS, RN-C, COHN-S, OHST, ASP, CHMM
Director of Environmental Health and Safety
University of Illinois at Chicago
Chicago, Illinois

Diane J. Knoblauch, JD, MSN, RN
Attorney
Rohrbachers Light Cron Zmuda & Trimble Co., L.P.A.
Toledo, Ohio

**Elizabeth Lawhorn, MSN, RN,
  COHN-S, CCM**
ExxonMobil Corporation
Medicine and Occupational
  Health-Americas
Houston, Texas

Jane Lipscomb, PhD, RN, FAAN
Associate Professor
University of Maryland School of Nursing
Baltimore, Maryland

**Sally L. Lusk, PhD, RN, FAAN,
  FAAOHN**
Professor and Director
Occupational Health Nursing Program
The University of Michigan School
  of Nursing
Ann Arbor, Michigan

Mary E. Miller, MN, RN, ARNP
Occupational Health Nurse Practitioner
Washington State
Department of Labor and Industries
Olympia, Washington

Karin Myerson, BSN, RN, COHN-S
Occupational Health Consultant
Myerson Occupational & Environmental
  Medicine, PC
Silver Spring, Maryland

Jane Parker-Conrad, PhD, RN, FAAOHN
Occupational Health Consultant
Conrad & Conrad Consultants
Knoxville, Tennessee

Jean Randolph, RN, COHN-S/CM, MPA
Employee Health Manager
Children's Healthcare of Atlanta
Atlanta, Georgia

Bonnie Rogers, DrPH, COHN-S, FAAN
Director, Occupational Health Nursing
  Program and
The Health Services Research in
  Occupational Safety and Health
  Program
School of Public Health
The University of North Carolina
  at Chapel Hill
Chapel Hill, North Carolina

**Mary K. Salazar, EdD, RN, COHN-S,
  FAAOHN**
Associate Professor
Director, Occupational Health Nursing
  Program
University of Washington School
  of Nursing
Department of Psychosocial and
  Community Health
Seattle, Washington

Barbara Sattler, DrPH, RN
Director, Environmental Health Education
  Center
Associate Professor
University of Maryland School of Nursing
Baltimore, Maryland

Kay Stepler, MA, BSN, CRRN, CCM
Process Expert, Operations Support
Crawford and Company
Atlanta, Georgia

**Patricia B. Strasser, PhD, RN,
  COHN-S/CM**
Owner
Partners in BusinessHealth Solutions, Inc.
Toledo, Ohio

Joy Wachs, PhD, RN, CS
Professor
East Tennessee State University
Mountain City, Tennessee

**Mary Lou Wassel, MEd, RN,
  COHN-S/CM, ARM**
Occupational Health Consultant
Fireman's Fund Insurance Company
Atlanta, Georgia

**Sandy Winzeler, MN, MPH, ANP,
  COHN-S**
Nurse Practitioner
Emory University Hospital
Atlanta, Georgia

FOREWORD

It is a great pleasure to welcome the reader to this second edition of the American Association of Occupational Health Nurses' (AAOHN) Core Curriculum for Occupational and Environmental Health Nursing. This edition of the Core Curriculum, expanded and more comprehensive than the first edition published in 1997, represents the latest body of knowledge pertinent to the field of occupational and environmental health nursing practice.

The business world is constantly changing, and we must adapt occupational health nursing practice to the needs of the populations and businesses we serve. Occupational health professionals are being challenged to demonstrate value, that is, the return on investment for their services and programs. Business drivers such as downsizing, right-sizing, outsourcing, "doing more with less," technology enhancements and improvements, and teleworking, all demand innovative approaches to delivering occupational health services. While many employees still report to a formal workplace, many others are now "virtual employees" in that they work where they live, and generally do not report to a formal workplace. The use of technology to communicate (e.g., by telephone, mobile, or handheld devices, email, intranet or internet) now demands that occupational health professionals communicate and deliver their services using the new technology to reach distant or "virtual" workforces.

We must position our practice for the 21st century to be competitive in the markets we serve. AAOHN, the professional association for occupational and environmental health nurses, defines the scope of practice and develops the standards that guide this specialty practice. This book provides the framework for the practice based on the scope and standards and reflects the changing and expanding roles of the profession.

The Core Curriculum will help you with your practice and will provide you with more than the "basics" of your business. We trust that you will find the newest edition of the Core Curriculum a valuable addition to your daily practice and library.

Sincerely,
Deborah V. DiBenedetto
President, AAOHN

PREFACE

The modern day workplace is inundated with constant and often dramatic changes that have the potential to affect the health and safety of workers and worker populations. Rapid advances in science and technology affect how work is done as well as the type of risks and dangers that are inherent in the work. The workforce is becoming more diverse, with an increasing number of older workers, workers with disabilities, and minority and female workers. More people are telecommuting or working at home, and the contracting and subcontracting of workers has become a prevalent practice among employers. Occupational and environmental health nurses must be knowledgeable about these and other forces and trends that affect organizational dynamics, and consequently, the health and safety of workers; and they need to possess business and political savvy so that they are well-prepared to deal with the complex interrelationships and environments that characterize most workplaces.

This edition of the Core Curriculum is intended to serve as a concise and comprehensive overview of the many dimensions of our specialty. As we developed this edition, we took special care to incorporate content that is relevant to the issues and concerns affecting the modern day workplace. There are several changes and additions that you will note as you examine this text. The first and most obvious is the expanded title that includes the words ". . . and environmental." These words have been used liberally throughout the text, as a reflection of a new direction in our practice in recent years. In addition to the updates and further development of the existing chapters, we have added four new chapters that focus on the following topics: information management systems, case management, psychosocial factors in the occupational setting, and, of course, environmental health.

Like the previous edition, this text is divided into three major sections:

The foundations of occupational and environmental health nursing practice, which provides a theoretical and conceptual overview of our practice;

Strategies and approaches to occupational and environmental health nursing practice, which focuses on the practical application of occupational health and safety principles to practice; and

Professionalism and future directions, which highlights issues and activities that contribute to the growth of our profession.

The appendixes were carefully selected to supplement the core content in the rest of the text. In addition to a list of resources to assist you in your practice, they also include a list of acronyms and a glossary, both of which can serve as quick references.

This text is the result of the collaboration of a great number of people. The authors and the reviewers who contributed to this text are known and respected occupational and environmental health nursing leaders. The content has been designed as a comprehensive resource for occupational and environmental health nurses from varying backgrounds and preparation, as well as a teaching tool for students who are emerging as our future leaders. We hope that you will find this text useful and practical, that it will result in your being better prepared to deal with a constantly changing work environment, and that it will enable you to achieve the highest level of excellence in your practice.

Mary K. Salazar
Managing Editor

ACKNOWLEDGMENTS

The completion of the second edition of AAOHN's core curriculum is the result of the contributions and the hard work of numerous individuals. First of all, I am so very grateful to all of the chapter authors for the excellence of their work, for the timeliness of their contributions, and for their patience and endurance through all stages of the text's development. It was my good fortune to work with such an exceptional and talented group of people!

In addition to all of the current authors, I would also like to thank all of the individuals who contributed to the first edition of the core curriculum, which served as a foundation for the development of this edition. These include:

Kay Arendasky, MSN, CRNP
Felicia J. Bayer, MSN, RN-C
Julia Faucett, PhD, RN
Jeannie K. Hanna, MSN, RN, COHN-S
Winifred Hayes, PhD, MS, CRNP
Christina Johnson, BSN, COHN-S
Diane Kjervik, JD, MS, RN, FAAN
Kleia Luckner, JD, MSN, CNM, RN
Susan Martyn, JD, BA
Judith S. Ostendorf, MPH, RN, COHN-S, CCM
Merey Price, MSN, RN
Jennifer B. Radford, MPH, RHV, SCM, COHN, Adv. Dip. TCDHE, FRSH
Genevieve B. Reed, MSN, RNC, COHN-S, OHNP
Betsy Eddins Richards, MSN, RN, COHN-S
Sharon Tanberg, MA, RN, COHN-S
Ann Keenan Widtfeldt, MPH, BSN, COHN-S, CCM

Thanks also to the following individuals who contributed to the review and production of this book. They are as follows:

AAOHN Staff
　Geraldine C. Williamson, MN, RN, CAE, Associate Executive Director
　Ann R. Cox, MN, RN, CAE, Executive Director
　Special Reviewers for Selected Portions of the Text
　Marilyn Edmondson, EdD, RN, AAOHN Project Coordinator, AAOHN/ATSDR Environmental Health Grant
　Elaine Papp, RN, CCM, COHN-S, Program Analyst, Director of Policy Division of Legislative Affairs
Publishers' Staff
　Thomas Eoyang
　Adrienne Simon
　Laura Selkirk
　Darlene Como
　Mike Ederer

Lastly, I wish to thank the members of the American Association of Occupational Health Nurses for their dedication and commitment to the health and safety of our nation's workers.

CONTENTS

SECTION ONE

Foundations of Occupational and Environmental Health Nursing Practice, 1

1 *Occupational and Environmental Health Nursing:*
An Overview   3
MARY E. DIRKSEN

   Introduction to Occupational Health and Safety   3
   Historical Perspective on Work and Occupational Health   4
   Evolution of Occupational Safety and Health   7
   History of Workers' Compensation   10
   The Occupational Safety and Health Act   11
   National Health Goals: Healthy People and
     Healthy Communities   11
   Occupational Health in the International Community   12
   The Workplace: Occupational Hazards and Their Impact
     on Workers   13
   Work-Related Injury and Illness   16
   Assessment and Prevention of Occupational and Environmental
     Injury and Illness   20
   History and Evolution of Occupational and Environmental
     Health Nursing   21
   The Practice of Occupational and Environmental
     Health Nursing   24
   Future Opportunities and Challenges   29

2 *Workers and Worker Populations*   33
SALLY LUSK, CATHERINE CONNON, MARY E. DIRKSEN, AND MARY E. MILLER

   Demographic and Social Trends   33
   Technologic Trends   35
   Females in the Work Force   36
   Minorities in the Work Force   38
   Age of Workers   39
   Children in the Work Force   41
   Contingent and Other Alternative Workers   45
   Workers in Labor Unions   48
   Disabled Workers   49
   Agricultural Workers   50
   Construction Workers   53
   Health Care Workers   56
   International (Expatriate) Workers   61

3 *Legal and Ethical Issues*   71
DIANE KNOBLAUCH, FRANCES CHILDRE, AND PATRICIA STRASSER

Sources of Law   71
Basic Legal Concepts Relevant to Occupational
    and Environmental Health Nursing Practice   72
Legal Responsibilities of the Occupational and Environmental
    Health Nurse   73
Occupational Safety and Health Act (Public Law 91-596)   73
Americans with Disabilities Act of 1990   77
Family and Medical Leave Act (FMLA) of 1993 (29CFR825.118)   79
The Department of Transportation   80
Documentation   81
Types of Records   83
Preservation of Employee Health and Exposure Records   85
Access to Employee Medical and Exposure Records   85
Overview of Workers' Compensation   87
Overview of Workers' Compensation Benefits   88
Professional Position on Ethics   89
Ethics: Definitions and Principles   90
Ethical Conflicts   90

4 *Economic, Political, and Business Forces*   95
DEBORAH V. DIBENEDETTO

Introduction to Economics   95
Economic State of the Nation   97
The Impact of Economics on the Individual   97
Changes in the National Economy   99
Factors Affecting National and Global Competitiveness   99
International Trade Status of the Nation   100
The Global Marketplace   101
Implications for the Occupational and Environmental
    Health Nurse   101
Business Trends   102
Major Business Issues   103
Implications for Occupational and Environmental
    Health Nursing   105
Health Care Reform and Managed Health Care   106
Overview of Managed Care   106
Quality Controls in Managed Care   107
Judging Standards of Care   108
Defining and Evaluating Quality Outcomes   108
Implications for Occupational and Environmental
    Health Nursing   109

5 *Scientific Foundations of Occupational and Environmental Health Nursing Practice*   111
JACQUELINE AGNEW

History of Nursing Science   111
Research–Theory–Practice Linkages   112
Early Nursing Theory   113
The Domain of Nursing   113
Modern Nursing Theory: Middle-Range Theories   114
The Practice of Occupational and Environmental
    Health Nursing   115
The Effects of the Environment on Health   115
Overview of Epidemiologic Terms and Principles   116
Measures of Association   117
Sources of Epidemiologic Data   118
Comparisons of Rates   118
Types of Rates   118
Inferential Statistics   119
Overview of Study Designs   120
Bias and Confounding in Epidemiologic Studies   121
Screening   122
Overview of Toxicologic Terms and Principles   123
Major Exposure Routes   124
The Dose-Response Relationship   125
Nature of Effects   125
The Fate of Toxins in the Body   126
Endogenous and Exogenous Host Factors   126
Examples of Work-Related Exposures and Their Effects   128
Overview of Industrial Hygiene   134
Sources of Information to Facilitate Hazard Recognition   134
Sampling Methods   135
Airborne Contaminants   135
Control Strategies for Occupational Exposures   136
Overview of Ergonomic Terms and Principles   136
Musculoskeletal Disorders   136
Risk Factors for Musculoskeletal Problems   137
High-Risk Jobs   138
Evaluating Risk Factors   138
Ergonomic Improvements   139
Occupational Injury Epidemiology   139
Countermeasures   140
Implications for Occupational and Environmental
    Health Nurses   141
Effects of Social Conditions and Behavior on Health   142
Health Promotion and Risk Reduction   143

6 Principles of Administration and Management   147
JOY WACHS

Leadership   147
Strategic Planning   148
The Management Process   150
The Organization: Its Culture, Climate, and Structure   152
Policies and Procedures   153
Fiscal Issues: Budgeting and Resource Management   154
Human Resources Issues   156
Communication   160
Project Management   161
Time Management   162
Critical Thinking   162
The Image of the Occupational and Environmental
    Health Nurse   163
Application of Ethics to Decision-Making   163
Outcomes Management   164
Benchmarking   164
Total Quality Management   165

7 Information Management in the Occupational Health Setting   171
MARY AMANN

Introduction to Nursing Informatics   171
Tools Available to the Occupational and Environmental
    Health Nurse   172
Selecting and Implementing Information Management Systems   173
The Internet   181
Intranets   183
Office Management Programs   184
Implications for Occupational and Environmental
    Health Nursing   185

SECTION TWO

Strategies and Approaches to Occupational and Environmental Health Nursing Practice, 189

8 Developing, Implementing, and Evaluating a Comprehensive Occupational Health and Safety Program   191
KARIN MYERSON AND JANE PARKER-CONRAD

Assessment   191
Program Planning   193
Program Implementation   194

The Evaluation Process   *196*
Structure, Process, and Outcome   *197*
Methods of Evaluation   *202*
Cost-Effective and Cost-Benefit Programs   *203*
Other Health and Safety Program Considerations   *204*

9 *Prevention of Occupational Injuries and Illnesses*   *209*
MARILYN HAU

Recognition and identification   *209*
  First Steps in a Prevention Program   *209*
  Methods of Identifying Hazards   *210*
Hazard evaluation and analysis   *218*
  Purpose of Hazard Evaluation and Analysis   *218*
  Industry Standards   *219*
  Exposure Monitoring   *221*
  Occupational Health Surveillance   *224*
  Worker Populations Analysis   *225*
Prevention and control   *228*
  Indentifying Appropriate Prevention and Control Approach   *228*
  Prevention and Control Approaches That Focus
    on Engineering Controls   *228*
  Prevention and Control Approaches That Focus
    on Administrative Controls   *234*
  Prevention and Control Approaches That Focus
    on Personal Productive Equipment   *239*

10 *Direct Care in the Occupational Setting*   *247*
BARBARA BURGEL

  Definition of Terms   *247*
  Overview of Direct Care   *248*
  Health History   *251*
  The Physical Evaluation   *255*
  Clinical Decision Making   *256*
  Practice Guidelines   *257*
  Application of Levels of Prevention to Direct Care Activities   *258*
  Evaluating Outcomes   *267*

11 *Disability Case Management*   *271*
MARY LOU WASSEL, JEAN RANDOLPH, KAY STEPLER,
AND SANDY WINZELER

  Case Management   *271*
  Important Case Management Terms   *271*
  Historical Perspective   *273*
  Practice Settings for Case Management Services   *275*
  Team Roles and Responsibilities   *275*

Steps in Program Development   *278*
Return to Work   *282*
Integrated Disability Management Programs   *288*
Federal Acts   *289*
Delivery Models   *289*

12 *Health Promotion and Adult Education*   *293*
KAY N. CAMPBELL

Overview of Health Promotion   *293*
National Health Promotion Objectives   *294*
Health Models   *295*
Behavior Change Theories and Models   *296*
Levels of Prevention   *298*
Framework for a Health Promotion Program   *298*
Lifestyle and Health Promotion   *302*
Employee Assistance Programs   *304*
Introduction to Adult Education   *307*
Philosophies of Adult Education   *310*
Motivating Adults to Learn   *310*
Teaching Methods and Techniques   *314*
Effective Presentations   *318*

13 *Managing Psychosocial Factors in the Occupational Setting*   *327*
MARY K. SALAZAR AND RANDAL D. BEATON

Overview of Psychosocial Factors   *327*
Psychosocial Hazards   *328*
Occupational Stress   *333*
Effects of Stress on Workers   *334*
Effects of Stress on Organizations   *335*
Occupational Stress Models   *335*
An Ecologic Approach to Occupational Stress   *336*
Managing Psychosocial Factors in the Workplace   *338*
Evaluating Interventions Targeting Adverse Effects
    of Psychosocial Factors   *340*

14 *Examples of Occupational Health and Safety Programs*   *343*
JANET DECARTERET, MARILYN HAU, AND MICHELLE KOM GOCHNOUR

International travel health and safety program   *343*
Purposes of an International Travel Health and Safety Program   *343*
Employer's Responsibilities to Traveling Employees   *343*
Occupational and Environmental Health
    Nurse's Responsibilities   *344*
Traveler's Responsibilities   *344*
Health and Safety Education for Travel   *345*

Control of Prevalent Communicable Diseases   346
Post-Travel Evaluation for Long-Term Travelers   348
Hearing-loss prevention program   349
Noise-Induced Hearing Loss   349
Purposes of a Hearing-Loss Prevention Program   349
Management's Role in an HLPP   350
The Role of the Hearing-Loss Prevention Coordinator   350
The Role of Workers   351
Program Requirements   351
Noise Assessment and Control   351
Worker Training and Education   352
Hearing Protection Devices   354
Audiometric Testing   355
Record Keeping   357
Program Evaluation   357
Hazard communication program   357
Purposes of a Hazard Communications Program   358
Management's Role   358
Description of the Program   358
Elements of the HazCom Program   359
Material Safety Data Sheets   360
Trade Secrets   360
Container Labeling and Warning Requirements   361
Record Keeping   361
Evaluation   361
Drug and alcohol testing program   361
Purposes of a Drug and Alcohol Testing Program   362
Preliminary Considerations   362
Program Components   363
Employee Assistance Programs   363
Training and Education   364
The Drug Free Workplace Act of 1998   364
Elements of a Drug and Alcohol Testing Program   365
Consequences of Drug and Alcohol Abuse   367
Emergency preparedness/disaster plan   367
Purposes of an Emergency Preparedness/Disaster Plan   367
The Scope of the Plan   368
Program Responsibilities   368
General Emergency Procedures   371
Specific Emergency Procedures   373
Recovery Procedures   374
Program Maintenance   375
Appendices to Include in a Written Plan   376
Ergonomics programs   377
Overview of Ergonomics   377
Work-Related Musculoskeletal Disorders   378
Ergonomic Regulation   378

Purposes of an Ergonomics Program   *379*
Program Components   *379*
Training and Education   *384*
Health Care Management   *385*
Documentation and Recordkeeping   *385*
Program Evaluation   *386*

SECTION THREE

Advancing Professionalism in Occupational and Environmental Health Nursing, *391*

15 *Environmental Health*   *393*
JANE LIPSCOMB AND BARBARA SATTLER

Introduction   *393*
Environmental Health Assessment   *395*
Children and Environmental Health   *396*
Environmental Justice and Advocacy   *398*
Risk Assessment, Risk Management, and Risk Communication *399*
Federal Agencies   *401*
Accessing Information and the "Right to Know"   *403*
Environmental health risks across settings   *404*
Environmental Health Risks in the Home   *404*
Environmental Risks in Schools   *406*
Environmental Risks in the Community   *406*
Environmental Risks at Work   *408*
Nurses' roles in environmental health   *408*
General Environmental Health Competency for Nurses   *408*
The Institute of Medicine's Recommendations on
    Nursing Practice, Education, Research, and Advocacy   *409*

16 *Research*   *411*
BONNIE ROGERS

Professional Mandates for Research   *411*
Research Roles of Occupational and Environmental Health
    Nurses by Education Level   *411*
Purposes of Research   *412*
Ethics in Research   *412*
Research Development   *413*
Research Dissemination   *418*
Research Utilization   *418*
Research Priorities   *418*
Evaluating Research   *419*
Funding Research   *421*

17 *Professional Issues: Advancing the Specialty* 425
ELEANOR MCCARTHY CHAMBERLIN AND ELIZABETH LAWHORN

Professional Associations 425

Professional Credentialing in Nursing 426

Competency in Occupational and Environmental
Health Nursing 427

Strategies for Advancing the Discipline and Practice 428

Role Expansion 433

Partnerships in Occupational and Environmental Health 434

APPENDIXES

APPENDIX I   Occupational and Environmental Health
and Safety Resources 437

APPENDIX II   Glossary 443

APPENDIX II   Acronyms 450

APPENDIX IV   Web Sites 455

APPENDIX V   Occupational Safety and Health
Administration Act of 1970 458

APPENDIX VI   American Association of Occupational Health Nurses
Code of Ethics 460

APPENDIX VII Occupational and Environmental Health
and Safety Legislation 461

SECTION ONE

Foundations of Occupational and Environmental Health Nursing Practice

~

CHAPTER

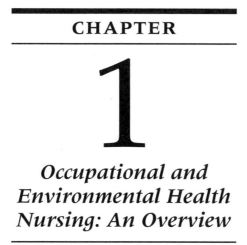

1

Occupational and Environmental Health Nursing: An Overview

MARY E. DIRKSEN

The primary focus of occupational and environmental health nursing practice is preventing work-related illnesses and injuries and promoting health and safety among workers and worker populations. Achieving these goals requires a clear understanding of the basic terminology used in this specialty and knowledge of the principles that underpin occupational and environmental health nursing practice, education, and research. This chapter presents an overview of the traditions and concepts inherent to the field, and a historical perspective of the development of the profession and practice.

I Introduction to Occupational Health and Safety

A The mission of occupational health and safety is "to assure so far as possible every working man and woman in the nation safe and healthful working conditions" (United States Congress, Occupational Safety and Health Act, 1970). (Appendix V).

B The primary objectives of occupational health and safety practice include the following:
1. Preventing work-related illnesses and injuries through a systematic process of assessment, data collection, planning, intervention, and evaluation
2. Evaluating and treating work-related injury or illness
3. Promoting health and safety behaviors among workers and worker populations
4. Implementing hazard prevention and abatement interventions that promote safe and healthy work environments while remaining consistent with organizational goals
5. Advocating organizational attention to environmental concerns on behalf of workers, their families, and the broader community

C The goals and objectives of occupational health and safety practice are achieved through the collaboration of multiple professional disciplines, which may include the following, depending on the needs of the work setting and the scope of the organization's occupational health program:
1. Occupational and environmental health nurses focus on promoting, protecting, restoring, and maintaining workers' health within the context of a safe and healthful work environment.

2. Occupational physicians focus on preventing, detecting, and treating work-related diseases and injuries.

3. Industrial hygienists identify, evaluate, and control toxic exposures and hazards in the work environment.

4. Safety engineers and other safety professionals focus on preventing occupational injuries and maintaining or creating safe workplaces and safe work practices.

5. Other professionals provide specific expertise as required by the occupational health and safety program needs of the organization; these could include epidemiologists, toxicologists, industrial engineers, ergonomists, health educators, occupational and physical therapists, and vocational rehabilitation specialists.

D **The workplace is characterized by multidimensional and complex environments that affect worker health and safety. These environments include the following (Figure 1-1):**

1. Social: the meaning of work, the social milieu of the worker (including the worker's baseline health status) and the structure of work

2. Cultural: beliefs, attitudes, and values related to work

3. Political: the prevalent ideology in a society; the distribution of power and level of governmental support for worker health and safety

4. Economic: the levels of unemployment, competition, and wage regulation, and the overall health of the local economy

5. Organizational: corporate mission, philosophy, and values; financial and structural viability of the organization; job security issues; and production structure and requirements

E **Occupational health and safety should be considered an integral part of all health services.**

1. Most Americans are directly or indirectly affected by hazards in the workplace.

2. Occupational health and safety services affect not only the worker, but also the worker's family, significant others, and community, and the larger society.

F **Occupational and environmental health sciences are in an early stage of development; much remains to be learned about the effect of the work environment on the health and safety of workers.**

II Historical Perspective on Work and Occupational Health

The concept and value of work is fundamental to every nation, race, culture, and time.

A **Earliest recorded history**

1. Hippocrates recognized clusters of specific diseases among craftsmen by 400 BC (Hunter, 1978).

2. Ancient miners were observed by Pliny the Elder (23-79 AD) to wear protective breathing devices to avoid inhaling toxic dusts and vapors.

B **The Middle Ages (roughly 500-1500 AD)**

1. Profitable work consisted primarily of crafts and arts using various metals, chemicals and minerals, the use of which was accompanied by observed adverse health effects.

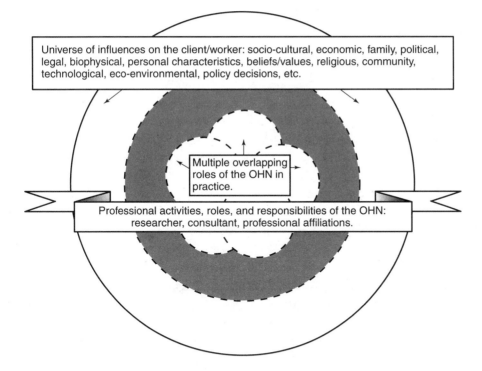

FIGURE 1-1 *A model for occupational and environmental health nursing.*

This model illustrates the interconnectedness and fluidity of the elements constituting and affected by the practice of occupational and environmental health nursing. The client, whether individual workers, aggregates of workers, or an organization's administration, is influenced by myriad work-related and external variables, all of which effect the individual, collective, or organizational state of health and safety. The roles and responsibilities of the occupational health nurse overlap. All interactions between the occupational health nurse and the client are bound together and guided by the professional responsibilities and activities engaged in by the occupational health nurse. The junction where the occupational health nurse and the client meet, each bringing their individual and collective experience to the interaction (as illustrated by the broken lines), represents the common ground where health and safety goals are mutually determined and realized. (Adapted from Dirksen, et al., 1994)

    2. Most manufacturing was conducted in rural homes, although some occurred in guild shops in towns.

    3. Increased competition resulted in increased production and escalating work hazards.

C **Preindustrial age**

    1. Georgius Agricola (1494-1555 AD) described the ailments of miners, such as joint, lung, and eye problems.

    2. Paracelsus (1493-1541 AD)

        a. Identified acute and chronic health effects in craftsmen exposed to metal smelting fumes

        b. Articulated the principle paradigm of toxicology, the dose/response ratio, when he wrote: "All substances are poisons; there is none which is not. Only the dose differentiates a poison from a remedy."

3. Bernardino Ramazzini (1633-1714 AD), considered the "father of occupational medicine"
   a. Published *De Morbis Artifactum Diatriba (The Diseases of Workmen)* in 1713, describing more than 100 different trade occupations, their associated hazards, and various methods of protection for tradespeople, including protective clothing, adequate ventilation, and proper working posture
   b. Noted that workers "who hoped for a subsistence . . . are too often repaid with the most dangerous diseases" (Ramazzini, 1993, p. 39)
   c. Encouraged physicians to inquire into their patients' occupations as part of their assessments

D **The industrial revolution (mid-18th to mid-19th century)**
1. Ordinary citizens' lifestyles in European and American societies were transformed by the shift from agrarian or home-based hand manufacturing to urban-based industrial processes.
2. Power-driven machinery introduced dramatic changes in production and work process.
   a. Mass factory production began in England in 1718 with the first mechanized silk-textile mill.
   b. Machine-driven jobs became specialized and work became monotonous.
3. The economic and social impact of work-related injury, illness, and death became evident with the high rates of factory workers affected.

E **America's response to the industrial revolution**
1. American economic focus shifted from agriculture to industry.
   a. Millions flocked to urban industrial centers for the promise of cash wages and an improved lifestyle.
   b. Company-owned housing districts became overcrowded, unsanitary centers of poverty and communicable disease.
   c. The abundant labor supply gave rise to massive exploitation of women, children, and non–English speaking immigrants; child labor and slavery were routine.
2. Trends toward division of labor, ownership of the means of production, and capitalism emerged.
   a. Accidents and workplace deaths were considered inevitable and acceptable consequences of progress.
   b. The industrial ethic of the time placed profit and property rights above human rights.
3. Working conditions were abysmal; machines were largely without protective devices and accidental-death rates were high.

F **The American workplace in the postindustrial era**
1. Throughout the early 1900s, responsibility for work-related injuries and illnesses was placed on the worker rather than on the hazards that caused injury and illness.
   a. Company-based industrial medicine programs focused on preemployment physical examinations.
   b. Primary causes of accidents were identified as lack of English language skills, inexperience, and worker carelessness.
   c. Prevention strategies were aimed at altering worker behaviors rather than controlling or preventing workplace hazard sources.
2. The economic and social conditions prevalent in the early 20th century led to a rise in the number of industrial nurses.

3. Alice Hamilton (1869-1970), considered the "matriarch of American occupational health":
   a. Was the first American physician to devote her life's work to industrial health
   b. Studied and documented the adverse human effects associated with occupational exposure to industrial toxins such as lead, arsenic, carbon monoxide, and solvents
   c. Published *Industrial Poisons in the United States* (1925) and *Exploring the Dangerous Trades* (1943)
   d. Served as editor of *The Journal of Industrial Hygiene*

III Evolution of Occupational Safety and Health

A **State and federal agencies and legislation focusing on workplace health and safety (Appendix VII)**
   1. Formal workplace regulation began in England with the Factory Acts; eight Acts were passed between 1802 and 1891.
   2. In the United States, Massachusetts created the first factory inspection department in 1867.
   3. State and federal reporting requirements for industrial accidents began in the late 1800s; the National Safety Council was organized in 1913 to collect and document occupational injury and illness data.
   4. The Federal Bureau of Labor, established in 1884 and reorganized as the United States Department of Labor (USDL) in 1913, was created "to foster, promote and develop the welfare of wage earners in the United States" (from William B. Wilson, first USDL secretary, 1913-1921) (http://www.blossburg.org/wb_wilson/thestory_6.htm)
   5. The U.S. Public Health Service (PHS), established in 1912, began to scientifically investigate and analyze the effects of toxins on individual workers.
   6. The New Deal of 1933 included occupational health reform statutes, and encouraged a renewed advocacy for workplace health and safety, efforts that had waned in the antilabor sentiment following World War I.
   7. The Division of Labor Standards was established in 1934 to collaborate with other organizations to develop safety codes and standards, disseminate information about chemical hazards to workers, and improve the efficacy of factory inspection processes.
   8. The National Labor Relations Act of 1935 and the Labor-Management Relations Act (Taft-Hartley Act) of 1947 were enacted to govern relations between workers and management which had, before that time, been confrontational, litigious, and sometimes violent.
   9. The Occupational Safety and Health Act (OSH Act) of 1970 established the Occupational Safety and Health Administration (OSHA) as an agency within the USDL.
   10. In 1970, the OSH Act established the National Institute for Occupational Safety and Health (NIOSH) as an institute within the PHS; it is currently positioned within the Centers for Disease Control and Prevention (CDC).

B **Organized labor's involvement in occupational health and safety (Box 1-1 presents a chronology of the labor movement.)**
   1. As workers began to assert their demands for workplace health and safety reforms, tensions between labor and management increased.

BOX 1-1

A chronology of the labor movement in the United States

1600s   • Agriculture was the major U.S. industry.

1739   • Boston shipyard workers formed the first political organization, called the "Caucus".

1750   • Trade associations developed among carpenters, tailors, and ironworkers.

1780s   • American and European economies shifted to a merchant/capitalist system.

1836   • The 10-hour workday was initiated.

1866   • The National Labor Union was established following an economic depression.

1876   • The Socialist Labor Party established its headquarters in New York.

1886   • The American Federation of Labor (AFL) was formed.

1913   • The U.S. Department of Labor was established.

1929   • The Great Depression resulted in nationwide unemployment, increasing by 12 million in 3 years.

1933   • The New Deal was introduced to stimulate the economy; millions found employment in federally sponsored works programs.
            • The Social Security Act was signed into law.

1937   • The Council of Industrial Organizations (CIO) organized strikes in all major industries.

1946   • The Full Employment Act was signed to increase national employment.

1947   • The Taft-Hartley Act was signed; intended to restrict union behavior to allow commerce to develop.

Sources: Encyclopedia of Work, The History of Occupations; lecture by Shirley Murphy, April 1992

2. The Knights of Labor, one of the earliest labor unions, began agitating for workplace safety laws in the 1870s (Levenstein et al., 1999).

3. Among the few early strategies effective in improving workplace conditions were labor strikes and lawsuits brought by injured workers against employers.

4. Labor unions are now the major organizations that represent and pursue the collective interests of workers in matters of health and safety, often in collaboration with occupational health and safety professionals.

   a. Unionized workers are more likely to be informed about the presence of health and safety hazards than are nonunion workers in the same jobs (Weil, 1992).

   b. The following are a few of the successful campaigns conducted by labor unions:

      1) The 8-hour work day, which was federally legislated in 1968

      2) Overtime compensation

      3) OHSA's Cotton Dust Standard of 1978

      4) OSHA's Occupational Tuberculosis Standard was proposed in 1997; plans to pass the standard are currently in progress.

BOX 1-1

A chronology of the labor movement in the United States—cont'd

1955	• The AFL/CIO unified.
1962	• Federal employees gained the right to organize and bargain collectively.
1969	• End of Kennedy/Johnson era aided development of depressed areas, urban renewal, and discrimination initiatives
1970	• The Occupational Safety and Health Act was signed into law.
1972	• Caesar Chavez organized agricultural workers, initially in California and eventually nationwide.
1960s-1970s	• Rise in debate began over environmental protection vis-à-vis jobs.
	• Theory X vs. Theory Y management initiatives were tested.
	• Affirmative Action and Equal Opportunity Acts were signed.
1980s	• Major industries were deregulated.
	• Theory Z gained favor, implementing "The Japanese Way," which included quality circles, consensual decision making, and outplacement programs.
1992	• By the end of the Reagan/Bush era, less than 18% of workers were affiliated with a labor union, compared with half the labor force following World War II.
1990s	• Technology began to surpass ethical guidelines. For example, inherited conditions may one day bar a choice of occupation; the use of random drug testing in non–safety sensitive occupations raises ethical and privacy questions.
	• Mistrust rises between employers and employees (e.g., flextime was allowed but the lack of "facetime" was feared).
	• Telecommuting increased.

---

    c. Although union membership in the United States represents approximately 15% of the work force, the influence of these organizations reaches far beyond their unionized workplaces (Silverstein, 1999).

C **Public pressure and social activism's influence on workplace health and safety**

  1. Increasing societal intolerance of the exploitation and abuse of women and children in the mid-19th century led to factory reform and inspection legislation, which included provisions for limited working hours and a minimum age for child employment.

  2. Public outrage contributed to the Coal Mine Health and Safety Act of 1969, after a mining accident had killed 78 miners in West Virginia the previous year (Levenstein, et al., 1999).

  3. Advances in occupational health regulation have often occurred in concert with major environmental protection laws.

    a. Social activism in the 1960s raised awareness of the link between environmental and occupational health concerns and work processes.

    b. After publication of *Silent Spring* (Carson, 1963), public attention was directed at the human health and environmental consequences of certain pesticides, leading to production and usage bans of some products.

  c. Increased societal awareness of the hazards of chemical exposure has led to pressure to implement comprehensive protective interventions aimed at both the workplace in general and the management of manufacturing by-products and waste.

  d. Environmental impact studies, aimed at protecting both the local ecology and the population, are now required in many jurisdictions before establishing new industrial enterprises.

4. In the 1970s, a growing wellness/health promotion movement encouraged employers to implement workplace wellness programs.

  a. The goal of these wellness programs was to reduce costs by enhancing awareness of self-care, decreasing absenteeism, improving worker morale, and increasing productivity.

  b. Critics of the movement maintained that these programs shifted blame from the work environment to the individual worker, repeating a trend from earlier years.

  c. Concerns were also raised about potential discrimination against populations at risk(e.g., smokers, obese workers, hypertensives).

IV History of Workers' Compensation

A Before the passage of workers' compensation laws, injured workers and the survivors of workers killed on the job could be compensated for their loss or medical costs only through litigation.

B Employers were historically protected from loss claims under three common legal defenses (Boden, 1999):

1. The *assumption-of-risk* defense assumed that workers were aware of occupational hazards and accepted the risk inherent to their jobs.

2. The *fellow servant rule* assumed that if a co-worker contributed to an accident or injury, that co-worker should be responsible for compensating the injured worker.

3. The concept of *contributory negligence* held that the employer was not liable if the employee contributed in any way to the injury; this defense strategy argued that physical harm would not have come to the worker had he or she been paying attention to the task, overriding the importance of a lack of protective devices.

C Workers' compensation legislation was intended to protect business from lengthy litigation and prevent injured workers from becoming wards of the state.

1. Workers' compensation laws were first enacted in Germany in 1884, and were widespread in Europe by the late 1890s.

2. In the United States, the first workers' compensation law was passed in Wisconsin in 1911 (Howard and Davies, 1985).

  a. Between 1911 and 1921, 25 states enacted workers' compensation laws.

  b. All 50 states and the District of Columbia now have workers' compensation laws; the last statute was enacted in Mississippi in 1948.

3. Each jurisdiction has administrative control over its own system, but there are several elements required of all statutes.

  a. Negligence or assumption of fault is not material to a claim, although it must be clear that the injury or illness occurred as a result of work-related processes.

     b. Benefits are made available by employers' payment of premiums to the established administrative system.

     c. Workers forfeit their right to sue their employer in exchange for prompt and reasonable compensation.

   4. Employers lose their immunity from litigation if any of the following conditions are present:

     a. An injury is caused by an employer's intentional act

     b. The employer is not in compliance with the state workers' compensation regulations

     c. Punitive action is taken against the employee in retaliation for filing a claim or otherwise pursing workers' compensation benefits

V The Occupational Safety and Health Act

A **Passage of the Occupational Safety and Health Act of 1970 (Appendix V) underscored two major points:**

   1. Many occupational hazards are controllable, and their resulting work-related injuries and illnesses are preventable.

   2. Primary responsibility for providing safe and healthful working environments rests with the employer.

B **Individual states may manage their own occupational health and safety programs with federal approval of the state plan, which is contingent upon a demonstrated ability to provide the essential elements required by the federal plan.**

C **The OSH Act of 1970 established three separate bodies with distinct functions (Chapter 3: Legal and Ethical Issues, presents a more detailed discussion):**

   1. The Occupational Safety and Health Administration (OSHA), positioned within the United States Department of Labor (USDL), promulgates, administers, and enforces workplace health and safety standards, and establishes reporting and recordkeeping procedures to monitor the number and type of job-related injuries and illnesses.

   2. The National Institute for Occupational Safety and Health (NIOSH) located in the U.S. Department of Health and Human Services (DHHS) as part of the Centers for Disease Control and Prevention (CDC), conducts occupational health and safety research, provides education, and makes recommendations to OSHA and the nation's employers.

   3. The Occupational Safety and Health Review Commission, a separate entity independent from OSHA, primarily arbitrates disputes between employers and OSHA regarding citations and proposed fines.

VI National Health Goals: Healthy People and Healthy Communities

A *Healthy People 2010* **(DHHS, 2000) outlines a comprehensive, nationwide health-promotion and disease-prevention agenda in 28 public-health focus areas, including occupational health and safety and environmental health;** *Healthy People 2010* **is designed to achieve two overarching goals:**

   1. Increase quality and years of healthy life

   2. Eliminate health disparities

B The underlying premise of *Healthy People 2010* is that "the health of the individual is almost inseparable from the health of the larger community."

C *Healthy People 2010* builds on initiatives and objectives pursued over the past two decades, aiming for measurable and achievable public health objectives. Interim evaluations in the occupational and environmental health and safety focus area have and will continue to result in the following:
1. New objectives to address emerging work-related concerns
2. Revision, replacement, or elimination of objectives that cannot be tracked reliably or have low relative value for monitoring improved outcomes in worker health and safety.

D The *Healthy People 2010* goal for Chapter 20, Occupational Safety and Health, is to "promote the health and safety of people at work through prevention and early detection" (http://www.health.gov/healthypeople/Publications/). Specific objectives related to occupational health and safety have been developed for the following areas:
1. Work-related injury deaths
2. Work-related injuries
3. Overexertion or repetitive motion
4. Pneumoconiosis deaths
5. Work-related homicides
6. Work-related assaults
7. Elevated blood lead levels from work exposure
8. Occupational skin diseases or disorders
9. Worksite stress reduction programs
10. Needlestick injuries
11. Work-related noise-induced hearing loss

E The *Healthy People 2010* goal for Chapter 8, Environmental Health, is to "promote health for all through a healthy environment." (http://www.health.gov/healthypeople/Publications/). Specific objectives related to environmental health have been developed for the following areas:
1. Outdoor air quality
2. Water quality
3. Toxins and wastes
4. Healthy homes and healthy communities
5. Infrastructure and surveillance
6. Global environmental health

F *Healthy Communities 2000: Model Standards* (American Public Health Association, 1991) was developed to help implement national health objectives for community populations, including working populations, by providing a "framework for incremental improvement in community health status through preventive health service programming."

VII Occupational Health in the International Community

A Occupational health and safety programs in developing countries face many societal, cultural and political challenges, including the following:
1. Poor general working conditions
2. Substandard wages
3. Inadequate workers' compensation, or no worker's compensation at all

4. Inadequate health and safety legislation; nonenforcement of existing laws
5. Exploitation of the labor force, including child labor
6. Lack of regulation related to environmental pollution and degradation
7. Inadequate supply of occupational health and safety expertise
8. Hazardous industries, operations, equipment, machinery, and products often imported from developed countries where they may be banned

B **The International Labour Organization (ILO) has estimated that in 1997 the overall economic losses resulting from work-related diseases and injuries were approximately 4% of the world's gross national product (World Health Organization [WHO], 1999).**

C International organizations committed to occupational health and safety include the following:
1. The WHO, which was established in 1948 to further international cooperation to improve health conditions
   a. The purpose of WHO is "to promote the attainment of the highest level of health by all people in the world" (WHO, 1994**).**
   b. Following the 1994 Declaration on Occupational Health for All, WHO developed a global strategy on occupational health (WHO, 1995).
   c. In 1990, WHO created a global network of Occupational Health Collaborating Centers.
2. The ILO, which was established in 1919 to protect the life and health of working men and women and to control occupational hazards. Its services include the following:
   a. Policy and advisory guidance through its International Program for the Improvement of Working Conditions and Environment
   b. Provision of information through its International Occupational Safety and Health Information Center in Geneva, Switzerland (known as CIS in the European Union)
3. The European Commission, which has developed directives aimed at harmonizing national occupational health and safety laws in European Union members
4. The International Commission on Occupational Health (ICOH), an international scientific society established in 1906, which is recognized by the United Nations as a nongovernmental organization
   a. The purpose of ICOH is to foster the scientific progress, knowledge, and development of occupational health in the international community.
   b. ICOH has a close working relationship with WHO, ILO, and other United Nations agencies.
   c. Since 1969, ICOH's Scientific Committee on Occupational Health Nursing has produced nine reports for occupational health nurses internationally.

VIII The Workplace: Occupational Hazards and Their Impact on Workers

The range of workplace hazards with actual or potential effects on worker health and safety is as broad and varied as work itself. The nature of occupational hazards changes with the evolution of work processes, but can be broadly categorized as follows:

A *Physical hazards* are agents or forces inherent to the nature of a work environment or process that may cause tissue damage or other physi-cal harm.

1. Environmental noise contamination is the single most prevalent occupa-tional hazard; its hazard potential is generally underestimated.
   a. Each year, more than 30 million workers are exposed to continuous or impulse noise at levels sufficient to cause measurable hearing loss (National Institute for Occupational Safety and Health [NIOSH], 1996).
   b. Environmental noise contamination can elicit physiologic and psycho-logic stress reactions resulting in neuro-endocrine stimulation capable of adversely affecting multiple body systems (Lusk, et al., 1996; Moll van Charante and Mulder, 1990; Suter, 1993).
2. Thermal stress experienced when working in conditions of excessive heat or cold can lead to multiple pathologies, including cardiovascular and metabolic disturbances, central and peripheral neurologic alterations, and mental status changes, resulting in impaired judgment and performance and increased risk of accidents.
3. Sustained or repeated body contact with vibrating surfaces has been associated with neurologic, neurovascular, and musculoskeletal changes and visual and gastrointestinal disorders.
4. Other examples of physical hazards include radiation, electric and magnetic fields, hyperbaric environments, lasers, and microwaves.

B Chemical hazards
1. Approximately 85,000 synthetic or natural chemicals appear on the Environmental Protection Agency's inventory of industrial chemicals (Goldman, 1999); more than six million synthetic chemicals have been registered by the American Chemical Association, and 1,000 new chemi-cals are introduced yearly (Levenstein, et al., 1999; Ottoboni, 1991).
2. Chemicals occur in various forms.
   a. The American National Standards Institute classifies chemicals as dusts/particulates, fumes, mists, vapors, and gases.
   b. Chemical formulations include solutions, metals, solvents, aerosols, pharmaceutics, oils, synthetic textiles, pesticides, and explosives.
   c. Commercial products are often formulated with various additives and stabilizers to render a useable form of substances that may also be toxic.
3. An estimated 32 million workers are annually exposed to one or more chemical hazards that may cause, contribute to, or exacerbate serious adverse health effects (http://www.osha-slc.gov/Preamble/Hazard_data/HAZCOMI.html)
4. NIOSH has identified 13,000 toxic substances and 2,000 carcinogens that pose threats to human health in the workplace.
5. Regulation of safe exposure limits for chemical substances requires clear scientific evidence of pathologic effects; the burden of proof lies with OHSA, which relies on evidence from NIOSH and other research entities.
6. Primary routes of chemical exposure are inhalation, transdermal absorp-tion, and ingestion; deleterious effects range from local reactions to systemic or end-organ damage.
7. Bio-pathologic effects of chemical exposures include the following:
   a. Acute effects—usually linked to a single high-dose incident with an identifiable offending substance.

    b. Chronic effects—evolve insidiously, presenting multiple challenges in establishing causal relationships to exposures.

    c. Allergic reactions—not consistent with the usual population dose-response curve.

NOTE: The toxicology of chemical exposure is discussed in Chapter 5.

C **Biologic hazards**

1. Biologic hazards found in the work environment include viruses, bacteria, fungi, molds, and parasites.

2. Exposure to biologic agents can be direct or indirect, and occurs through one of three routes of transmission: airborne, droplet, or contact.

3. Many occupations are at risk of exposure to biohazards

    a. The occupational risk of exposure to infectious agents among employees in health care and related fields is well documented (see Table 2-3 in Chapter 2).

    b. Workers who have contact with animals or animal products may be at risk for zoonotic diseases.

    c. Workers whose jobs involve contact with soil are at risk for parasitic diseases and bacterial or fungal infections.

4. Prevention and control methods include immunization, isolation of the agent, engineering control measures (e.g., effective ventilation mechanics), personal protective gear, and hand washing.

5. Challenges to prevention and control include the following:

    a. Emerging infectious agents (CDC, 1998b)—more than 30 new infectious processes have been detected in the past two decades, including Lyme disease, Legionnaire's disease, human immunodeficiency virus/acquired immunodeficiency syndrome, necrotizing fasciitis, avian influenza, hantavirus, and Ebola fever.

    b. Drug resistance and organism mutation because of overuse of antibiotics and lapses in treatment regimens

D **Mechanical hazards**

1. *Mechanical hazards* are elements of the workplace that lead to stress or injury through an incompatibility between the design of the workplace or work processes and human physiology.

    a. Such hazards might also be termed *biomechanical,* as they represent not only an interface between equipment and humans, but also the physiologic mechanics required to perform work duties.

    b. The effect of this incompatibility is most often exacted on the musculoskeletal and peripheral nervous systems, but other body systems may be effected as well.

2. The identification, analysis, and abatement of biomechanical hazards are often a function of *applied ergonomics* (Chapter 14 presents an example of an ergonomics program).

3. Several subdisciplines of ergonomic science are concerned with occupational health and safety (Rom, 1998).

    a. *Human factors engineering,* sometimes called *engineering psychology,* is concerned with the perceptual, cognitive, and psychomotor aspects of work.

    b. *Work physiology* is concerned with the physiologic stresses, primarily those of the musculoskeletal, pulmonary, and cardiovascular systems, that occur in response to the metabolic demands of work, whether sedentary or physically demanding.

    c. *Biomechanics* is concerned with the mechanical properties of human tissue and the response of tissue to mechanical stresses.

    d. *Anthropometry* is concerned with the measurement and statistical characterization of body size, which is important when designing protective clothing, machinery, tools, and furniture that allows all workers to perform their duties in a safe and non–biomechanically stressful manner.

4. Effects of biomechanical stresses may be temporary or result in permanent disability.

    a. Acute effects include musculoskeletal injuries resulting from overexertion, slips, falls, or other accidents; muscular strain or fatigue resulting from forceful exertion or awkward positioning; and visual fatigue.

    b. Chronic effects include Raynaud's syndrome resulting from the use of vibrating power tools; cumulative trauma injuries stemming from repeated or sustained motions resulting in neurologic and musculoskeletal disorders; and chronic back pain resulting from improper lifting or awkward, abrupt movements.

    c. Biomechanical injuries may impair mobility, strength, tactile capabilities, or motor control; recovery is often long-term and may be incomplete.

5. Prevention and control of biomechanical pathologies is best achieved through engineering designs which focus on manipulating the elements of the work facilities and processes to accommodate the characteristics, capabilities, and expectations of the worker.

E **Psychosocial hazards**

1. Psychosocial workplace stress has become a nationally recognized problem of epidemic proportions.

2. Psychosocial hazards are often difficult to identify and even more difficult to quantify because of their intangible and insidious nature and the variable responses among individuals.

3. Sources of workplace psychosocial distress stem from multiple sources internal and external to the organization (Chapter 13).

4. Psychosocial stress hazards that occur in the workplace may have the following characteristics:

    a. They may be manifested physically, psychologically, or behaviorally, with outcomes detrimental to the individual, co-workers, and general workplace morale and productivity.

    b. They may have economic implications to the organization, including lost productivity, costs related to medical benefits, temporary help, and employee turnover, and losses related to the impact of stressed employees on customer relations (Lee, 1997; Reichheld, 1996).

    c. They may be symptomatic of widespread organizational problems rather than isolated incidents, indicating a need for systematic solutions (Lee, 1997).

IX Work-Related Injury and Illness

A **OSHA definitions:**

1. An *occupational injury* is any injury, such as a cut, fracture, sprain, amputation, etc., that results from a single instantaneous exposure or incident in the work environment.

2. An *occupational illness* is any abnormal condition or disorder, other than one resulting from an occupational injury, caused by exposure to environmental factors associated with employment, including acute or chronic illnesses that may be caused by inhalation, absorption, ingestion, or direct contact.

B **Challenges in accurately defining the extent of occupational and environmental injury and illness**
   1. Statistical data on occupational injury and illness rates are dependent upon thorough and accurate incident reporting
      a. Statistical accuracy may be compromised when the differentiation between illnesses or injuries is not clear (e.g., chronic disorders such as back pain, multiple chemical sensitivity, or cumulative trauma disorders may result from single or repeated injurious events).
      b. There is no national reporting system for occupation-related chronic disease or death.
   2. Underreporting of work-related incidents is a well-recognized phenomenon, and occurs on several levels:
      a. Governmental surveillance criteria do not require gathering data on certain categories of workers.
      b. Employees may not report nonacute incidents or those not requiring medical attention, or may not recognize the work-relatedness of a disorder.
      c. The organizational culture may discourage reporting incidents or filing workers' compensation claims.
      d. Death certificates may lack work-relatedness; only 67% to 90% of all occupational fatalities resulting from injury can be identified through the death certificate (CDC, 1998a).
   3. Work-related illnesses are more difficult to quantify than injuries and are more likely to be underreported.
      a. Diseases related to occupational exposures are indistinguishable from those caused by non–work-related sources.
      b. The onset of illness resulting from occupational exposure is often subtle, occurring years after the exposure.
      c. Health care providers may not recognize the relationship of a worker's presenting symptoms to past or present occupations or may find the determination of relative causation of work-related hazards to a disorder difficult because of genetic or behavioral variables.

C **Economic impact of occupational and environmental injury and illness**
   1. The total cost of work-related injuries is conservatively estimated to range from $125.1 billion to $145 billion annually (Leigh, et al., 1997; National Safety Council (NSC), 1999), and includes such costs as wage and productivity losses, medical costs, and administrative expenses such as time spent investigating injuries and writing accident reports.
   2. It is estimated that 125 million days of productive work time were lost in 1998; future time loss from disabling occupational injuries and deaths that occurred in 1998 is estimated at 60 million days (NSC, 1999).
   3. In 1996, $42.4 billion was paid out through workers' compensation for income benefits and medical costs (NSC, 1999).
   4. Economic estimates of loss do not include the impact on communities and families, such as pain and suffering, lowered workplace morale because of

the loss of a co-worker, the strain of taking care of a disabled family member, or the loss of the injured employee's contributions to community activities.

D Occupational injuries

1. Estimates of nonfatal workplace injuries resulting in temporary or permanent disability range from 3.6 million to 3.8 million annually (Rosenstock, Olenec, and Wagner, 1998). Table 1-1 presents the most common of those injuries.
2. Independent researchers estimate the total number of occupational injuries at more than 13 million cases annually (Leigh, et al., 1997).
3. Injury rates tend to be higher in mid-sized organizations with 50-249 employees than in either smaller or larger organizations.
4. Workplace fatalities resulting from accidents and injuries have declined from 21 per 100,000 full-time workers in 1912, when surveillance began, to an estimated 3.8 per 100,000 in 1998 (NSC, 1999).
   a. An estimated 17 persons die daily from injuries sustained at work (USDL Bureau of Labor Statistics [BLS], 1999).
   b. The three most hazardous industries in terms of fatalities are mining, agriculture, and construction, with rates reported at 27.4, 22.1, and 13.9 per 100,000 full time workers, respectively; although agricultural mortality rate has been estimated at more than 50 per 100,000 (NSC, 1999).
5. Underlying or root causes of workplace accidents stem from the human-hazard interface, and injuries are often the result of deficiencies in adhering to safety precautions, either at an administrative level or by the individual worker.

E Occupational illness

1. Work-related illness morbidity and mortality figures are more difficult to quantify and more likely to be underreported than are injuries. Table 1-2

TABLE 1-1

Nonfatal work injuries involving days away from work—1997

Type of injury	Percent of private industry total[a]
Overexertion	27.7
Overexertion while lifting	*(16.2)*
Contact with objects or equipment	27.0
Struck by object	*(13.1)*
Caught in, under, or between object	*(4.4)*
Struck against object	*(7.0)*
Fall to same level, including slips and trips	10.8
Fall from elevation to lower level	5.4
Exposure to harmful substances	4.6
Transportation accidents	4.0
Slips, trips	3.1
Assaults; violent acts by person	1.2
Fires, explosions	0.2
All other	11.9
	95.9[b]

Source: National Safety Council, 1999

[a] Figures for all industries combined; excludes farms with fewer than 11 employees.

[b] Total excludes repetitive motion, discussed in occupational illness section.

summarizes the number of cases and the incident rate of occupational diseases reported to the BLS in 1997.

2. The most common occupational illnesses are associated with repeated trauma.

   a. More than 276,000 cases of repeated trauma were reported or diagnosed in 1997, accounting for over 64% of all reported work-related illnesses (NSC, 1999).

   b. The incidence of repeated trauma disorders more than tripled between 1987 and 1994.

3. Skin disorders are the second most prevalent work-related illness, and the most common non–trauma related illness (National Center for Health Statistics, 1996; NSC, 1999; DHHS, 2000).

   a. Skin disorders represent over 13% of all reported occupational disease.

   b. Manufacturing has the greatest number of cases, but the highest rate for new case diagnosis is in agriculture, forestry, and fishing.

4. The prevalence of occupation-related chronic respiratory disease is difficult to determine; it has been estimated that less than 5% of chronic respiratory disease is correctly identified as associated with work exposure (Christiani and Wegman, 1999).

   a. The proportion of chronic obstructive pulmonary disease attributable to workplace respiratory exposure, factoring out the contribution of smoking, may be 14% (NIOSH, 1996).

   b. Up to an estimated 28% of the 10 million cases of asthma in the general population is thought related to workplace exposure (NIOSH, 1996).

5. Hazardous occupational exposures are considered substantial contributors to many other disease processes, affecting nearly every body system.

6. New disorders have emerged with evolving technologies and work processes that present new challenges to occupational health and safety professionals, including sick-building syndrome, multiple-chemical sensitivity, and cumulative trauma disorders.

F Sources of information and data on occupational injury and illness include the following:

1. U.S. Department of Labor, Bureau of Labor Statistics

TABLE 1-2

Reported occupational illnesses, United States: 1997

Occupational or environmental illness	All private sector industries combined[a]	
	Number of cases[b]	Incidence rate[c]
All illnesses	429.8	49.8
Disorders associated with repeated trauma	276.6	32.0
Skin diseases, disorders	57.9	6.7
Respiratory conditions due to toxic agents	20.3	2.4
Disorders due to physical agents	16.6	1.9
Poisoning	5.1	0.6
Dust diseases of the lungs	2.9	0.3
All other occupational diseases	50.4	5.8

National Safety Council, 1999

[a]Private sector includes all industries except government, and excludes farms with fewer than 11 employees. [b]Number in thousands. [c]Incidence rate per 10,000 full-time workers.

2. National Safety Council
3. Workers' compensation records
4. State and federal occupational health and safety administrations
5. National Institute for Occupational Safety and Health

X Assessment and Prevention of Occupational and Environmental Injury and Illness

A **Theoretically, all occupational and environmental injuries and illnesses are preventable.**

1. Prevention measures include modifying hazardous workplace conditions, preventing contact between the hazard and the worker, and educating and training workers regarding safe work practices.
2. The efficacy of prevention strategies is dependent upon the accurate assessment of the following:
   a. Hazardous workplace conditions
   b. Actual or potential risk of employee exposure, previous similar exposures, and preexisting health conditions that may impact the severity of the exposure

B **Hazards in the workplace can be assessed by the following approaches (Chapter 9 presents a more detailed discussion):**

1. Actual or potential hazards are identified through site surveys, record audits, accident investigations, chemical inventory analyses, or other methods.
2. Exposure monitoring quantitatively assesses exposures to known, suspected, or reasonably predicted hazards such as chemicals, noise, or atmospheric conditions.
3. Process safety analysis focuses on assessing the hazards inherent to specific work processes such as ergonomic analysis or production line safety.
4. Population analysis takes an epidemiologic approach to identifying work-related hazards.

C **Assessment of occupational and environmental illness**

1. There are no specialized diagnostic procedures to identify the work-relatedness of a disorder, making the occupational and environmental exposure history the crucial tool to accurate diagnosis and appropriate treatment recommendations.
2. The key components of the occupational and environmental exposure history include the following (Levy and Wegman, 1999):
   a. Descriptions of all jobs held
   b. Environmental (work/home/school/community) exposures, and protective mechanisms and interventions in use
   c. Temporal relationship between symptoms and work schedule or between symptoms and exposure
   d. Epidemiology of similar symptoms or illnesses among peers
   e. Incidental exposures—descriptions of nonemployment activities
3. The accurate determination of the work-relatedness of an illness provides benefits to the following:
   a. The individual worker, who receives an accurate diagnosis, relevant treatment recommendations, and meaningful prevention measures to reduce or eliminate the source of the exposure

b. The population of workers, who, through an investigative assessment of the hazard, benefit from the implementation of prevention strategies aimed at groups of workers in work environments similar to the effected employee

c. The organization, which avoids the costs of unnecessary diagnostic procedures, medications, or referrals

XI History and Evolution of Occupational and Environmental Health Nursing

The evolution of industrial nursing paralleled the growth of industry.

A Industrial nursing, with its roots in 19th century Great Britain, emerged as a new specialty field during the era of rapid industrialization (McGrath, 1946; American Association of Industrial Nurses, 1976).

1. The philosophy of care of industrial nursing was based on the concepts and principles of public health nursing.
2. Early industrial nurses were public health nurses employed by mining and manufacturing companies and department stores to:
   a. Provide primary and community health services to employees and their families
   b. Focus on preventing and treating communicable diseases
3. Earliest recorded industrial nurses included the following:
   a. Phillippa Flowerday, who was hired in 1878 by the J.J. Coleman Mustard Company in England to provide home care to workers and their families
   b. Betty Moulder, who is often considered the first American occupational health nurse; it has been reported that she was hired by a group of coal mining companies to care for miners and their families in the late 1880s
   c. Ada Mayo Stewart, who, in 1895 was hired by the Vermont Marble Company; in 1896, she became the superintendent of the company-built hospital in Proctor

B As the profession developed into the early 20th century, the focus remained with public and community health services.

1. In 1909, the Milwaukee Visiting Nurse Association placed a nurse in a plant to offer public health services in order to demonstrate the economic value of the service.
2. For the most part, industrial nurses remained visiting nurses until workers' compensation laws were instituted, at which time first-aid stations were opened in plants.
3. In 1916, Florence Wright, in an address to the National Safety Council, described the valuable work done by the industrial nurse as follows:
   a. Promotes pleasant industrial relations
   b. Reduces time lost through accident and illness
   c. Minimizes the results of accidents by providing first aid and subsequent care under the direction of the surgeon
   d. Searches out the causes of illness and accidents through cooperation with employers and outside agencies in the community and the home
   e. Makes possible the healthy, happy, thrifty home life in the families of those visited, preventing waste of life and health and increasing the efficiency of each member

4. In 1916, Ella Phillips Crandall described the roles of occupational health nurses as follows:
   a. First aid and dispensary service
   b. Hospital duty
   c. Making rounds in industrial plants to inspect conditions and observe employees
   d. Consultation—chiefly for women
   e. Teaching health and hygiene classes
   f. Making home visits to provide nursing and social services, including domestic education in food economics, cookery, and budgeting
   g. Keeping records of occupational diseases and injuries, and of the relationship of employment to disease and mortality

C Occupational health nursing organizations have defined the profession,

---

BOX 1-2

Historical development of occupational and environmental health nursing organizations

- 1913: The first industrial nurse registry was opened in Boston for the purpose of supplying emergency room nurses to factories.
- 1915: The Boston Industrial Nurses' Club was formed, the forerunner of the New England Association of Industrial Nurses.
- 1916: The Factory Nurses' Conference was formed, admitting only graduate, state-registered nurses who belonged to the American Nurses' Association.
- 1917: Boston University's College of Business Administration offered the first industrial nurse educational course.
- 1922: The Factory Nurses' Conference changed its name to the American Association of Industrial Nurses (AAIN) to more closely identify with the industrial physician's group.
- 1933: The AAIN merged with the New England Association of Industrial Nurses.
- 1938: The fist annual joint conference of the industrial nurses' associations of New England, New

Jersey, New York, and Philadelphia met in New York City.
- 1942: On April 19, at the Philadelphia conference, the AAIN became a national organization; Catherine R. Dempsey was its first president.
- 1943: The first annual meeting of the new AAIN was held in New York City.
- 1944: AAIN prepared an "Outline of Basic College Courses for Industrial Nurses" and distributed it to colleges and universities in the United States.
- 1944: *Industrial Nursing* became the official publication of AAIN.
- 1949: Publishing of *Industrial Nursing* was halted because of increased publishing costs; a newsletter was substituted.
- 1953: *Industrial Nurses Journal* was re-established, winning several awards in the years that followed.
- 1964: AAIN copyrighted its publication as the *American Association of Industrial Nurses Journal, The Journal of Occupational Health Nursing*.
- 1966: A committee consisting of

guided its development, and established its professional foundations (Box 1-2).

1. In 1942, the American Association of Industrial Nursing (AAIN) was formed.
2. In 1943, at its first annual meeting in New York City, AAIN described its purposes and objectives as follows:
   a. To develop sound standards of education and practice in industrial nursing
   b. To cooperate with physicians, management, safety professionals, and other allied groups in conserving the health of industrial workers
   c. To promote mutual understanding of the goals of occupational health and safety programs among these groups
   d. To interpret the objectives and ideals of industrial nurses to the professional and lay world

---

BOX 1-2

Historical development of occupational and environmental health nursing organizations—cont'd

members from AAIN, the American Industrial Hygiene Association, the Industrial Medical Association, and the American Academy of Occupational Medicine was established to study the formation of an American Board of Certification for Occupational Health Nurses.

- 1969: The name of the journal became *Occupational Health Nursing*, the Official Journal of the American Association of Industrial Nurses.
- 1971: The American Board for Occupational Health Nurses was established as a separate organization whose purpose was certification of occupational health nurses.
- 1977: To better reflect the nature of practice, the name AAIN, Inc. was changed to the American Association of Occupational Health Nurses, Inc. (AAOHN).
- 1983: The official headquarters of AAOHN moved from New York City to Atlanta, Georgia.
- 1986: The journal became known

as the *AAOHN Journal*, the Official Journal of the American Association of Occupational Health Nurses.

- 1988: Occupational health nursing celebrated its centennial year.
- 1992: AAOHN celebrated its 50th anniversary with 12,500 members.
- 1996: AAOHN was awarded a cooperative agreement by Agency for Toxic Substances and Disease Registry to develop and provide environmental health information to AAOHN members, other nursing professionals, and community groups.
- 1997: *AAOHN Core Curriculum for Occupational Health Nursing* was published.
- 1998: To reflect the broader scope of practice, the words "occupational and environmental" were included in the mission statement, by-laws, and standards of practice.
- 2001: The *Core Curriculum for Occupational and Environmental Health Nursing* was published.

e. To bring industrial nursing participation into the plans for advancing industrial and community health

3. The official publication of AAIN was originally called *Industrial Nursing*.

4. In 1971, the American Board for Occupational Health Nurses was established; its purpose is to certify occupational health nurses.

5. In 1977, the American Association of Industrial Nurses' name was changed to the American Association of Occupational Health Nurses (AAOHN) to reflect the broader scope of practice of its members.

6. In 1986, the journal became known as the *AAOHN Journal, The Official Journal of the American Association of Occupational Health Nurses.*

7. Through a cooperative agreement awarded to AAOHN by the Agency for Toxic Substances and Disease Registry (ATSDR) and extending from 1996-1999, AAOHN developed and provided environmental health information to its members, other nursing professionals, and community groups. AAOHN and ATSDR have an ongoing partnership under a second cooperative agreement.

8. Since 1998, the importance of environmental health concerns to occupational health nurses has also been reflected through the addition of the term "occupational *and environmental* health nursing" to AAOHN's mission statement, by-laws, professional standards, and other AAOHN publications.

XII The Practice of Occupational and Environmental Health Nursing

A **Occupational and environmental health nursing is the specialty practice that provides health and safety services to employees, employee populations, and community groups (AAOHN, 1999).**

1. The practice focuses on promoting and restoring health, preventing injury and illness, and protecting workers from occupational and environmental hazards.

2. The research-based foundation of occupational and environmental health nursing derives its theoretic, conceptual, and factual framework from a multidisciplinary scientific base.

3. Guided by the AAOHN Code of Ethics (AAOHN, 1998) (Appendix VI), occupational and environmental health nurses encourage informed decision making regarding health care concerns, adhere to strict confidentiality practices, and advocate on behalf of employees and community groups for safe and healthy environments in which to work and live.

B **Standards of Practice define, guide, and advance professional practice, providing a framework for evaluation while remaining dynamic to reflect the evolving and changing scope of practice and the development of new knowledge. AAOHN has identified 11 Standards of Practice for Occupational and Environmental Health Nursing (AAOHN, 1999).**

1. Standard I: Assessment
The occupational and environmental health nurse systematically assesses the health status of the individual client or population and the environment.

2. Standard II: Diagnosis
The occupational and environmental health nurse analyzes assessment data to formulate diagnoses.

3. Standard III: Outcome Identification
   The occupational and environmental health nurse identifies outcomes specific to the client.
4. Standard IV: Planning
   The occupational and environmental health nurse develops a goal-directed plan that is comprehensive and formulates interventions to attain expected outcomes.
5. Standard V: Implementation
   The occupational and environmental health nurse implements interventions to attain desired outcomes identified in the plan.
6. Standard VI: Evaluation
   The occupational and environmental health nurse systematically and continuously evaluates responses to interventions and progress toward the achievement of desired outcomes.
7. Standard VII: Resource Management
   The occupational and environmental health nurse secures and manages the resources that support an occupational health and safety program.
8. Standard VIII: Professional Development
   The occupational and environmental health nurse assumes accountability for professional development to enhance professional growth and maintain competency.
9. Standard IX: Collaboration
   The occupational and environmental health nurse collaborates with employees, management, other health care providers, professionals, and community representatives.
10. Standard X: Research
    The occupational and environmental health nurse uses research findings in practice and contributes to the scientific base in occupational and environmental health nursing to improve practice and advance the profession.
11. Standard XI: Ethics
    The occupational and environmental health nurse uses an ethical framework as a guide for decision making in practice.

C **Primary responsibilities**
1. The scope of practice described by AAOHN (AAOHN, 1999) outlines the essential elements of this specialty practice and represents a coordinated multidisciplinary approach to delivering safe, quality, and comprehensive occupational health and safety services that include the following:
   a. Clinical and primary care for occupational and nonoccupational illnesses and injuries
   b. Case management for occupational and nonoccupational illnesses and injuries
   c. Health hazard assessment and surveillance of employee populations, workplaces, and community groups
   d. Investigation, monitoring, and analysis of illness and injury events and trends
   e. Development, implementation, monitoring, and analysis of health and safety interventions
   f. Maintaining legal, regulatory, and ethical compliance for employee and environmental health and safety

      g. Management and administration
      h. Knowledge and use of health promotion and prevention principles
      i. Counseling, health education, and training
      j. Participating and contributing to occupational and environmental health and safety research
  2. Additional responsibilities required for a successful occupational health and safety program include the following:
      a. Development of professional rapport with employees and employers
      b. Development of collegial and cooperative relationships with members of the interdisciplinary health and safety team
      c. Establishing a liaison with community referral agencies and resources
      d. Establishing a network of professional resources
      e. Maintenance and enhancement of professional competence in occupational and environmental health and related subspecialties through continuing education and other professional development activities
  3. Broader environmental issues are increasingly being recognized as within the domain of occupational health practice (Rogers and Cox, 1998; Salazar and Primomo, 1994), partly because of the following (Chapter 15 presents a more detailed discussion):
      a. A recognition of the link between environmental conditions and human disease
      b. A greater understanding of the impact of industry and its byproducts on the environment
      c. The occupational health nurse's unique, integrated body of scientific knowledge that can be drawn upon to advocate for practices that impact workers, the community, and environmental health

D **Occupational and environmental health nursing is a unique, complex, and multidimensional practice (Figure 1-1).**
  1. The occupational and environmental health nurse is professionally accountable to workers, employers, communities, their profession, and are responsible for their own professional development.
  2. Multiple work-related and external variables influence the health of workers and workplaces and the outcomes of the occupational and environmental health and safety program.

E **Practice settings for occupational and environmental health nurses are as diverse as the many types of businesses in existence, and include:**
  1. Industrial, business, or corporate settings
      a. Organizations with more than 250 employees are most likely to employ occupational and environmental health nurses.
      b. Firms with relatively high occupational injury and illness rates are more likely to employ occupational health nurses.
      c. The most common employer-based sites include manufacturers, service providers, and the transportation, communication, and utility industries.
      d. At the organizational administrative level, the occupational and environmental health nurse may be primarily focused on policy development and program oversight.
  2. Insurers and third-party administrators (TPAs)
      a. Occupational and environmental health nurses monitor and manage the work-related injury and illness of patients for whom insurers and TPAs provide workers' compensation insurance coverage.

      b. Insurers and TPAs provide occupational health and safety consultation to their clients, including:

         1) Employee and supervisor training

         2) Program and regulatory compliance audits

         3) Health screening and surveillance

         4) Management support

         5) Case management protocol development

         6) Injury and illness trend analysis

3. Government and regulatory agencies

      a. Government agencies employ occupational health nurses as consultants, analysts, program developers, and compliance officers; they also provide occupational health services for government employees.

      b. Governmental and regulatory agencies focus their services and activities on populations rather than individual clients.

      c. Agencies may be federal (e.g., PHS, OSHA, NIOSH); state (e.g., state health and safety administrations, state health departments); or local (e.g., city or county health departments).

4. Utilization review and case management firms

      a. Occupational and environmental health nurses may work directly with employees and employers, through insurers and third party administrators, or in managed care settings.

      b. Health care services and return-to-work interventions are monitored and managed by occupational and environmental health nurses individually with the employee or as an oversight service for the organization.

      c. The ultimate objectives are to provide cost-effective, quality health care and facilitate the employee's return to an optimally expected level of work.

      d. A utilization review and case management firm may exist in a range of organizations, from an independent nurse practice to a large multimillion-dollar firm.

5. Consulting firms

      a. Consulting services provided to client employers encompass evaluation and audit activities, training, trend analysis, program and system development, and management support.

      b. Consulting firms may be:

         1) Independent occupational and environmental health and safety consulting firms

         2) Finance-oriented consulting firms, such as insurance or accounting firms

         3) An independent practice owned and managed by one or more occupational health nurses

6. Occupational and environmental health nurses may also work for research or academic organizations.

F **Functional roles of the occupational and environmental health nurse**

The breadth and depth of occupational/environmental health and safety programs and the practice of the occupational and environmental health nurse vary in accordance with the needs and resources of the work setting.

    1. Specific functions are determined by a number of factors, including the nature of the work and its associated hazards, the number of employees, the organizational structure, and the organization's administrative and financial support for the program.

2. Functional roles of the occupational and environmental health nurse have been defined by AAOHN as follows (AAOHN 1997):
   a. Clinician—Primary responsibilities aimed at preventing work-related and non–work-related health problems and restoring and maintaining health
   b. Case manager—Coordinates health and rehabilitation services for an individual worker from the onset of an injury or illness to an optimal return to work status or a satisfactory alternative
   c. Occupational health services coordinator—Functions as the single occupational health nurse for a business or organization
   d. Health promotion specialist—Develops and manages a comprehensive, multilevel, broad range health promotion program that supports organizational business objectives
   e. Manager—Directs, administers, and evaluates an occupational and environmental health and safety service and its policies, maintaining consistency with organizational goals and objectives
   f. Nurse practitioner—Uses additional specialized preparation meeting state requirements for advanced practice nursing to critically evaluate the health status of workers through health histories, physical assessments, and diagnostic tests
   g. Corporate director—Responsible for the total occupational and environmental health and safety program at the policy-making level
   h. Consultant—Serves as an advisor for developing, selecting, implementing, and evaluating occupational and environmental health and safety services
   i. Educator—Assumes programmatic and administrative responsibilities for curricula and/or clinical experiences in occupational and environmental health nursing
   j. Researcher—Identifies occupational and environmental health problems, develops researchable questions with consideration for research priorities, assesses study feasibility, and initiates and conducts research studies using all elements of the research process

3. Many occupational and environmental health nurses work in more than one of these roles simultaneously; for example, a nurse whose primary role is a clinician may also serve as a health promotion specialist, educator, and case manager.

G **Occupational and environmental health nurses who have pursued additional specialized education or training have expanded their roles to various nontraditional areas, including:**

1. Risk management
   a. Responsibilities include anticipating and controlling potential causes of human and financial loss related to occupational health and safety incidents.
   b. Risk managers help manage insurance coverage for workers' compensation and other health- and disability-related insurance products.
2. Occupational and environmental health nurses may also be responsible for an organization's safety program.

a. A primary responsibility of the safety officer is maintaining organizational regulatory compliance.

b. Functional activities may include some tasks usually performed by industrial hygienists or other safety professionals.

3. Occupational and environmental health nurses may provide counseling services for work-related or non–work-related concerns, many of which may adversely impact the employee's work effort.

a. The occupational health nurse counselor addresses the worker's psychosocial needs, wellness/health promotion concerns, and other health or work-related concerns.

b. The occupational health nurse counselor may assume primary responsibility for managing the employee assistance program (EAP); in workplaces where this service is outsourced, the occupational health nurse may be the first contact for referral to the EAP.

4. Occupational and environmental health nurses are increasingly called upon to manage benefit programs and advise management regarding the development of integrated benefit plans.

5. An increasing number of occupational and environmental health nurses are self-employed, working as independent contractors in many of these roles.

XIII Future Opportunities and Challenges

A Globally, workplaces and work forces are changing as a result of demographic, social, and technologic changes.

1. Changes in the United States include the following:

a. The demographics of the country, and consequently the work force, are changing.

b. Managed care is replacing "free choice" as the predominant system for the delivery of health care in this country; employers have a major role in the provision of health care packages for employees.

c. The information, technology, and service industries are expanding; the manufacturing industry is shrinking as a result of company closures, global economics, and increased automation.

d. Increasingly, businesses are choosing such cost-cutting measures as hiring part-time and temporary workers and using subcontractors for specialized work.

e. Technology is affecting communication patterns and the nature of work for many Americans.

f. Telecommuting is becoming increasingly common, transferring occupational hazards to the home setting.

2. Immigration and the development of multinational corporations have increased the likelihood that occupational and environmental health nurses will be working with an ethnically and racially diverse work force.

a. Culturally based norms, beliefs, and behaviors affect work ethics, practices, and health-related values.

b. Multilingual work forces are increasingly common, creating communication challenges.

B Implications for occupational and environmental health nurses

1. Health and safety services provided must be adjusted to accommodate a changing work force and its changing needs.

2. Occupational and environmental health nurses have a professional responsibility to keep abreast of changes in the field by reading professional literature and participating in continuing education and other forms of professional development.

3. Increasing opportunities exist for global and international practice, teaching, and research.

4. Occupational and environmental health nurses should participate in an effort to ensure that industries exported to developing countries incorporate adequate occupational and environmental safeguards.

5. Continual expansion of the occupational and environmental health nurses' functional roles, especially those relating to direct clinical interventions and management/administrative responsibilities, is creating additional opportunities to affect the health and safety of working populations.

BIBLIOGRAPHY

Agency for Toxic Substances and Disease Registry (ATSDR). (1992). *Taking an exposure history* (monograph). Atlanta, GA: DHHS.

American Association of Industrial Nurses, Inc. (AAIN). (1976). *The nurse in industry.* New York: AAIN.

American Association of Occupational Health Nurses, Inc. (AAOHN). (1997). *Guidelines for developing job descriptions in occupational and environmental health nursing.* Atlanta, GA: AAOHN.

American Association of Occupational Health Nurses, Inc. (AAOHN). (1998). *AAOHN code of ethics and interpretative statements.* Atlanta, GA: AAOHN.

American Association of Occupational Health Nurses, Inc. (AAOHN). (1999). *Standards of ocupational and environmental health nursing.* Atlanta, GA: AAOHN.

American Public Health Association (APHA). (1991). *Healthy communities 2000: Model standards* (3rd ed.). Washington, DC: APHA.

Ashford, N.A. (1995). Government regulation of occupational health and safety. In B.S. Levy & D.H. Wegman (Eds.), (1999). *Occupational health: Recognizing and preventing work-related disease and injury* (4th ed.) (pp. 211-236). Boston: Little, Brown and Company.

Boden, L.I. (1999). Workers' compensation. In B.S. Levy & D.H. Wegman (Eds.), *Occupational health: Recognizing and preventing work-related disease and injury* (4th ed.) (pp. 237-256). Boston: Little, Brown and Company.

Carson, R. (1963). *Silent spring.* Boston: Houghton Mifflin.

Centers for Disease Control and Prevention. (1996). Clarification. *MMWR Morbidity and Mortality Weekly, 45,* 495.

Centers for Disease Control and Prevention (CDC). (1998a). Fatal occupational injuries—United States, 1980-1994. *MMWR Morbidity and Mortality Weekly, 47,* (15).

Centers for Disease Control and Prevention (CDC). (1998b). Preventing emerging infectious diseases: A strategy for the 21st century overview of the updated CDC plan. *MMWR Morbidity and Mortality Weekly, 47 (RR15),* 1-14.

Chin, J. (Ed.). (2000). *Control of communicable diseases manual* (17th ed.). Washington, DC: American Public Health Association.

Christiani, D.C., & Wegman, D.H. (1999). Respiratory disorders. In B.S. Levy & D.H. Wegman (Eds.), *Occupational health: Recognizing and preventing work-related disease and injury* (4th ed.) (pp. 477-502). Boston: Little, Brown and Company.

Dirksen, M.E., Boni, P., Cassler, J., Hussey, P., Ivy, S.O., Schiffren, C., Olson, N.K., & Viges, J. *A model for occupational health nursing practice.* Unpublished.

Gerberding, J.L., & Holmes, K.K. (1994). Microbial agents and infectious diseases. In L. Rosenstock & M.R. Cullen (Eds.). *Textbook of clinical occupational and environmental medicine* (pp. 699-716). Philadelphia: Saunders.

Goldman, L.R. (1999). Environmental health and its relationship to occupational health. In B.S. Levy and D.H. Wegman (Eds.). *Occupational health : Recognizing and preventing work-related disease and injury* (4th ed.) (pp. 51-96). Boston: Little, Brown, and Company.

Grossman, J. (1973). *The Department of Labor.* New York: Praeger.

Howard, P.H., & Davies, W.S. (1985). Workers' compensation: An overview. *AAOHN Update Series, 2* (3), 1-8.

Hunter, D. (1978). *The diseases of occupations* (6th ed.). London: Hodder & Stroughton.

Karasek, R., & Theorell, T. (1990). *Healthy work: Stress, productivity, and the reconstruction of working life.* New York: Basic Books.

Kasl, S.V. (1984). Stress and health. *Annual Review of Public Health, 5,* 319-341.

LaDou, J. (1981). *Occupational health law: A guide for industry.* New York: Marcel and Dekker.

Lee, D. (1997). The high price of employee stress: How much is it costing your organization? *John Liner Review, 11* (3), 33-38.

Leigh, J.P., Markowitz, S.B., Fahs, M., Shin, C., & Landrigan, P.J. (1997). Occupational injury and illness in the United States: Estimates of costs, morbidity, and mortality. *Archives of Internal Medicine, 157 (14),* 1557-1568.

Levenstein, C., Wooding, J., & Rosenberg, B. (1999). Occupational health: A social perspective. In B.S. Levy & D.H. Wegman (Eds.), *Occupational health: Recognizing and preventing work-related disease and injury* (4th ed.) (pp.27-38). Boston: Little, Brown and Company.

Levy, B.S. & Wegman, D.H. (1999). Occupational health: An overview. In B.S. Levy & D.H. Wegman (Eds.), *Occupational health: Recognizing and preventing work-related disease and injury* (4th ed.) (pp.3-26). Boston: Little, Brown and Company.

Lusk, S.L., Gillespie, B., Ziemba, R.A., Caruso, C.C., & Hagerty, B.M. (1996). *Noise effects on cardiovascular and stress related diseases.* (Final Report to The United Auto Workers/ General Motors National Joint Committee on Health and Safety and its Occupational Health Advisory Board).

McGrath, D.J. (1946). *Nursing in commerce and industry.* New York: The Commonwealth Fund.

Moll van Charante, A.W., & Mulder, P.G. (1990). Perceptual acuity and the risk of industrial accident. *American Journal of Epidemiology, 131 (4),* 652-663.

National Center for Health Statistics. (1996). *Healthy people 2000 review, 1995-96.* Hyattsville, MD: U.S. Public Health Service.

National Institute for Occupational Safety and Health (NIOSH). (1996*). National occupational research agenda (NORA).* U.S. Department of Health and Human Services, Public Health Service, Centers for Disease Control and Prevention (Publication No. 96-115). Cincinnati, OH: NIOSH.

National Safety Council (NSC). (1996). *Accident facts, 1996 edition.* Itasca, IL: NSC.

National Safety Council. (1999). *Injury facts, 1999 edition.* Itasca, IL: NSC.

Ottoboni, M.A. (1991). *The dose makes the poison.* New York: Van Nostrand Reinhold.

Ramazzini, B. (1993). *The diseases of workmen* (Translated from the Latin *De morbis artificium diatriba of 1713,* by Wilmer Care Wright*).* Thunder Bay, Ontario: OH&S Press.

Reichheld, F.F. (1996). Learning from customer defections. *Harvard Business Review, 74 (2),* 56.

Rogers, B., & Cox, A. (1998). Expanding horizons: Integrating environmental health in occupational health nursing. *American Association of Occupational Health Nurses Journal, 46 (1),* 9-13.

Rom, W.N. (1998). *Environmental and occupational medicine* (3rd ed.) Philadelphia: Lippincott-Raven.

Rosenstock, L., & Cullen, M.R. (Eds.). (1994). *Textbook of clinical occupational and environmental medicine.* Philadelphia: Saunders.

Rosenstock, L., Olenec, C., & Wagner, G.R. (1998). The national occupational research agenda: A model of broad stakeholder input into priority setting. *American Journal of Public Health, 88 (3),* 353-356.

Salazar, M.K., & Primomo, J. (1994). Taking the lead in environmental health: Defining a model for practice. *American Association of Occupational Health Nurses Journal, 42 (7),* 317-324.

Silverstein, M. & Mirer, F.E. (1999). Labor unions and occupational health. In B.S. Levy & D.H. Wegman (Eds.), *Occupational health: Recognizing and preventing work-related disease and injury* (4th ed.) (pp. 715-728). Boston: Little, Brown and Company.

Suter, A.H. (1993). *Hearing conservation manual: Council for Accreditation in Occupational Hearing Conservation* (3rd ed.). Milwaukee, WI: Council for Accreditation in Occupational hearing Conservation.

U.S. Department of Health and Human Services (DHHS). (2000). *Healthy People 2010* (Conference Edition, in two volumes). Washington, DC: U.S. Government Printing Office.

U.S. Department of Labor (USDL), Bureau of Labor Statistics (BLS). (1999). *National census of fatal occupational injuries, 1998* (USDL 99-208). Washington, DC: U.S. Department of Labor.

Weil, D. (1992). Reforming OSHA: Modest proposals for major change. *New Solutions, 2,* 26.

World Health Organization (WHO). (1994). *Declaration on occupational health for all.* Geneva, Switzerland: WHO.

World Health Organization (WHO). (1999). *Occupational health: Ethically correct, economically sound* (Fact Sheet No. 84, revised June 1999). Geneva, Switzerland: WHO.

World Health Organization. (1995*). Global strategy on occupational health for all—The way to health at work.* Geneva, Switzerland: WHO.

CHAPTER

2

Workers and Worker Populations

Sally Lusk, Catherine Connon, Mary E. Dirksen, and Mary Miller

Workers and workplaces are affected by changes and trends that occur in the larger society. It is essential that occupational and environmental health nurses be knowledgeable about the potential effects that these changes have on the work force. This chapter provides an overview of current demographic, social, and technologic trends and describes some of the many worker populations that characterize the modern workplace.

I Demographic and Social Trends

A Supportive and explanatory data
1. Work force changes reflect changes in the general population.
    a. Assuming no change in immigration laws and fertility rates, the U.S. population will increase by nearly 50% from 2000 to 2050 (U.S. Department of Labor [USDL], September 1999).
    b. From 1998 to 2008, the size of the labor force is expected to increase by 17 million, a growth rate of about 1.2% per year, roughly the same as for 1988-1998 (Bowman, 1999).
    c. The work force will experience an increase in the proportion of women workers, an increase in the average age of workers, and continued, though variable, growth of all ethnic groups. The Hispanic labor force will expand about four times faster than the rest of the labor force (Bowman, 1999).
2. Society is placing a higher priority on family relationships, leisure time, and recreational activities.
    a. Many white-collar workers are unwilling to continue to work long hours, and many blue-collar workers are opposed to overtime (Lewin, 1995).
    b. Work and career goals may have a diminished importance (Lewin, 1995; Stone, 1995).
    c. Many professional-level workers are unwilling to accept transfer because of its effects on their families (Capell, 1995).
    d. Flextime and job sharing are work options increasingly used to help workers handle competing demands of work and family (Scott, 1995; Olmsted and Smith, 1994).
3. Workers may arrive at work more fatigued because of long commutes (Burke, 1995).

4. Virtual offices, or offices without walls, are increasingly used as telecommuting options to reduce office costs and commuting time (Dent, 2000; McNerney, 1995).
   a. The numbers telecommuting via computer from home to business drastically increased from 4 million in 1990 to 11 million in 1997.
   b. In 1992, nearly one-half of the 17 million small businesses in the United States were home-based.
   c. In 1990, the majority of those who worked at home were self-employed (54%), but a significant proportion (36%) were employed by private sector companies (U.S. Census Bureau, [US DOC]; March 1998).
   d. By 2006, nearly one half of all U.S. workers will be employed in industries that produce or intensively use information technology, products, and services (USDL, 1999).
5. Health care benefits provided at work sites are undergoing rapid changes.
   a. Health care options are increasingly being restricted with implementation of managed care systems (Burke & Jain, 1995).
   b. Workers are increasingly being required to pay more out-of-pocket expenses and may have reduced choice of providers (Service, 1995; Burke & Jain, 1995).
6. Stress and psychologic problems are increasingly seen as common problems, and the workplace is the greatest single source of stress (Dear, 1995).
   a. Layoffs and corporate downsizing are occurring with greater frequency (Lambert, 1995; National Institute for Occupational Safety and Health [NIOSH], 1996a).
   b. The organization of work is a major contributor to workplace stress (NIOSH, 1996a); work organization refers to the following:
      1) Scheduling of work (work-rest schedules, number of hours of work, shift work)
      2) Job design (complexity of tasks, skill and effort required, degree of worker control)
      3) Interpersonal aspects of work (relationships with supervisors and co-workers)
      4) Career concerns (job security and growth opportunities)
      5) Management style (participatory versus autocratic)
      6) Organizational characteristics (climate, culture, communications)
   c. Longer hours, compressed workweeks, shift work, reduced job security, and part-time and temporary work are realities of the modern workplace (NIOSH, 1996a).
   d. The shift from manufacturing to service continues, with service sector jobs now employing 70% of workers (NIOSH, 1996a); because service sector jobs require more interaction with people, they are more likely to involve stress, confrontation, and violence.
7. Violence in the workplace is on the increase; it is often associated with situations involving disputes and problem resolution (Dear, 1995; Stone, 1995).
   a. The physical security of workers is an increasing problem because of work-site burglaries, robberies, assaults, and homicides; armed robberies are a growing concern, especially in small retail and manufacturing businesses.
   b. Health care workers are at particularly high risk for violent situations because of the prevalence of handguns, the decrease in care for the

mentally ill, and the increasing use of hospitals for care of disturbed persons (Dear, 1995).

c. Taxicab drivers have the highest rate of workplace homicides, a rate 60 times higher than the national average (http://www.cde.gov/niosh/riolfs.html)

d. Women and older workers are at highest risk for assault in the workplace (Kraus & McArthur, 1996).

B **Implications for occupational and environmental health nurses**

1. Occupational and environmental health nurses will need to take into account the changing population and work force when designing and implementing work-site programs.

2. Changes in health care benefits may influence the type of services available to workers from their primary providers; this then may influence the choice of services provided at work sites.

3. Workers may need assistance in handling conflicting demands.

4. Workers who are transferred will benefit from assistance with family concerns (Capell, 1995).

5. Occupational and environmental health nurses may have less opportunity for face-to-face communication with workers; thus they will have to develop less-personal methods of communication with off-site workers.

6. Occupational and environmental health nurses need to be alert to the potentially dangerous effects of fatigue on work-site health and safety.

7. Programs are needed to help employers identify and prevent potentially dangerous or explosive personal reactions because of stress or mental illness (American Psychological Association, 1995; Stone, 1995; Harvey & Cosier, 1995).

8. Appropriate violence prevention and control measures should be developed for the work setting.

II Technologic Trends

A **Explanatory and supportive data**

1. The service sector is the most rapidly growing job sector in the United States.

   a. Computer technology, health care, and other professional services top the list of fastest growing occupations (Bowman, 1999).

   b. From 1994 to 2005, nearly all job growth will be in the service sector; manufacturing's share of total jobs will decline (USDL, BLS, 1995a).

   c. From 1998 to 2000, the fastest rate of increase and the greatest job growth was in professional specialty occupations; faster-than-average growth will continue for executive, administrative, managerial, technical support, marketing, and sales roles (Bowman, 1999).

2. Although there will continue to be new jobs for all levels of education from 1994 to 2005, the largest growth (29%) will occur in occupations requiring a master's degree, and the smallest growth (5%) will occur in those requiring moderate (1 to 12 months) on-the-job training.

3. Educational requirements for jobs are shifting:

   a. Occupations requiring an associate degree or higher education accounted for 25% of all jobs in 1998.

   b. An associate degree or higher education will be required for 40% of the job growth from 1998-2008.

      c. Large numbers of new jobs will require no education beyond high school (57% of the job growth from 1998-2008) (Bowman, 1999).

      d. Occupations requiring a bachelor's degree will grow almost twice as fast as the overall average and all of the 20 highest paying occupations require at least a bachelors' degree (USDL, September 1999).

4. Equipment using increasingly high technology will be used in all work settings.

      a. Advances in technology have increased the speed of production and the subsequent demands on workers.

      b. Computer equipment is increasingly being used at home for household tasks, purchases, and recreation.

      c. Automation (robots, robotic systems, and automated machinery) eliminates certain types of jobs, so fewer workers are responsible for complex systems (Levy & Wegman, 1999).

B **Implications for occupational and environmental health nurses**

1. New technologies will present new hazards that will need to be considered in occupational disease surveillance and prevention; the additive effect of home and recreational use of the technologies will also need to be evaluated.

2. Occupational stress related to job ambiguity, role uncertainty, and job insecurity may become increasingly apparent as technologic changes are implemented.

III Females in the Work Force

An increasing proportion of workers are female.

A **Supportive and explanatory data**

1. Demographics

      a. In 1998, 60% of women age 16 and older were in the labor force, up from 51% in 1977, (USDL, Women's Bureau [WB], April 1999), and by 2008 women are expected to constitute 48% of the labor force, up from 46% in 1994 [Bowman, 1999]).

      b. The proportion of female workers increased from 42.5% in 1980 to 45.6% in 1994 (USDL, WB, April 1999).

      c. Among white, African American, and Hispanic females, African American women had the highest rate of participation in the labor force in 1999 (62.8%); white and Hispanic women participated at 59.4 and 55.6%, respectively (USDL, WB, 1994).

      d. The participation rate of women with children is affected by the age of their children: (USDL, WB, April 1999)

         1) Mothers with children age 14 to 17: 79% participation

         2) Mothers with children age 6 to 13: 78% participation

         3) Mothers with children under age 6: 65% participation

         4) Mothers with children under age 3: 62% participation

      e. Between 1969 and 1999, the number of working married women with children increased by 84%. By 1998, two-thirds of all mothers in married couple families were employed (USDL, September 1999).

      f. From 1996 to 2006, growth in labor-force participation will be noticeable among 45 to 64 year olds, who will be more likely to work than were middle-aged women in the past (USDL, September 1999).

g. Seventy-one percent of working mothers with children at home reported they worked to support the family (USDL, WB, 1994).
2. Social factors
   a. Women are disproportionately represented in the lower-paying service sector occupations; job segregation by gender continues.
   b. Women have greater responsibilities for care of dependents, both children and the elderly; more women are single custodial parents than men; 72% of caregivers of the elderly are women (USDL, WB, 1998).
   c. "In an effort to meet family and work responsibilities, women may neglect self-care behaviors that promote and maintain their own health" (Killien, 1999, p. 472).
   d. In 1997, the aggregate cost of care-giving in lost production to U.S. business was estimated at $11.4 billion per year (USDL, 1999).
3. Work-related factors
   a. Females are often shorter, lighter, and not as physically strong as males; as a result, they may be more at risk for certain types of injuries.
   b. Higher rates of work-related musculoskeletal disorders have been reported in females as compared with males; risk factors may include differences in stature and physiology and the nature of jobs performed by women.
   c. Lung cancer rates are increasing faster in females than in males.
   d. Work-site exposures that present reproductive hazards are a serious consideration for female workers.
(Note: Reproductive hazards are also a serious consideration for male workers.)
   e. Almost 60% of working women identify stress as the number-one problem (Dear, 1995).

B Implications for occupational and environmental health nurses
1. Work-site programs should address the specific needs and problems of females. These programs may include education, support groups, referral to community resources, and other strategies that promote health and safety.
   a. Programs on prenatal care, women's health, and menopause concerns should be increased.
   b. Programs for early detection of breast, uterine, and ovarian cancer should be offered.
   c. Support for caregiver roles assumed outside of work may be required.
   d. Work-site day care for children and dependent adults may be needed.
   e. Women should be targeted for smoking cessation programs in view of their increasing smoking rates.
2. Work-site adjustments will need to be made to accommodate biologic characteristics of female workers.
   a. Work stations should be adjusted to accommodate females' stature.
   b. Ergonomic programs should be targeted to females to prevent work-related musculoskeletal disorders.
   c. Surveillance for potential reproductive hazards should be conducted.
   d. Personal protective equipment that fits females should be provided.
   e. Because job stress can result from a variety of working conditions, attention should be directed toward the following (Swanson, 2000):
      1) Eliminating sex discrimination and harassment
      2) Developing coping skills
      3) Promoting participation in decision making
      4) Expanding opportunities for advancement
      5) Providing family support programs

IV Minorities in the Work Force

An increasing proportion of the population consists of minority groups. Minority populations in the United States are defined as blacks (African-American), Hispanics, Asians and Pacific Islanders, and American Indians and Alaskan Natives (DHHS, 1991).

A **Supportive and explanatory data**
1. Demographic and social factors
   a. Because of immigration and the growth of resident minority populations, the United States is becoming increasingly a multiracial, multiethnic society.
   b. By 2013, Hispanics will replace African-Americans as the largest minority group (Jarratt, et al., 1994).
   c. By 2025, minorities will increase to almost one-half of the population (USDL, BLS, 1994).
   d. Because of limited opportunities and, in some cases, language and cultural barriers, some minority groups may have poorer education outcomes and lower household incomes (Jarratt, et al., 1994); low socioeconomic status is related to higher rates of illness and premature death.
   e. "Excess deaths," defined as the number of deaths occurring in relation to the number expected based on the death rate for the white population, occur in minority populations (DHHS, 1991).
   f. Leading causes of death differ by minority group; for example, hypertension is more common among African-Americans, diabetes among Native Americans, and chronic liver disease among Hispanics.
2. Employment factors
   a. Hispanic men will compose the largest share of the nonwhite work force in 2005 (6.4%); African-American women will be the second largest share (5.6%) (USDL, BLS, 1994).
   b. The African-American labor force is projected to grow more rapidly than the overall labor force (USDL, BLS, 1994).
   c. Minorities tend to work disproportionately in high-risk occupations, thus they suffer a disproportionate burden of morbidity and mortality (Frumkin, et al., 1999).
   d. Nonwhite workers experience higher unemployment rates than white workers (Taylor & Murray, 1999).
   e. Minority workers are more likely than white workers to hold jobs with lower pay and lower status (Taylor & Murray, 1999).
   f. Changes in labor-force composition include continued growth in women's participation, a decline in men's, and continued growth by all racial groups (white, black, Hispanic, Asian, and other) (USDL, BLS, 1994).

B **Implications for occupational and environmental health nurses**
1. Because of the increasing number of minority workers, occupational and environmental health nurses will need to have greater knowledge of and make greater use of multicultural approaches.
2. Occupational and environmental health nurses will need increased knowledge of diseases that are common in certain minorities.
3. For workers with fewer educational opportunities, remedial programs offered at the work site will present avenues to learn new skills and knowledge.

4. To ensure participation, work-site health and safety programs will need to consider the special needs of workers who are non–English speaking or who have low literacy levels.

V Age of Workers

The average age of the work force is increasing.

A **Supportive and explanatory data**

1. Demographic and social factors
   a. The U.S. population is growing older; in 1990 the median age was 32.8; it is projected to climb to 38.0 by the year 2020 (Jarratt, et al., 1994).
   b. The numbers and proportion of older adults in the population is increasing; by 2030, 20.0% of the U.S. population may be over 65 years of age (Wegman, 1999).
   c. With greater longevity and healthier lives, retirees at age 65 can look forward to as many as 30 more productive years (Fyock, 1990).
   d. More elderly workers are returning to or remaining in the work force.
   e. "In 1995 there were 3.4 workers per retired person and in the year 2030 there will be only 2.0 workers per retired person" (Jones, 1995, p. 3).
   f. A study of retired men found that almost one third returned to work, typically within the first year of retirement, with two thirds of these taking full-time jobs (Mergenhagen, 1994).
   g. Savings for retirement for middle-aged workers who suffer a reduction in salary or disruption of employment will be seriously affected.
   h. "Baby-boomers," the population of workers born between 1946 and 1964, indicate interest in early retirement, but may not be able to afford it (Mergenhagen, 1994).

2. Employment and work-related factors
   a. U.S. law has changed; there is no longer a mandatory retirement age for workers in nearly all job categories.
   b. The middle-aged and older worker is more likely to have responsibilities for a dependent elderly parent or spouse.
   c. Some older workers would like to work, but they think no work is available to them: the needs for money and life satisfaction are the chief reasons cited for returning to work (McNaught, et al., 1989).
   d. Labor-force projections for 1990-2005 estimate increases in participation by workers age 55 and older, with a gain of 2.5% for men and 5.7% for women (Fullerton, 1999).
   e. A study of available middle-aged nonworkers found that most considered themselves involuntarily retired (McNaught et al., 1989); many may embark on second and third careers after age 65 (Fyock, 1990).
   f. Retired workers represent an important worker pool (Herz, 1995).
   g. Middle-aged and older workers may experience increased musculoskeletal problems and decreased vision, hearing, and agility.

B **Implications for occupational and environmental health nurses**

1. Occupational and environmental health nurses should consider the following strategies to address the special needs and problems of older workers:
   a. Programs to prevent and treat musculoskeletal disorders related to poor ergonomics

     b. Increased light at work sites to improve visibility, because light requirements increase with age

     c. Increased attention to measures to ensure adequate hearing ability

     d. Increased support for caregiver roles assumed outside of work

     e. Promotion of work-site or community day care facilities for dependent adults

     f. More programs focusing on the illnesses more common in middle age, such as cardiovascular disease and cancer

     g. More programs to prepare workers for retirement

2. Interactions with older workers should allow for possible decreases in their ability to hear, process information, and handle new technology (Box 2-1).

3. Disease prevention programs may become increasingly important to employers as a means of decreasing health care costs, including the costs of supplemental health care insurance.

4. As corporations attempt to improve their profit picture by reducing employment of mid-level middle-aged workers, programs will be needed to assist workers with job and career transitions.

5. Occupational and environmental health nurses should ensure that wellness programs take into consideration the needs and interests of older workers.

6. Health promotion by mail has been successful in reducing health care costs of retirees and decreasing health-risk behaviors; this approach represents an opportunity for occupational and environmental health nurses to implement a cost-savings program (Lusk, Ronis, and Kerr, 1995).

BOX 2-1

Recommendations for training programs for older workers

Training programs for older workers should:

- Allow self-paced learning
- Use training materials with high-contrast colors and bold typeface
- Avoid posting training materials above eye level
- Speak clearly and distinctly during training sessions
- Use adult learning principles to train older adults in new skills
- Provide a friendly, supportive environment
- Eliminate jargon from the work site, or at least explain it from the start
- Use multiple training methodologies
- Use older workers to teach other older adults
- Group older workers in the learning process
- Build upon valuable life experiences
- Link learning with rewards
- Give older learners something in writing to help reinforce learning

Source: Adapted from Fyock, 1990.

VI Children in the Work Force

Children represent a significant portion of the work force; the number of working children has been increasing.

A **Supportive and explanatory data**

1. Demographics

    a. Children and adolescents under the age of 18 are legally considered minors and are regulated differently from adults in the workplace.

    b. The minimum age for youth employment is 14 years, except for certain agricultural jobs in which 12- and 13-year-olds are permitted to work; children working on family farms are exempt from regulations and typically work at a much younger age.

    c. The minimum age for hazardous job activities is 18 years of age in nonagricultural settings, but 16 years of age in agriculture.

    d. Children who work in exploitative situations like sweatshops, largely out of view of regulators or the public, account for a small fraction of those engaged in work in the United States (Castillo, Davis, & Wegman, 1999).

    e. In 1997, it was estimated that nearly 3 million 16- and 17-year-olds were employed (USDL, BLS, 1998); it is estimated that these data miss at least 11% of workers under the age of 18. In addition, USDL figures exclude 14- and 15-year-olds and do not include various job activities, such as news carriers and family businesses, including farming (National Research Council, 1998).

    f. The percentage of 16- and 17-year-olds working at some point during high school ranges between 50% and 80%, with most working from 16 to 21 hours per week (Parker, Carl, et al., 1994a; National Research Council, 1998); many report working more than 20 hours per week (Resnick, et. al., 1997).

    g. Most minors are employed in the retail trade, primarily restaurants and grocery stores, and in service industries (Miller & Kaufman, 1998; Windau, Sygnatur, & Toscano, 1999).

    h. Low-income and minority children are less likely to be employed and, when employed, work in more hazardous jobs than high-income youths (National Research Council, 1998).

2. Injury and illness data

    a. Occupational injuries experienced by children and adolescents, including disabilities and fatalities, occur with alarming frequency (NIOSH, 1995; National Research Council, 1998).

    b. Although most adolescents work part-time, their injury rate may actually be two to three times greater than for adults, based on the number of hours worked or exposure time on the job (Brooks & Davis, 1996; Miller & Kaufman, 1998).

    c. The National Institute for Occupational Safety and Health (NIOSH, 1995) estimates that 70 adolescents die from injuries at work each year, and nearly 200,000 suffer nonfatal injuries, a substantial number of which require hospitalization.

    d. Most occupational injuries occur in retail industries (e.g., restaurants and grocery stores), service jobs, agriculture, construction, and manufacturing (Banco et al., 1992; Belville, Pollack, Godbold, & Landrigan,

1993; Miller & Kaufman, 1998; Parker, Clay, et al., 1991); more than half of work-related injuries occur in restaurants, the majority of which are fast-food establishments (Hendricks & Layne, 1999).

   e. Many nonfatal injuries involve working with knives, hot oil, and cooking appliances; working on wet and greasy floors leading to falls; and overexertion from hazardous manual lifting (NIOSH, 1995); lacerations, strains and sprains, contusions, and burns occur most often (Banco et. al., 1992; Hendricks & Layne, 1999; Miller & Kaufman, 1998; Center for Disease Control and Prevention [CDC] 1996; Parker, Carl, et. al., 1994b).

   f. Chemical exposures, although less common, typically involve cleaning compounds, caustics, bleach, paints and solvents; routes of exposures include inhalation, splashes to the eye and skin, and ingestion (Woolf & Flynn, 2000).

   g. Adolescent males have been found to have injury rates up to twice as high as females (Banco, et al., 1992; Belville, et. al., 1993; Brooks & Davis, 1996; Miller & Kaufman,1998; Parker, Carl, et. al., 1994a, 1994b).

   h. The occupational fatality rate for 16- and 17-year-olds is 5.0 per 100,000 full-time workers, similar to that found in adults (Castillo, Landen, & Layne, 1994; Windau, Sygnatur, & Toscano, 1999).

   i. Most fatal occupational injuries to minors involve working in and around motor vehicles, operating tractors and other heavy equipment, working near electrical hazards, and working in jobs with a high risk of homicide (Castillo & Jenkins, 1994; NIOSH, 1995).

   j. Occupational homicide was the fourth leading cause of death for 16- and 17-year-olds from 1980-1987 (Castillo, Landen, & Layne, 1994); from 1992-1997, occupational homicide exceeded highway incidents as the leading cause of death, primarily in the retail trade (Windau, Sygnatur, & Toscano, 1999).

   k. The youngest workers (under 16 years of age) have a higher proportion of injury claims, and with greater severity, in agricultural work than in other industries (Heyer, et al., 1992; Layne, et al., 1994; Miller & Kaufman, 1998).

   l. Transportation-related events, primarily involving tractors, account for at least one half of fatalities to young workers in agriculture (Castillo, Adekoya, & Myers, 1999); this same study found a work-related fatality rate for youth in agriculture in 1992-1993 to be 12.2 deaths per 100,000 full-time equivalents (FTE)—2.4 times greater than for all industries and ages combined.

3. Work-related factors
   a. Federal and state child labor laws regulate youth employment and establish the permitted hours of work, prohibited work activities, and administrative requirements.

   b. Many fatal and nonfatal work-related injuries involve activities prohibited by federal and state child labor regulations (NIOSH, 1995; Knight, Castillo, & Layne, 1994; Suruda & Halperin, 1991).

   c. The Fair Labor Standards Act (FLSA) of 1938, the federal law regulating youth employment, has not been revised to reflect changes in the patterns of work for young people, the nature of work and accompanying hazards, and knowledge about the health and safety risks young workers face; some state laws differ in their level of protection.

  d. Agricultural work, on family farms and in employment settings, expose younger workers to hazards not allowed in nonagricultural settings, including the operation of hazardous machinery, exposure to pesticides, poor sanitary conditions, trauma from animals, and falls from ladders.

  e. Industries that are known to hire youths, such as restaurants, grocery stores, and services, are also known to have a high risk for work-site violence, largely because of the exchange of money that takes place in these settings (Castillo, Lander, & Layne, 1994; Jenkins, et al., 1993).

  f. More than half (54%) of teens receiving care in emergency departments for work-related injuries reported not having received any health and safety training at work (Knight, et al., 1994).

  g. Little research has been done to evaluate children for acute, chronic, or latent effects from exposure to toxic chemicals, such as pesticides, or to physical hazards, such as noise; the long-term effects of injuries sustained during early work experiences is also unknown.

4. Social factors

  a. The failure to prevent work-related injuries and provide adequate protection to children in the workplace is a serious public health problem.

  b. The United States leads all other industrialized nations in the employment of youth (Wegman & Davis, 1999).

  c. Children who work have two jobs—education and employment—but typically their work is not connected to their educational needs and goals.

  d. Contributing factors for the increase in the number of children working include social pressure, high level of consumerism, acceptance of child employment, availability of low-skilled jobs, lower wages, growing poverty, relaxation in law enforcement, and increasing immigration.

  e. The health and safety problems of child and adolescent workers typically fall outside the scope of pediatric public health programs, and most occupational health and safety efforts focus primarily on adult workers.

  f. Teens are inexperienced workers and less likely to recognize hazards or understand their legal rights on the job; teens may not feel capable of speaking up to an adult supervisor or refusing to do a task that is inappropriate or dangerous, especially if they desire to be treated more like adults than children.

  g. The number of hours worked by teens may affect academic performance and lower educational attainment, diminish participation in peer and family activities, and increase the risk of substance abuse and other minor deviant behaviors (Carskadon, 1990b; Greenberger & Steinberg, 1986; National Research Council, 1998).

  h. Adolescents have a physiologic need for more sleep than adults; longer and later work hours may lead to sleep deprivation and thus to increased levels of stress, anxiety, and depression (Carskadon, 1990a; Kelman, 1999; Steinberg & Dornbusch, 1991).

  i. In addition to possible disability leading to lost work time, work-related injuries contribute to missed school time (Parker, Carl, et al., 1994b).

  j. Children and adolescents are not just small adults; differences in physical, cognitive, and psychologic development, including maturity, experience, and judgment, put them at greater risk of injury on the job.

k. Risk-taking behavior is a typical characteristic of adolescents as they explore their capabilities, but they often fail to perceive their limitations and vulnerability.

l. Protecting young workers can hopefully contribute to a change in the culture of health and safety and lead to greater protection of our future adult work force.

B **Implications for occupational and environmental health nurses**

1. Advocacy

   a. Reinforce that teens have the right to a safe and healthy work environment.

   b. Participate in partnerships with diverse members of the community to develop a comprehensive educational approach that addresses the health and safety needs of young workers, preferably integrated into existing initiatives aimed at protecting youth; such programs should include parents, employers, educators, health care providers, teens, and others (NIOSH, 1999).

   c. Encourage parents to take an active role in their children's employment decisions, including decisions about specific job assignments and work intensity (i.e., the number of hours of work per week).

   d. Encourage educators, who play a role in approving work permits or authorization forms that allow teens to work, to use this opportunity to monitor the planned work activities and hours of work, and ensure they do not interfere with the student's education.

   e. Reinforce to employers that they are responsible for providing a safe and healthy work environment and must provide adequate (i.e., extra) supervision and training for young workers and assign only age-appropriate activities; work practices should also be modified to accommodate the particular abilities, skill levels, and developmental needs of adolescents.

   f. Educate primary care and adolescent health care providers to inquire about their patients' work activities and provide appropriate anticipatory guidance.

   g. Promote job opportunities that provide both educational opportunities and a balanced schedule for youths to allow participation in family and peer activities.

   h. Encourage teens to be involved in the development and delivery of health and safety training programs; such programs increase acceptance among peers and enhance their own investment in protecting themselves and understanding their rights.

   i. Advocate that enforcement of existing regulations should be strengthened; existing child labor regulations should also be evaluated for their appropriateness in the current work environment and updated accordingly; agricultural regulations should become more consistent with nonagricultural restrictions for hazardous activities.

2. Education and outreach

   a. Public health professionals and injury control experts should be educated regarding the risk of occupational injury for children and adolescents.

   b. Occupational health and safety professionals should become knowledgeable about the hazards faced by young workers.

    c. Workplace health and safety training programs (e.g., hazard communication, injury and illness prevention, safe task performance) should be age appropriate; teen workers should be encouraged to ask questions and refuse to perform activities that they have not been trained to do or that are too dangerous.

    d. Front-line supervisors and adult co-workers who directly interact with young workers should receive extra training about the special needs of young workers.

    e. Education about occupational health and safety issues, including rights and responsibilities in the workplace, should be provided in all high schools; occupational health and safety curricula has been shown to be successful in secondary education (Lerman, et. al., 1998).

    f. Farm families should be involved in educational and prevention activities to increase awareness of the risk of injury in the home and farm work environment.

3. Research

    a. More research is needed to examine the association of factors, such as work experience, gender, work setting, and pace of work, with the occurrence of hazardous exposures and injuries among adolescents.

    b. Research leading to a better understanding of age-appropriate work activities in agricultural and nonagricultural settings is crucial.

    c. Intervention research projects should be developed to evaluate the effectiveness of training programs (i.e., apprenticeship and other vocational education programs), integration of occupational health and safety curriculum in high schools, federal and state child labor regulations, and other preventive strategies for adolescent workers.

    d. Research of the long-term impacts of early work-related exposures and injuries should be done, including evaluation of disability outcomes and psychosocial responses, attitudes toward work and the risk of occupational hazards, biologic effects of toxic exposures, and changes in career options as a result of injury.

    e. More surveys of teens regarding their beliefs and attitudes about safety on the job should be undertaken.

VII Contingent and Other Alternative Workers

The use of contingent and alternative workers is markedly increasing. These workers may be floaters, regular part-time workers, formal intermittents, limited-duration hires, informal intermittents, casuals, contract labor–service workers, independent contractors, leased workers, or temporary workers (Mayall, 1995). The Bureau of Labor Statistics (USDL, BLS, 1999) defines contingent work as any job in which an individual does not have an explicit or implicit contract for long-term employment.

A Supportive and explanatory data

1. Demographics

    a. In 1999, 8.2 million workers were identified as independent contractors, 2.0 million worked "on-call," 1.2 million worked for temporary agencies, 769,000 worked for contract firms, and 5.6 million held contingent jobs (USDL, BLS, 1999).

    b. The number of people employed full time by Fortune 500 companies shrunk from 19% of the work force in the early 1970s to less than 10% in the 1990s (Castro, 1993).

c. Wage differentials between temporary and permanent work are much larger for blue-collar workers, but nearly zero for those in professional or managerial positions (Segal & Sullivan, 1995).

d. The model selected for using contingent workers is influenced by the following factors (Mayall, 1995):
   1) Volume, periodicity, and duration of work
   2) Skill required for the work
   3) Labor supply
   4) Cost of hiring, benefits, job security
   5) Legislation and unions

e. The number of part-time female workers is increasing dramatically; from 1980 to 1991 there was a 16% increase in female part-time workers and only a 3% increase in male part-time workers (USDL, WB, 1994); 44% of contingent workers work part-time (USDL, BLS, 1999).

f. All types of workers may be employed as temporary workers (e.g., doctors and nurses, bank officers, attorneys, and corporate executives) (Castro, 1993).

g. Contingent workers are over represented in professions, with teachers accounting for more than 10% of all contingent workers (Polivka, 1996).

h. The trend among large corporations is to outsource their occupational health services, with the following results:
   1) Occupational health nursing positions may be eliminated.
   2) Nurses with inadequate occupational health and safety preparation may deliver work-site services.

i. Contingent workers, as compared with noncontingent workers, are:
   1) More likely to be female and black and in construction and services industries (Hipple, 1998)
   2) More than twice as likely to be aged 16 to 24 than noncontingent workers and thus more likely to be enrolled in school (USDL, BLS, 1999), generally earning lower incomes and less likely to have health insurance and pension benefits through the employer (Hipple & Stewart, 1996).

2. Work-related factors (Lenz, 1994)

a. Alternative workers may be co-employed. *Co-employment* is the term used to describe ". . . a relationship between two or more employers in which each has actual or potential legal rights and duties with respect to the same employee or group of employees" (Lenz, 1994, p. 13).

b. Co-employment influences civil rights, workers' compensation, labor relations and practices, workers' benefits, reasonable accommodation for the disabled, work-site safety, and job training.
   1) Liability is generally determined by the employer's relationship with or actions toward the worker.
   2) Workers' compensation and unemployment insurance laws related to co-employment vary by state in terms of single or joint responsibility.
   3) Generally, health and pension benefits, if any, are provided by the staffing agency (that is, the agency that provides workers for an employer); although few workers receive these benefits now, they may increase as work assignments become more long-term.

    4) Both staffing agencies and the work-site employer can be held liable for infringements of civil rights (Lenz, 1994).

  c. The Americans with Disabilities Act (ADA) requires reasonable accommodation on the part of the staffing agency and the work-site employer, but it is not clear regarding specific responsibilities related to alternative workers, making cooperation essential.

  d. Under ADA, staffing companies have the right to ask relevant health questions before considering a worker for a specific job assignment.

  e. Work-site employers, rather than staffing agencies, are required to maintain OSHA records of workers' illnesses and injuries and to provide work-site safety programs; however, staffing agencies are responsible for workers' compensation coverage.

  f. A greater use of staffing agencies is expected in the future.

  g. The increased use of contingent workers is estimated to account for about one half of the decline in permanent jobs in manufacturing (Segal & Sullivan, 1995).

  h. Temporary workers may be less willing to report illnesses or injuries because of fear that doing so may interfere with the possibility of being hired as a permanent employee (Morris, 1999).

  i. Use of temporary employees offers a business the opportunity to more carefully screen and evaluate potential employees (Segal & Sullivan, 1995).

3. Health considerations

  a. Contingent or alternative workers are less likely to have health insurance than noncontingent or nonalternative workers, and for those who do have coverage, it is less likely to have been provided by their employers (USDL, BLS, 1995b).

  b. The lack of job security may increase contingent and alternative workers' stress.

  c. Assignment to hazardous work without adequate training increases temporary workers' risk of illness and injury (Castro, 1993).

  d. Tensions may exist between contingent workers and regular workers in a given job site (Caudron, 1994).

  e. The lack of an emotional and psychologic attachment to a place of employment may have a negative effect on a worker's health.

B Implications for occupational and environmental health nurses

1. Occupational and environmental health nurses in some organizations will be serving an increasing number of temporary workers.

2. Because alternative workers are less likely to have health insurance, they will be constrained in their follow-up of recommendations for preventive care and ongoing treatment of chronic problems.

3. Occupational and environmental health nurses must be familiar with state and federal laws governing the obligations of work-site employers and staffing agencies regarding civil rights, disabilities, safety education, and job training.

4. Occupational and environmental health nurses may be involved in negotiating arrangements between the staffing agency and the work-site employer regarding selection criteria, care of injured workers, disability adjustments, and safety education.

5. Because the majority of temporary workers are female, all implications for female workers apply to this group as well. (Section III. B)

6. Stress reduction programs may be particularly important at work sites with large numbers of contingent workers.
7. Alternative workers may need extra help in assessing jobs for hazards and direction regarding job training and job safety.
8. As corporations outsource their health care services, more occupational and environmental health nurses may experience the challenges of being temporary workers; occupational and environmental health nurses may need to move into entrepreneurial roles to sell their services to industry.

VIII Workers in Labor Unions

A decreasing proportion of workers are represented by labor unions.

A Supportive and explanatory data

1. In contrast with other developed countries, American unions have seen a decline in membership from a high of 35% of workers in the 1950s to less than 14% in 1999 (USDL, BLS, 2000a).
2. The number of union workers increased by more than 265,000 in 1999, the largest annual increase in 20 years. The percentage remained the same, at 13.9%, stopping a trend of decline (USDL, BLS, 2000a).
3. The percentage of workers belonging to unions varies by type of employer, as illustrated by the following (USDL, BLS, 2000a):
   a. Government—37%
   b. Public utilities—26%
   c. Transportation—26%
   d. Construction—19%
   e. Manufacturing—16%
4. Union membership is highest among local-government workers (service groups that include police and firefighters) at 43%. (USDL, BLS, 2000a).
5. The highest unionization rate across demographic groups is for employed African American men; a little more than 20% are members of unions (USDL, BLS, 2000a)
6. From 1983 to 1999, union membership has declined more among men (25% to 16%) than women (15% to 11%) (USDL, BLS, 2000a).
7. Factors contributing to the decline in union membership include the following (Ziegler, 1994):
   a. International competition
   b. More diversified and specialized production techniques
   c. Deregulation of industries
   d. Increased use of part-time and temporary workers
   e. Failure of unions to focus on recruitment
   f. Disenchantment with union leadership
   g. Lack of enforcement of labor laws

B Implications for occupational and environmental health nurses

1. In work sites without union contracts, occupational and environmental health nurses may serve as the primary advocate for the promotion of occupational health and safety programs and activities.
2. In work sites without unions, occupational and environmental health nurses may have the primary responsibility for ensuring that workers are informed and knowledgeable about health and safety hazards in the workplace.

3. Occupational and environmental health nurses need to involve worker representatives in program planning and implementation, whether they are from the union or other work-team structures.

IX Disabled Workers

There are increased numbers of disabled workers who require accommodation.

A **Supportive and explanatory data**
1. Terms and definitions regarding disabilities from the ADA (Chapter 3 presents more information about the ADA.)
   a. The ADA defines disability as one of the following: (ADA, 1990)
      1) A physical or mental impairment that substantially limits one or more of the major life activities of such individual
      2) A record of such an impairment
      3) Being regarded as having such an impairment
   b. A physical or mental impairment is "any physiological disorder, or condition, cosmetic disfigurement, or anatomical loss affecting one or more body systems [specified]; or, any mental or psychological disorder such as mental retardation, organic brain syndrome, emotional or mental illness, and specific learning disabilities" (ADA, 1990)
   c. A qualified individual with a disability is an individual with a disability who, with or without reasonable accommodation, can perform the essential functions of the job (ADA, 1990)
   d. The ADA defines reasonable accommodation as follows (ADA, 1990):
      1) Modification of work processes or existing facilities used by workers such that they be readily accessible to and usable by individuals with disabilities
      2) [Reasonable accommodation] may include job restructuring, modified work schedules, modified equipment, job reassignment, and training
   e. It is important to distinguish between work disability and work-related disability; not all work disabilities are work-related.
2. Demographics and social factors
   a. In 1999, 17 million persons (9.7% of the working-age population [ages 16 to 64]), had work disabilities (U.S. Census Bureau, 1999a).
   b. In 1999, among persons aged 16 to 64 years, 68% of all work disabilities were severe (U.S. Census Bureau, 1999a).
   c. Work disability increases with age, as follows (U.S. Census Bureau, 1999a):
      1) 3.8% of persons 16 to 24 years of age
      2) 5.6% of persons 25 to 34 years of age
      3) 8.8% of persons 35 to 44 years of age
      4) 12.9% of persons 45 to 54 years of age
      5) 22.3% of persons 55 to 64 years of age
      6) 23.6% of persons 65 to 69 years of age
   d. In 1998, more females had work disabilities than males (10.1% vs. 9.8%), and more African-Americans had work disabilities than Caucasians (14.7% vs. 9.3%) (U.S. Census Bureau, 1999b).
   e. Educational level is inversely associated with work disability, as shown by the following figures for ages 16 to 65 (U.S. Census Bureau, 1999a):
      1) 24.8%, for those with less than 12 years of education

2) 11.6%, for those with high school education

3) 6.7%, for those with college education

   f. Persons aged 16 to 64 with a disability who completed 16 or more years of education are nearly twice as likely to be employed compared with those with 12 years of education (47.3% vs. 24.7%) (U.S. Census Bureau, 1999a).

3. Work-related factors

   a. From 1995 to 1997, the number of disabling injuries occurring on the job increased from 3.6 million to 3.8 million, whereas the number of worker deaths on the job decreased from 5,300 to 5,000 for the same period. These deaths and disabling injuries accounted for 80 million days of production time lost (U.S. Census Bureau, 1999b).

   b. The unemployment rate for persons aged 16 to 64 with work disabilities is estimated at 10.9%, whereas the unemployment rate for persons of the same age group without work disabilities is less than half of that (4.4%) (U.S. Census Bureau, 1999a).

   c. By 1997, more disabling injuries occurred to persons employed in services, trade, manufacturing, and construction than in other industry groups (U.S. Census Bureau, 1999b).

   d. Women with disabilities are concentrated in the service and retail sectors, and men in service and manufacturing sectors (Kraus & Stoddard, 1991).

B **Implications for occupational and environmental health nurses**

1. Increased attention will need to be given in the workplace to specific needs of disabled workers (Harber & Fedoruk, 1994; West, 1995).

2. Work-site adjustments will be needed to accommodate physical limitations of disabled or functionally impaired workers; these include (Pruitt, 1995):

   a. Modification of equipment

   b. Installation of mechanic aids

   c. Job restructuring

   d. Work-schedule modifications

   e. Additional training or conditioning

3. Job requirements, including job tasks, will need to be clearly defined.

4. Case management, as a strategy to ensure attainment of timely health services and supportive work-site accommodations for workers with disabilities or functional impairment, will become an increasingly important role for occupational and environmental health nurses (Martin, 1995).

5. Program efforts need to be directed at preventing work-related disabling conditions or functional impairments.

6. Comprehensive surveillance programs, including hazard and health surveillance, should be incorporated into existing health monitoring systems (Baker & Matte, 1992).

X Agricultural Workers

A **Supportive and explanatory data**

1. Characteristics of the population

   a. Agriculture ranks among the most hazardous industries

   b. Including unpaid workers and family members, nearly 8 million persons work in agriculture (NIOSH, 1996a, July).

   c. Farm workers are classified into three categories:

      1) Resident farm workers

      2) Nonresident farm workers

      3) Migrant farm workers who travel north and south for seasonal harvesting

   d. All three categories of farm workers often include children as workers.

   e. Migrant workers are subject to all hazards described for resident farm workers, plus those associated with frequent moves, poor housing, poverty, social and cultural isolation, lack of health insurance, and work-related musculoskeletal disorders caused by the postures required for harvesting (Smith, 1986).

   f. The majority of nonresident farm workers are local persons with lower levels of education and wages and, often, only seasonal work with no benefits; the nonresident farm worker is one of the lowest paid and least protected workers in the United States (Morrison, 1990).

   g. Nonresident farm workers may experience the same problems as migrant workers except for the frequent moves.

   h. All farm workers, including resident farm workers, are likely to be underinsured for health care.

2. Illnesses and injuries

   a. Agricultural production workers have one of the highest incidences of occupational injuries and illnesses—8.4 cases per 100 full-time workers vs. 6.7 for all private industry (USDL, BLS, 1999).

   b. In 1998, 115,000 agricultural work injuries and 831 agricultural work-related deaths occurred (USDL, BLS, 1999).

   c. Approximately one half of the injuries and deaths involved farm residents; one half involved nonresidents working on farms or in other industries classified as agricultural (fishing, agricultural services, and forestry, excluding logging) (National Safety Council [NSC], 1999).

   d. Every day about 500 agricultural workers incur disabling injuries; about one half result in permanent impairment (NIOSH, 1996a, July).

3. Causes of injury and illness

   a. Farm machinery is the most common cause of injury and death in children and adolescents (Merchant, 1991). Causes include the following (Wright, 1993):

      1) Rollovers of tractors or harvesting equipment that cause crushing or amputation injuries; one half of deaths are caused by tractors

      2) Power–take off equipment (machinery with a long, powered, rotating shaft) that can twist the worker around the shaft, causing suffocation, scalping, and avulsion injuries

      3) Machinery running in enclosed spaces that can cause carbon monoxide poisoning

   b. Farm machinery may cause noise-induced hearing loss (NIHL).

      1) NIHL may occur at an earlier age and be more severe among farm workers (Thelin, et al., 1983; Wright, 1993).

      2) Approximately 25% of male farm workers in one study had a hearing loss affecting communication by age 30, and 50% by age 50 (Karlovich, et al., 1988).

      3) Hearing loss has been documented in high school students involved in farm work, suggesting that the hearing loss seen in adult farmers may begin in childhood (Broste, et al., 1989).

      4) Noise-induced hearing loss can be prevented through engineering changes to equipment to reduce the noise levels and by workers' use of hearing protection (Lusk, Ronis, & Kerr, 1995).

c. Safety features in farm equipment
   1) New equipment may have built-in safety features; however, much of the machinery in use is older.
   2) Even new machines may be altered to circumvent safety features that are perceived as interfering with efficiency.
d. Agricultural workers are exposed to a number of hazardous materials (Table 2-1).
e. Exposure can be prevented through proper work practices and use of personal protective equipment.

4. The NIOSH Agricultural Initiative, developed in 1990, is a comprehensive research-based intervention program to reduce injury and disease among agricultural workers and their families.
   a. The Agricultural Initiative is designed to accomplish the following (Cordes and Rea, 1991):
      1) Assign nurses to rural areas to talk about prevention and distribute information about injury and illness prevention to farmers.
      2) Assess incidence of injury and illness
      3) Provide cancer screening and assess cancer rates
      4) Evaluate farms for safety hazards and determine the incidence of illness among farm family members
      5) Award academic grants to establish new centers and support applied research
   b. An Occupational Health Nurse in Agricultural Communities (OHNAC) program was initiated with 31 nurses in rural hospitals, clinics, and health departments in 10 states to provide surveillance of illnesses and injuries related to agricultural work (Connon, et al., 1993).

TABLE 2-1

Hazards to agricultural workers

Hazardous substance	Health effects
Anhydrous ammonia fertilizer	Contact can cause irritation, burns, or asphyxiation (Wright, 1993).
Insecticides and herbicides	Used to increase crop productivity, they can cause coma and death; insecticides and herbicides have been associated with increased incidence of cancer (Blair & Zahn, 1991; Wright 1993).
Fungal spores and moldy grains	These cause "farmer's lung," a chronic debilitating condition (Wright, 1993).
Nitrogen oxides	These oxides, found in silos, can cause chemical pneumonitis and pulmonary edema (Wright, 1993).
Methane gases	Gases formed in manure holding tanks and livestock confinement buildings can cause asphyxiation (Wright, 1993).
Extreme heat and cold	Because they work outside, agricultural workers may suffer heat exhaustion or frostbite. Because of their extensive exposure to the sun, they have higher rates of skin cancer and melanoma (Brown, 1991; Blair & Zahn, 1991).
Occupational infections	These infections, acquired from working with soil, animals, and animal wastes, affect thousands of farm workers each year, causing disability (Kligman, Peate, & Cordes, 1991).

B **Implications for occupational and environmental health nurses**

1. Agricultural workers generally do not receive services focused on their occupational health and safety needs.
2. There is an opportunity and need for collaboration between community health services and occupational health nurses to meet the needs of agricultural workers, including the following:
   a. Improved recordkeeping and a national monitoring and surveillance system for agricultural occupational illnesses and injuries
   b. Input regarding occupational health and safety illnesses and injuries into federally sponsored programs, such as migrant worker programs
   c. Improving farm families' understanding of and ability to appropriately respond to hazards that may result in their children's illness or injury
3. NIOSH's OHNAC program begins to address the needs of agricultural workers, but it is available to only a small proportion of agricultural workers.
4. Although the role of the agricultural health nurse has been described (Randolph and Migliozzi, 1993), studies are needed to determine the effectiveness of interventions to prevent illness and injury related to agriculture.
5. Intervention programs may include improved engineering standards for equipment, advocacy for legislation related to agricultural health and safety, and education of agricultural workers (Cordes and Rea, 1991).
6. Nurses not trained in occupational health nursing nonetheless need information regarding agricultural hazards in order to assess and treat rural residents.

XI Construction Workers

A **Supportive and explanatory data**

1. Characteristics of population
   a. There are approximately 7 million workers in the construction trades in the United States, representing 4.3% of all non–farm workers (NIOSH, 1996b, July).
   b. Of 636,000 construction companies, 90% employ fewer than 50 workers. Few have formal health and safety programs.
   c. Construction workers are a diverse and mobile population that comprises numerous specialists and skilled and semiskilled workers on job sites that are varied and changeable (Lusk, Ronis & Hogan, 1997).
   d. Subcontractors and laborers may work for several employers on different job locations in the space of only a few days (Lusk, 1993).
   e. According to trade association executives, the construction industry has ". . . one of the worst histories for attracting women and minorities . . ." (Dunbar, 1992, p. 12).
   f. Workers in the skilled and semiskilled trades tend to identify more with their trade than with the employer and are often self-supervised.
   g. Approximately one fifth of all construction workers are self-employed (NIOSH, 1996b, July).
   h. A higher proportion of construction workers are without health insurance (28%) compared with the total for all industries (16%) (Center to Protect Workers' Rights, 1998).

2. Work characteristics
   a. A significant portion of construction work is done outdoors, and indoor activities occur in relatively small spaces.
   b. Job sites are temporary; workers may work on several different job sites in a single day.
   c. The variability of the job sites, job conditions, tools used, and patterns of employment inhibit the use of environmental and engineering controls to reduce hazards (Lusk, 1993).
   d. Better general safety practices exist among unionized workers than among nonunionized workers (Dedobbeleer, et al., 1990).
3. Injury and illness data
   a. In 1998, national injury and illness rates for the construction industry were 8.8 cases per hundred workers, a rate higher than that for mining (4.9) and agricultural, forestry, and fishing (7.9) (USDL, BLS, 1999).
   b. Because injury rates are calculated with numbers of workers rather than hours worked as the denominator, the rates of construction worker fatalities is underestimated because many construction workers are employed part-time.
   c. "In two decades, the rates of lost-time injuries and lost work time per injury have remained fairly constant" (Ringen, et al., 1995).
   d. Fatalities and injuries in the construction industry are often a result of falls; 3,491 construction workers fell to their deaths between 1980 and 1989 (NIOSH, 1996b, July).
   e. 1,000 construction workers are killed on the job each year—more fatal injuries than in any other industry (NIOSH, 1996b, July).
   f. Because of the large amount of time spent outdoors, construction workers are at increased risk from the effects of heat, cold, and sun exposure.
   g. Construction health hazards have been characterized as ranging "from A to Z" (Table 2-2).
   h. Exposure to hazardous materials may spread to family members when construction workers carry home toxic substances on their clothing and tools.
   i. Some believe that construction workers are not afforded the same level of protection from health hazards as their counterparts in general industry (Rekus, 1994).
4. Standards for hearing-conservation programs are less stringent for construction than for manufacturers even though construction workers are exposed to excessive noise in many of their job sites.
   a. No requirement exists for periodic noise monitoring, dosimetry, periodic audiometric testing, or worker education.
   b. Beginning in 1991, U.S. legislators began to seriously consider extending more-stringent standards to the construction industry (Dumas, 1991).
   c. "Many hazardous exposures result from inadequacies in access to information, measurement technology, and personal protective equipment" (Ringen, et al., 1995).
   d. OSHA has issued three regulations for the construction industry:
      1) Hazardous Waste Operations and Emergency Response Standard (29CFR1926.65)

TABLE 2-2

Examples of construction hazards A to Z

Hazardous substance	Sources of exposure
Asbestos	Pipe insulation, asbestos concrete building materials, roofing felts
Beryllium	Beryllium-copper alloys
Carbon monoxide	Gasoline-powered engines and power tools
Diesel emissions	Portable power tools, heavy equipment
Electromagnetic radiation	X-radiography, UV from welding,
Formaldehyde	Plywood, particleboard, carpet
Gasoline	Operating and refueling equipment
Heat stress	Roofing, carpentry
Insect bites	Ticks or other insects
J-Band radio energy	Construction around radar sites
Ketones	Adhesives, glues, mastics
Lead	Fumes from hot work on painted structural elements
Metal fumes	Welding, cutting, and burning metal
Noise	Heavy equipment, portable power tools
Overexertion	Handling materials, lifting
Polynuclear aromatics	Combustion products
Q-switched lasers	Surveying, aligning sewer pipe
Repetitive trauma	Laying carpet, tying rebar
Styrene	Plastic materials
Tar	Roofing materials, coatings and linings for underground tanks and pipelines
Urethane paints	Decomposition products, including hydrogen cyanide
Vibration	Pneumatic tools
Welding fumes	Lead, copper, cadmium, iron, chrome, nickel
Xylene	Paints, glues, adhesives, mastics
Zinc	Fumes from cutting galvanized metals

Source: Rekus, 1994

   UV, Ultraviolet.

2) Process Safety Management of Highly Hazardous Chemicals Standard (29CFR1926.64)

3) Lead Exposure and Construction: Interim Final Rule (29CFR1926.62)

B **Implications for occupational and environmental health nurses**

1. Construction workers are underserved by occupational health and safety programs; therefore there is a need for new programs to reach this segment of the worker population.

2. Programs should focus on the major hazards of the construction industry—falls, machinery, chemicals, and noise.

3. Because construction workers work for multiple employers, there may be opportunities for entrepreneurial nurses to provide occupational health and safety services.

4. Ensuring health and safety in construction is complex, involving short-term work sites, changing hazards, and multiple crews working in close proximity (NIOSH, 1996b, July)

5. Because of the strong identification with the trade, trade union groups represent potential avenues for providing occupational health and safety services to construction workers.

XII Health Care Workers

A Supportive and explanatory data

1. Demographics and trends
    a. Health care and related services is one of the largest industries in the nation, employing about 11.3 million in 1998, of which more than two million were registered nurses and nearly a half million were self-employed (Kelenson and Tate, 2000; USDL, BLS, 2000b).
    b. The health industry employs a diverse population in a variety of occupational segments; it includes workers from all socioeconomic strata with varying levels of education, training, and English language skills, including the following:
        1) Professional specialties such as physicians, registered nurses, social workers, and therapists
        2) Service occupations such as nurse aides, medical assistants, dietary aides, janitors and housekeepers, and personal care and home health aides
        3) Technicians and support personnel such as health information and laboratory technicians, dental hygienists, clerical staff, and others
        4) Executive and administrative personnel
    c. More than 460,000 establishments make up the health industry, varying greatly in terms of size, staffing, and organization (USDL, BLS, 2000b).
        1) Hospitals constitute less than 2% of all private health service establishments, but employ nearly 40% of all workers in the industry; when government hospitals are included, the proportion rises to nearly half of all workers.
        2) Nearly two thirds of hospital employees work in establishments with more than 1,000 workers.
        3) Two thirds of all private health establishments are physician or dentist offices.
        4) More than half of all nonhospital health establishments employ fewer than five workers.
    d. Much of the health industry work force is employed part-time; many of these workers are students, parents of young children, dual jobholders, and older workers.
    e. Health care professionals tend to be older than workers in other industries, particularly in specialties requiring higher levels of education and training.
    f. Growth in the health industry is expected to exceed that of other industries for at least another decade (USDL, BLS, 1999, 2000b).
        1) Between 1986 and 1996, nearly one out of every nine new jobs created by the economy was in the health industry.
        2) Between 1998 and 2008, approximately 14% of all new jobs will be in the health industry, adding about 2.8 million new jobs.
        3) Employment in the health industry is projected to increase 26% through 2008, compared with an average of 15% for all industries; the greatest growth will be concentrated outside the inpatient hospital sector.
        4) By 2008, 12 of the 30 fastest growing occupations will be in the health industry.
    g. The changing landscape of the health industry and the evolving national

demographics will continue to redistribute the work force (Kelenson and Tate, 2000; USDL, BLS, 2000b):

1) Advancing medical technology enables increasingly sophisticated treatments and procedures to be provided in ambulatory clinics, provider offices, residential care facilities, and private homes.

2) The aging of the general population will require more home care and personal care services and residential nursing facilities; these segments of the industry will increase by 58% to 80% between 1998 and 2008.

3) As advances in medical technology increase the survival rate of severely ill or traumatically injured patients, more extensive therapy and rehabilitation facilities will be required.

2. Work environment

a. The USDL categorizes eight work environments in the health industry:
   1) Hospitals
   2) Nursing and personal-care facilities (inpatient convalescence and rehabilitation facilities; residential assisted-living facilities)
   3) Offices and clinics of physicians and osteopaths (including free-standing urgent care centers and ambulatory surgical centers)
   4) Home health care services
   5) Offices and clinics of dentists
   6) Offices and clinics of other health practitioners
   7) Health and allied services not elsewhere classified (such as kidney dialysis centers, drug treatment clinics, blood banks, and others)
   8) Medical and dental laboratories

b. Many who are employed in the health industry have little or no direct health care delivery functions, yet may be exposed to the same occupational hazards.

c. Most segments of the health services industry were not heavily unionized; in 1998, 14.9% of hospital workers and 10.7% of workers in nursing and personal care facilities were covered by union contracts.

d. Very few hospital-based facilities offer comprehensive health promotion programs for employees (Rogers, 1994).

e. Personnel who provide home care are exposed to many of the hazards traditionally associated with acute-care settings in addition to those unique to residential environments (e.g., traffic accidents, falls inside and outside homes, and increased risk of overexertion injuries). Mechanic lifting devices are rarely available in patients' homes (Smith & White, 1993; USDL, BLS, 2000b).

f. Occupational injury and illness incidence rates for health care workers (HCWs) in 1997, per 100 full-time equivalents (FTEs), compared to the rate for all service industries at 5.7, are as follows (NSC, 1999):
   1) Nursing and personal care facilities: 16.2
   2) Hospitals: 10.0
   3) HCWs providing residential care: 9.9

g. Needlestick and other sharps injuries present a significant risk of bloodborne pathogen infection to direct caregivers and others working in the health care environment.
   1) OHSA has responded to this risk by issuing a revised Bloodborne Pathogen Compliance Directive (1999) emphasizing the importance of implementing safer medical technologies, such as needleless

systems, among other administrative, engineering, and training requirements.

2) Several states have introduced or passed legislation aimed at requiring health care establishments to evaluate and make available safer medical devices.

h. HCWs and others in the industry who regularly don latex gloves are at increased risk for developing latex allergy; an estimated 10% to 17% of HCWs are allergic to latex, compared to less than 1% of the general population (Liss and Sussman, 1999; Yassin, Lierl, Fischer, O'Brien, Cross, and Steinmetz, 1994).

i. Workers in health care delivery environments are routinely exposed to biologic hazards at rates far exceeding the exposure to the general population, including the following general categories (Table 2-3 lists the most significant biologic hazards):

1) Blood-borne pathogens
2) Airborne pathogens
3) Vaccine-preventable communicable diseases

TABLE 2-3

Selected biologic occupational hazards to health care workers

Biologic/infectious agent	Major sources of exposure
Hepatitis A, E	Feces
Hepatitis B (HBV), Hepatitis C	Blood and body fluids
Hepatitis D (found only in patients with HBV)	Blood and body fluids
Human immunodeficiency virus	Blood and body fluids
Cytomegalovirus	Blood and body fluids
Rubeola (hard measles, red measles, 10-day)	Respiratory secretions (direct contact, droplet)
Mumps	Saliva (droplet, direct contact)
Rubella (German measles, 3-day)	Respiratory secretions (direct/indirect contact, droplet, airborne); virus shed in urine and stool
Influenza	Respiratory secretions, airborne droplet
Varicella zoster virus:	Indirect contact with freshly soiled articles
• Chickenpox	Respiratory secretions (direct contact, airborne)
• Shingles	Secretions of lesions, saliva
Herpes simplex virus	Secretions of lesions, saliva
Tuberculosis (pulmonary)	Airborne droplet
Salmonella, Shigella, Campylobacter	Feces
Parvovirus B19	Airborne droplet
Adenovirus	Airborne droplet, possibly by contact
Respiratory syncytial virus	Respiratory secretions (direct/indirect, droplet)
Pertussis	Airborne droplet, respiratory secretions
Scabies	Direct skin contact with infected lesions
Methicillin resistant staph aureus	Contact with purulent lesion, airborne (rare)
Fungal infections: dermatitis, parenychia	Frequently moist skin; direct contact

Chin, 2000; DiBenedetto, 1995; Sepkowitz, 1996

     j. Workers in health care facilities are often exposed to chemical hazards, which may contribute to sensitization or allergy, such as the following:
1) Anesthetic gases
2) Chemotherapeutic and antineoplastic agents
3) Disinfectants, detergents
4) Sterilizing agents
5) Solvents
6) Latex proteins
7) Tissue fixatives and reagents

    k. Workers in health industries are regularly exposed to multiple physical and environmental hazards (Box 2-2).

    l. Psychologic and emotional hazards in health care fields stem from the following sources and may result in the effects listed in Box 2-3.
1) Dealing directly with human suffering
2) Ethical dilemmas regarding client care decisions
3) Work overloads, staff shortages, hectic work schedules
4) Cyclic job insecurity
5) Verbal and physical aggression
6) Working rotating or nighttime shifts

B Implications for occupational and environmental health nurses
  1. Collaborative relationships between occupational health and safety professionals and administrative personnel can effectively facilitate the prevention, control, and abatement of occupational hazards, thereby reducing a number of risks.

BOX 2-2

Physical and environmental hazards in health care settings

- Needlesticks are the most commonly reported injury among HCWs.
- Over one-half of all reported back injuries occur within the health care field.
- Radiation:
  —Ionizing radiation has cumulative detrimental effects to all living tissue, including fetal tissue.
  —Nonionizing radiation poses thermal and light hazards to skin and eyes.
- Workers in health care are at greater risk for violent incidents than in other industries.
- Noise levels in housekeeping, dietary, laboratories, engineering, laundry, some nursing units, and other departments are often recorded at 80 dBA or higher.
- Ergonomic hazards in health care include cluttered hallways, patient rooms crowded with equipment, wet floors, the need to maneuver multiple pieces of equipment, awkward patient transfers, and the fast pace of emergent situations.
- Verbal and physical aggression is increasing in health care work environments.
- Lasers, a type of electromagnetic radiation increasingly used in health care settings, pose a risk of tissue trauma, particularly to vulnerable tissue, such as the eye.

BOX 2-3

Adverse effects of psychologic stress in health care workers

- Higher incidence of depression than in the general population
- Higher incidence of chemical substance addiction than in the general population
- Career burnout
- Psychologic and physical effects of shift work:
  —Chronic fatigue
  —Alterations in mood and personality
  —Strained interpersonal relationships; decreased socialization
  —Disorders of sleeping, eating, and elimination

—Decreased alertness; higher rates of accidents
—Increased rates of infertility or decreased fertility and other adverse reproductive outcomes among workers who rotate shifts
- Anxiety-related disorders, including altered work performance, related to actual or potential exposures to biologic, chemical, or other occupational hazards

---

2. As occupational hazards become known (e.g., latex allergies) and new technologies emerge (e.g., safer needle systems), occupational and environmental health nurses have a responsibility to advocate for organizational policies that address these issues.
3. The wide variety of workers in health industries, with their varying educational levels and job tasks, requires that occupational health and safety services and information be customized to the audience.
4. Comprehensive employee health services need to be made available to all health care workers including those who work off-site, those who provide home care services, night shift workers, and workers with no patient-care responsibilities.
5. There is a need for health establishments to offer more comprehensive health promotion programs to employees.
6. There may be increased opportunities for occupational and environmental health nurses to offer health and safety services to independent and alternative practitioners, as the public increases its demand for such professional services as acupuncture, naturopathy, hypnosis, chiropractic, and others.
7. As health establishments reorganize and merge, occupational and environmental health nurses will increasingly be responsible for the health and safety of employees in satellite and ambulatory clinics and associated service facilities, such as long term care facilities, that are affiliated with health care consortiums.
8. Health and safety services for home care workers need to be expanded to include assessments of the client's living environment; occupational and environmental health nurses may be able to advocate for temporary equipment to reduce the risk of injury.
9. Organizational policies and procedures to prevent, and a crisis plan to handle, violent incidents should be developed (USDL, OSHA, 1996).

10. Attention to the health and safety concerns of workers of childbearing age, particularly with respect to reproductive hazards, continues to be needed.

XIII International (Expatriate) Workers

A Supportive and explanatory data

1. Demographics and trends
   a. More than 60 million international workers are employed by more than 100,000 U.S. business concerns abroad (Marquardt & Engel, 1993).
   b. Ninety percent of U.S. expatriates are male; the percentage of female expatriates is increasing.
   c. New capitalistic and developing nations enthusiastically recruit business enterprises and skilled labor from the United States and other developed nations.
   d. The numbers of Americans and foreign nationals working in U.S. concerns abroad is increasing because of the following factors:
      1) The globalization of the marketplace
      2) Economic and regulatory incentives
      3) Trade policy reforms
2. The international workplace
   a. Approximately 80% of U.S. companies with expatriate workers provide predeparture orientation regarding health issues; of these, only 42% offer orientation to all expatriate workers (Solomon, 1994).
   b. Health systems abroad vary widely; some may not be able to offer the quality or quantity of services to which U.S. workers are accustomed.
   c. Occupational health and safety services in developing countries are generally poorly funded and often staffed with inadequately trained occupational health professionals (Levy, 1996); only 5% to 10% of workers in developing countries and 20% to 50% of workers in industrialized countries (with a few exceptions) are estimated to have access to adequate occupational health services (WHO, 1999).
   d. Local business, cultural, and social norms abroad may differ significantly from those in the U.S. workplace; a lack of understanding of norms may lead to interpersonal conflict and workplace stress among expatriate workers.
   e. Economic and environmental regulatory incentives that help recruit multinational companies to foreign locations may also contribute to unsafe, unhealthy, and repressive working conditions for local workers (Ballinger, 1995; Coats, 1995; Levy, 1995).
   f. A number of member countries in the European Union have adopted occupational health and safety regulations that are more advanced than those in the United States.
   g. Many developing countries continue to use the labor of children, despite local and international prohibitions against this practice; of the estimated 250 million children between the ages of 5 and 14 working in developing countries, nearly 70% work under hazardous conditions (WHO, 1999).
   h. The special needs of women, who constitute approximately 42% of the global work force, are seldom adequately addressed (WHO, 1999).
   i. Hazardous industries relocated in developing and newly industrialized

countries are often without adequate worker health and safety precautions (Johanning, et al., 1994; LaDou, 1992; Levy & Rest, 1996).

j. Although international guidelines for selected toxicants exist, efforts to develop international uniform occupational exposure limits have been unsuccessful; political and social forces often influence scientific decisions about exposure limits (Levy & Rest, 1996).

k. The most common health threat abroad is contamination of water supplies and food, particularly outside of urban centers in developing countries (http://www.cdc.gov/travel/foodwatr.htm)

B **Implications for occupational and environmental health nurses**

1. The breadth and depth of predeparture orientation related to the health issues of U.S. nationals planning to work abroad will need to be increased. (Chapter 14 presents an example of an international travel program).

2. U.S. nationals who are dispatched to work abroad need appropriate vaccinations against infectious agents endemic to the destination country.

3. Contingency plans for accessing local emergency services and for emergency evacuation should be developed.

4. Occupational health and safety programs need to be sensitive to regional management practices and cultural norms.

5. Occupational and environmental health nurses can be advocates for ethical practices related to child labor, women's health, and other workplace health and safety issues.

6. Occupational and environmental health nurses responsible for the health and safety of expatriate workers can gain valuable advice and insight from such international resources as the WHO, ILO, and International Safety Council.

BIBLIOGRAPHY

American Psychological Association. (1995, May–June). Society: Violence in the workplace. *The Futurist, 29,* 51-52.*Americans with Disabilities Act of 1990.* Public Law 101-336. 42 USC, 12101-12134.

Baker, E.L., & Matte, T.P. (1992). Surveillance of occupational illness and injury. In W. Halperin & E.L. Baker (Eds.), *Public health surveillance* (pp. 178-194). New York: Van Nostrand Reinhold.

Ballinger, J. (1995). Just do it—Or else. *Multinational Monitor, 16(6),* 7-8.

Banco, L., Lapidus, G., & Braddock, M. (1992). Work-related injury among Connecticut minors. *Pediatrics, 89(5),* 957-960.

Belville, R., Pollack, S., Godbold, J., & Landrigan, P. (1993). Occupational injuries among working adolescents in New York State. *Journal of the American Health Association, 269(21),* 2754-2759.

Benenson, A.S. (Ed.). (1995). *Control of communicable diseases manual* (16th ed.). Washington, DC: American Public Health Association.

Biefang, S., & Potthoff, P. (1994). Screening process to discover insured persons in need of rehabilitation. *International Journal of Rehabilitation Research, 17(3),* 215-229.

Blair, A., & Zahn, S.H. (1991). Cancer among farmers. In D.H. Cordes & D.F. Rea (Eds.), *Occupational medicine: Health hazards of farming. State of the art reviews, 6(3)* 335-354. Philadelphia: Hanley & Belfus, Inc.

Bowman, C. (1999, November). Employment outlook: 1998-2008: BLS projections to 2008: A Summary. *Monthly Labor Review,* 122 (11), 3-4.

Brimsek, T.A., & Bender, D.R. (1995). Making room for the virtual office. *Association Management, 47(12),* 71-86.

Brooks, D., & Davis, L. (1996). Work-related injuries to Massachusetts teens, 1987-1990. *American Journal of Industrial Medicine, 29,* 153-160.

Broste, S.K., Hanson, D.A., Strand, R.L., & Stueland, D.T. (1989). Hearing loss among high school farm students. *American Journal of Public Health, 79,* 619-622.

Brown, W.D. (1991). Heat and cold in farm workers. In D.H. Cordes & D.F. Rea (Eds.), *Occupational medicine: Health hazards of farming. State of the art reviews, 6(3)* 371-390. Philadelphia: Hanley & Belfus, Inc.

Burke, R.J. (1995). Commuting to work. *Perpetual and Motor Skills, 80(1),* 49-50.

Burke, T.P., & Jain, R.S. (1995). Employee benefits survey: *ABLSReader.* USDL Bulletin No. 2459, 90-96.

Capell, P. (1995, November). The stress of relocating. *American Demographics, 17,* 15-16.

Carskadon, M. (1990a). Patterns of sleep and sleepiness in adolescents. *Pediatrician, 17,* 5-12.

Carskadon, M. (1990b). Adolescent sleepiness: Increased risk in a high risk population. *Alcohol, Drugs and Driving, 5(4), 6(1),* 317-327.

Castillo, D., & Jenkins, E. (1994). Industries and occupations at high risk for work-related homicide. *Journal of Occupational Medicine, 36(2),* 125-132.

Castillo, D., Adekoya, N., & Myers, J. (1999). Fatal work-related injuries in the agricultural production and service sectors among youth in the United States, 1992-1996. *Journal of Agromedicine, 6(3),* 27-41.

Castillo, D., Davis, L., & Wegman, D. (1999). Young workers. *Occupational medicine: State of the art reviews, 14(3),* 519-536.

Castillo, D., Landen, D., & Layne, L. (1994). Occupational injury deaths of 16- and 17-year-olds in the United States. *American Journal of Public Health, 84(4),* 646-649.

Castro, J. (1993, March 29). Disposable workers. *Time, 141(13),* 43-47.

Caudron, S. (1994, July). Contingent work force spurs HR planning. *Personnel Journal,* 52-60.

Center to Protect Workers' Rights (CPWR). (1998). *The construction chart book: The U.S. construction industry and its workers* (2nd ed). Washington, DC: CPWR.

Centers for Disease Control and Prevention (CDC). (1990). Protection against viral hepatitis: Recommendations of the Immunization Practices Advisory Committee. *Morbidity And Mortality Weekly Report, 39(RR-2),* 1-26.

Centers for Disease Control and Prevention (CDC). (1991). Recommendations for preventing transmission of human immunodeficiency virus and hepatitis B virus to clients during exposure-prone invasive procedures. *Morbidity And Mortality Weekly Report, 40(RR-8),* 1-9.

Centers for Disease Control and Prevention (CDC). (1994). Guidelines for preventing the transmission of mycobacterium tuberculosis in health care facilities. *Federal Register, 59(208),* 54242-54303.

Centers for Disease Control and Prevention (CDC). (1996). Work-related injuries and illnesses associated with child labor—United States, 1993. *MMWR Morbidity and Mortality Weekly, 45(22),* 464-468.

Chin, J. (Ed.). (2000). *Control of communicable diseases manual* (17th ed.). Washington, DC: American Public Health Association.

Coats, S. (1995). Organizing and repression. *Multinational Monitor, 16(6),* 17-19.

Connon, C.L., Freund, E., & Ehlers, J.K. (1993). The occupational health nurse in agricultural communities program: Identifying and preventing agriculturally related illnesses and injuries. *AAOHN Journal, 41,* 422-428.

Cordes, D.H., & Rea, D.F. (1991). Farming: A hazardous occupation. In D.H. Cordes & D.F. Rea (Eds.), *Occupational medicine: Health hazards of farming. State of the art reviews, 6(3)* 327-334. Philadelphia: Hanley & Belfus, Inc.

Dear, J.A. (1995, November 1). Work stress and health '95: Creating healthier workplaces. *Vital Speeches of the Day, 62,* 39-42.

Dedobbeleer, N., Champaign, R., & German, P. (1990). Safety performance among union and nonunion workers in the construction industry. *Journal of Occupational Medicine, 32,* 1099-1103.

Dent, Jr., H.S., (2000) *The roaring 2000s.* New York: Simon & Schuster.

DiBenedetto, D.V. (1995). Occupational hazards of the health care industry: Protecting health care workers. *AAOHN Journal 43(3),* 131-137.

Ditlea, S. (1995). Home is where the office is. *Nation's Business, 83(11),* 41-44.

Dumas, K. (1991). House panels vote measures on worker health, safety. *Congressional Quarterly Weekly Report, 49,* 2081.

Dunbar, M. (1992, November/December). Women & minorities in construction. *Michigan Construction Users Council Newsletter,* 12.

Felton, J.S. (1990). *Occupational health management.* Boston: Little, Brown.

Frumkin, H., Walker, E.D., & Friedman-Jimenez, G. (1999). Minority workers and communities. *Occupational medicine, State of the art review. 14(3),* 495-517.

Fullerton, H.N. (1999, November). Employment outlook: 1998-2008: Labor force projections to 2008: steady growth and changing composition. *Monthly Labor Review,* 19-32.

Fyock, C.D. (1990). *America's work force is coming of age.* Lexington, MA: Lexington Books.

Greenberger, E., & Steinberg, L. (1986). *When teenagers work: The psychological and social costs of adolescent employment.* New York: Basic Books, Inc.

Harber, P., & Fedoruk, M.J. (1993). Personal risk assessment under the Americans with Disabilities Act: A decision analysis approach. *Journal of Occupational Medicine, 35(10),* 1000-1010.

Harber, P., & Fedoruk, M.J. (1994). Work placement and worker fitness: Implications of the Americans with Disabilities Act for pulmonary medicine. *Chest, 105(5),* 1564-1571.

Harvey, M.G., & Cosier, R.A. (1995, March-April). Homicides in the workplace: Crisis or false alarm? *Business Horizons, 38,* 11-20.

Hendricks, K., & Layne, L. (1999). Adolescent occupational injuries in fast food restaurants: An examination of the problem from a national perspective. *Journal of Occupational and Environmental Medicine, 41(12),* 1146-1153.

Herz, D.E. (1995, April). Work after early retirement: An increasing trend among men. *Monthly Labor Review,* 13-20.

Heyer, N., Franklin, G., Rivara, F., Parker, P., & Haug, J. (1992). Occupational injuries among minors doing farm work in Washington. *American Journal of Public Health, 82(4),* 557-560.

Hipple, S. (1998, November) Contingent work: Results from the second survey. *Monthly Labor Review,* 22-35.

Hipple, S., & Stewart, J. (1996, October). Earnings and benefits of contingent and noncontingent workers. *Monthly Labor Review,* 22-30.

Jarratt, J., Coates, J.F., Mahaffie, J.B., & Hines, A. (1994). *Managing your future as an association: Thinking about trends and working with their consequences 1994-2020.* Washington, DC: American Society of Association Executives.

Jenkins, E., Kisner, S., Fosbroke, D., Layne, L., Stout, N., Castillo, D., Cutlip, P., Cianfrocco, R., et al. (1993). *Fatal injuries to workers in the United States, 1980-1989: A decade of surveillance. National profile,* (DHHS publication NIOSH 93-108). Washington, DC: U.S. Government Printing Office.

Johanning, E., Goldberg, M., & Kim, R. (1994). Asbestos hazard evaluation in South Korean textile production. *International Journal of Health Services, 24(1),* 131-144.

Johnston, W.B., & Packer, A.E. (1987). *Workforce 2000: Work and workers for the twenty-first century.* Indianapolis, IN: Hudson Institute.

Jones, T.W. (1995, November). A warning on the future of U.S. pensions. *The Participant,* 3.

Karlovich, R.S., Wiley, T.L., Tweed, T., & Jensen, D.V. (1988). Hearing sensitivity in farmers. *Public Health Reports, 103(1)*, 61-71.

Kelenson, J.W., & Tate, P. (2000). The 1998-2008 job outlook in brief. *Occupational Outlook Quarterly*, (Spring, 2000). http://www.bls.gov.oco

Kelman, B. (1999). The sleep needs of adolescents. *Journal of School Nursing, 15(3)*, 14-19.

Killien, M. (1999). Women's work, women's health: In A. Hinshaw, S. Feetham, & S. Shawn (Eds.), *Handbook of clinical nursing research* (pp. 459-484). Thousand Oaks, CA: Sage Publications.

Kligman, E.W., Peate, W.F., & Cordes, D.H. (1991). Occupational infections in farm workers. In D.H. Cordes & D.F. Rea (Eds.), *Occupational medicine: Health hazards of farming. State of the art reviews, 6(3)*, 429-446. Philadelphia: Hanley & Belfus, Inc.

Knight, E., Castillo, D., & Layne, L. (1995). A detailed analysis of work-related injury among youth treated in hospital emergency departments: A nationally representative sample. *American Journal of Industrial Medicine, 27*, 793-805.

Kraus, J.F., & McArthur, D.L. (1996) Violence in the workplace: Epidemiology of violent injury in the workplace. R. Harrison (Guest Ed.) In *Occupational Medicine: State of the Art Reviews, 11(2)*, 201-218. Philadelphia: Hanley & Belfus, Inc.

Kraus, L.E., & Stoddard, S. (1991). *Chartbook on work disability in the United States. An InfoUse report.* Washington, DC: U.S. National Institute on Disability and Rehabilitation Research.

LaDou, J. (1992). The exposure of hazardous industries to newly industrialized countries (editorial). *Polish Journal of Occupational Medicine and Environmental Health, 5(3)*, 223-226.

Lambert, V. (1995). Give your company a checkup. *Personnel Journal, 74*, 143-149.

Layne, L., Castillo, D., Stout, N., & Cutlip, P. (1994). Adolescent occupational injuries requiring hospital emergency department treatment: A nationally representative sample. *American Journal of Public Health, 84(4)*, 657-660.

Lenz, E.A. (1994). Employer liability issues in staffing services arrangements. *Co-employment* (2nd ed.). Alexandria, VA: National Association of Temporary Staffing Services.

Lerman, Y., Feldman, Y., Shnaps, R., Kushnir, T., Ribak, J. (1998). Evaluation of an occupational health education program among 11th grade students. *American Journal of Industrial Medicine, 34*, 607-613.

Levy, B.S. (1995). Health and social effects of worldwide economic transformation: Focus on occupational and environmental health. *Social Justice, 22*, 77-84.

Levy, B.S. (1996). The context of hazards in the international setting, with a focus on developing countries, In L. Fleming, J. Herzstein, & W. Bunn (Eds.). *International occupational and environmental health.* Beverly, MA: OEM Publishing.

Levy, B.S., & Rest, K.M. (1996). Policies to protect and promote workers' health are necessary for sustainable human development. In G. Shahi, B.S. Levy, A. Binger, T. Kjellstrom, & R. Lawrence (Eds.), *International perspectives in environment, health and development: Toward a sustainable world* (pp. 486-496). New York: Springer.

Levy, B.S., & Wegman, D.H. (1999). *Occupational health: Recognizing and preventing work-related disease and injury,* (4th ed.). Boston: Little, Brown and Company.

Lewin, T. (1995, October 29). Workers of both sexes make trade-offs for family, study shows. *The New York Times: National,* p. 25.

Liss, G., & Sussman, G. (1999). Latex sensitization: occupational versus general population prevalence rates. *American Journal of Industrial Medicine, 35(2)*, 196-200.

Lusk, S.L. (1993). *Preventing noise induced hearing loss in construction workers.* Grant proposal funded by National Institute for Occupational Safety & Health. Grant No. R01 OH03136-03.

Lusk, S.L. (1995). Linking practice & research: Health promotion by mail. *AAOHN Journal, 43(6)*, 346-348.

Lusk, S.L., Ronis, D.L., & Hogan, M.M. (1997). Test of the health promotion model as a causal model of construction workers' use of heavy protection. *Research in Nursing and Health, 20*, 183-194.

Lusk, S.L., Ronis, D.L., & Kerr, M.J. (1995). Predictors of hearing protection use among workers: Implications for training programs. *Human Factors, 37(3),* 635-640.

Marquardt, M.J., & Engel, D.W. (1993). *Global human resource development.* Englewood Cliffs, NJ: Prentice-Hall.

Martin, K.J. (1995). Workers' compensation: Case management strategies. *AAOHN Journal, 43(5),* 245-250.

Mayall, D. (1995). Temporary work and labor market detachment: New mechanisms and new opportunities. In D.B. Bills, *The new modern times: Factors reshaping the world of work* (pp. 163-192). Albany, NY: State University of New York Press.

McNaught, W., Barth, M.C., & Henderson, P.H. (1989). The human resource potential of Americans over 50. *Human Resource Management, 28,* 455-473.

McNerney, D.J. (1995). Telecommuting: An idea whose time has come. *HR Focus, 72(11),* 1, 4-5.

Merchant, J.A. (1991). Agricultural injuries. In. D.H. Cordes & D.F. Rea (Eds.), *Occupational medicine: Health hazards of farming. state of the art reviews, 6(3)* 529-539. Philadelphia: Hanley & Belfus, Inc.

Mergenhagen, P. (1994, June). Rethinking retirement. *American Demographics,* 28-34.

Miller, M. (1995, March). *Occupational injuries among adolescents in Washington State, 1988-1991: A review of workers' compensation data* (Technical Report Number 35-1-1995). Safety and Health Assessment and Research for Prevention. Olympia, WA: Washington State Department of Labor and Industries.

Miller, M., & Kaufman, J. (1998). Occupational injuries among adolescents in Washington State, 1988-1991: A review of workers' compensation data. *American Journal of Industrial Medicine, 34,* 121-132.

Morris, J. (1999). Injury experience of temporary workers in a manufacturing setting. Factors that increase vulnerability. *AAOHN Journal, 47(10),* 470-478.

Morrison, P.A. (Ed.) (1990). A taste of the country: A collection of Calvin Beale's writings. University Park, PA: The Pennsylvania State University Press.

Morrow, L. (1993, March 29). The temping of America. *Time,* 40-47.

National Institute for Occupational Safety and Health (NIOSH) *Facts,* (1996a, July). Agriculture safety and health. http:1//www.cdc.gov/niosh/agfc.html.

National Institute for Occupational Safety and Health (NIOSH) *Facts.* (1996b, July). Construction safety and health.http://www.cdc.gov/niosh.constfc.html

National Institute for Occupational Safety and Health (NIOSH). (1996). *National occupational research agenda.* Atlanta: U.S. Department of Health and Human Services.

National Institute for Occupational Safety and Health (NIOSH). (1997). *Alert: Preventing allergic reactions to natural rubber latex in the workplace.* (DHHS [NIOSH] Publication No. 97-135). Available: http://www.cdc.gov/niosh/latexalt.

National Institute for Occupational Safety and Health (NIOSH) (1999). *Promoting safe work for young workers: A community-based approach,* (DHHS [NIOSH] Publication No. 99-14. Cincinnati, OH: U.S. Department of Health and Human Services.

National Institute for Occupational Safety and Health (NIOSH). (1995, May). *NIOSH Alert: Request for assistance in preventing deaths and injuries of adolescent workers,* (DHHS [NIOSH] Publication No. 95-125). Cincinnati, OH: U.S. Department of Health and Human Services.

National Institute of Occupational Safety and Health (NIOSH) (1999). *Promoting safe work for young workers: A community-based approach,* (DHHS [NIOSH] Publication No. 99-14. Cincinnati, OH: U.S. Department of Health and Human Services.

National Research Council and Institute of Medicine (1998). *Protecting Youth at Work: Health, Safety, and Development of Working Children and Adolescents in the United States.* Washington, DC: National Academy Press.

National Safe Worksite Institute. (1992). *Sacrificing America's youth: The problem of child labor and the response of government.* Chicago, IL: National Safe Worksite Institute.

National Safety Council (NSC). (1999). *Injury facts, 1999 edition.* Itasca, IL: NSC.

Olmsted, B., & Smith, S. (1994). *Creating a flexible workplace: How to select and manage alternative work options.* New York: American Management Association, (2nd ed.)

Palchak, R.B., & Schmidt, R.T. (1996, February). *Protecting the health of employees abroad. Occupational Health & Safety, 65(2),* 53-56.

Parker, D., Carl, W., French, L., & Martin, F. (1994a). Nature and incidence of self-reported adolescent work injury in Minnesota. *American Journal of Industrial Medicine, 26,* 529-541.

Parker, D., Carl, W., French, L., & Martin, F. (1994b). Characteristics of adolescent work injuries reported to the Minnesota Department of Labor and Industry. *American Journal of Public Health, 84(4),* 606-611.

Parker, D., Clay, R., Mandel, J., Gunderson, P., & Salkowicz, L. (1991). Adolescent occupational injuries in Minnesota: A descriptive study. *Minnesota Medicine, 74,* 25-28.

Polivka, A.E. (1996, October). A profile of contingent workers. *Monthly Labor Review,* 10-21.

Polivka, A.E., & Nardone, T. (1989, December). On the definition of contingent work. *Monthly Labor Review,* 9-16.

Pruitt, R.H. (1995). Preplacement evaluation: Thriving within the ADA guidelines. *AAOHN Journal, 43(3),* 124-130.

Randolph, S.A., & Migliozzi, A.A. (1993). The role of the agricultural health nurse: Bringing together community and occupational health. *AAOHN Journal, 41,* 429-433.

Rekus, J.F. (1994, May). Chronic risks in construction. *Occupational Health and Safety,* 103-104, 106-108, 129.

Resnick, M., Bearman, P., Blum, R., Bauman, K., Harris, K., Jones, J., Tabor, J., Beuhring, T., Sieving, R., Shew, M., Ireland, M., Bearinger, L., & Udry, R. (1997). Protecting adolescents from harm: Findings from the national longitudinal study on adolescent health. *Journal of the American Medical Association. 27(10),* 823-832.

Richter, E., & Jacobs, J. (1991). Work injuries and exposures in children and young adults: Review and recommendation for action. *American Journal of Industrial Medicine, 19,* 747-769.

Ringen, K., Englund, A., Welch, L., Weeks, J.L., & Seegal, J.L. (1995). Perspectives of the future. Ringen, et al. (Eds.), *Occupational medicine: Construction safety and health. State of the art reviews, 10(2),* 445-451. Philadelphia: Hanley & Belfus, Inc.

Rogers, B. (1994). *Occupational health nursing: Concepts and practice.* Philadelphia: W.B. Saunders.

Russi, M. (1993). Environmental health issues for travelers. In F.J. Bia (Ed.) *Travel medicine advisor* (pp. TCI. 1–TCI. 8) Atlanta, GA: American Health Consultants, Inc.

Schober, S., Jandke, J., Halperin, W., Moll, M.., & Thun, M. (1988). Work-related injuries in minors. *American Journal of Industrial Medicine, 14,* 585-595.

Scott, M.B. (1995). Focus on work and family: Work/family programs: Their role in the new workplace. *Employee Benefit Plan Review, 50,* 32-33.

Segal, L.M., & Sullivan, D.G. (1995, March-April). The temporary labor force. *Ergonomic Perspectives,* 2-19.

Sepkowitz, K.A. (1996). Occupationally acquired infections in health care workers, Part 1. *Annals of Internal Medicine, 125(10),* 826-834.

Service, M. (1995, March 20-28). Why health costs got smaller in 1994. *Business & Health, 13,* 20-22, 26, 28.

Smith, K.G. (1986). The hazards of migrant farm work: An overview for rural public health nurses. *Public Health Nursing, 3(1),* 48-56.

Smith, W.A., & White, M.C. (1993). Home health care: Occupational health issues. *AAOHN Journal, 41(4),* 180-185.

Solomon, C.M. (1994). Global operations demand that HR rethink diversity. *Personnel Journal, 73(7),* 40-50.

Steinberg, L., & Dornbusch, S. (1991). Negative correlates of part-time employment during adolescence: Replication and elaboration. *Developmental Psychology, 27,* 304-313.

Stone, R.A. (1995 March-April). Workplace homicide: A time for action. *Business Horizons, 38*, 3-10.

Suruda, A., & Halperin, W. (1991). Work-related deaths in children. *American Journal of Industrial Medicine, 19*, 739-745.

Swanson, N.G. (2000). Working women and stress. *Journal of the American Medical Women's Association, 55(2)*, 76-79.

Tanzillo, K. (1995). Georgia Power workers use remote centers for telecommuting. *Successful Telecommuting, 32(12)*, 14.

Taylor, A.K., & Murray, L.R. (1999). Minority workers. In B.S. Levy & D.H. Wegman (Eds.) *Occupational health: Recognizing and preventing work-related disease and injury* (pp. 679-688). Philadelphia: Lippincott Williams & Wilkins.

Thelin, J.W., Joseph, D.J., Davis, W.E., Baker, D.E., & Hosokawa, M.C. (1983). High-frequency hearing loss in male farmers of Missouri. *Public Health Reports, 98(3)*, 268-272.

Trape, M. (1998). Workplace violence: Occupational safety and health administration guidelines for workers in health care and social services. *Connecticut Medicine, 62(6)*, 333-336.

U.S. Census Bureau. (1998, March). *Census brief: Increase in at-home workers reverses earlier trend.* Pub. No. CENBR/98-2. Washington, DC: U.S. Government Printing Office.

U.S. Census Bureau. (1999a). *March 1999 current population survey. Table 1. Selected characteristics of civilians 16 to 74: 1999*, accessed on 4/10/2000. http://www.census.gov.

U.S. Census Bureau. (1999b). Statistical abstract of the United States: 1999. *The national data book.* (119th ed.). U.S. Department of Commerce, Washington, DC (pp. 396, 450).

U.S. Department of Health and Human Services (DHHS). U.S. Public Health Service. (1991). *Healthy people 2000: National health promotion and disease prevention objectives: Full report with commentary.* (National Institutes of Health Publication No. 91-50212). Washington, DC: U.S. Government Printing Office.

U.S. Department of Labor, Bureau of Labor Statistics (USDL BLS). (1995b). *Employee benefits survey: A BLS reader,* (Bulletin 2459, February 1995). Washington, DC: U.S. Government Printing Office, pp. 97-109.

U.S. Department of Labor, Occupational Safety and Health Administration (USDL OSHA). (1996). *Guidelines for preventing workplace violence for health care and social service workers* (OSHA 348). Washington, DC: U.S. Government Printing Office.

U.S. Department of Labor, Women's Bureau (USDL WB). (1994). *1993 handbook on women workers: trends and issues.* Washington, DC: U.S. Government Printing Office.

U.S. Department of Labor, Bureau of Labor Statistics (USDL BLS). (2000a, January 19). *Union members in 1999.* http://stats.bls.gov/newsrels.html.

U.S. Department of Labor, Bureau of Labor Statistics (USDL BLS). (1995a). *BLS releases new 1994-2005 employment projections,* (Bulletin 95-485, December 1995). Washington, DC: U.S. Government Printing Office.

U.S. Department of Labor, Bureau of Labor Statistics (USDL BLS). (199). *Employment and earnings,* 8 Issue 1. Washington, DC, U.S. Department of Labor.

U.S. Department of Labor, Bureau of Labor Statistics (USDL BLS). (1999, December 16*). Workplace injuries and illnesses in 1998.* http://stats.bls.gov/news.release/osh.nws.html

U.S. Department of Labor, Bureau of Labor Statistics (USDL BLS). (2000b). *Career guide to industries: Health services.* http://www.bls.gov/oco/cg

U.S. Department of Labor, Bureau of Labor Statistics (USDL BLS). (1994). *The American workforce: 1992-2005,* (Bulletin 2452, April 1994). Washington, DC: U.S. Government Printing Office.

U.S. Department of Labor, Women's Bureau (USDL WB). (1998, May*). Work and elder care: Facts for caregivers and their employers.* http://dol.gov/dol/wb/public/wb pugs/elderc.html

U.S. Department of Labor, Women's Bureau (USDL WB). (1999, April). *Facts on Working Women: 20 facts on women workers.* http://col.gov/dol/wb/public/wb_pubs/fact98.html.

U.S. Department of Labor. (1999, September). Futurework: Trends and challenges for work in the 21st century. http://www.dol.gov/dol/asp/public/futurework/report/main.htm.

Verbrugge, L.M., & Wingard, D.L. (1987). Sex differentials in health and mortality. *Health Matrix 5 (2), 3-19.*

Wegman, D., & Davis, L. (1999). Protecting Youth at Work. *American Journal of Industrial Medicine, 36,* 579-583.

Wegman, D.H. (1999). Older workers. *Occupational Medicine State of the Art Review. 14(3),* 537-57. Review.

West, M.D. (1995). Aspects of the worksite and return to work for persons with brain injury in supported employment. *Brain Injury, 9(3),* 301-313.

Windau, J., & Toscano, G. (1994). *Workplace homicides in 1992.* Washington, DC: U.S. Government Printing Office (U.S. Department of Labor, Bureau of Labor Statistics.).

Windau, J., Sygnatur, E., & Toscano, G. (1999, June). Profile of work injuries incurred by young workers. *Monthly Labor Review,* 3-10.

Woolf, A., & Flynn, E. (2000). Workplace toxic exposures involving adolescents aged 14 to 19 years. *Archives of Pediatrics and Adolescent Medicine, 154(3),* 234-239.

World Health Organization (WHO). (1999). *Occupational health: Ethically correct, economically sound.* (Fact Sheet No. 84, revised June 1999). Geneva, Switzerland: WHO.

Wright, K.A. (1993). Management of agricultural injuries and illness. *Nursing Clinics of North America, 28,* 253-266.

Yassin, M.S., Lierl, M.B., Fischer, T.J., O'Brien, K., Cross, J., & Steinmetz, C. (1994). Latex allergy in hospital employees. *Annals of Allergy, 72(3),* 245-249.

Ziegler, R.H. (1994). *American workers, American unions.* Baltimore: John Hopkins University Press (pp. 193-205).

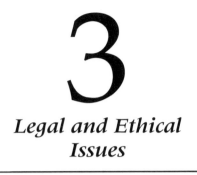

CHAPTER

3

Legal and Ethical Issues

DIANE KNOBLAUCH, FRANCIS CHILDRE, AND PATRICIA STRASSER

Legal and ethical issues often arise in the occupational setting. It is essential that occupational and environmental health nurses be familiar with state and federal regulations that affect employees in their work settings and that they clearly understand their professional responsibility with regard to those regulations. Furthermore, they must be prepared to respond effectively to the various ethical concerns that may arise in a competitive environment, which often breeds conflicting opinions and moral dilemmas. The information in this chapter provides a broad overview of government regulations and ethical principles that can serve as a guide to occupational and environmental health nursing practice.

I Sources of Law

A *Common law* **is based upon judicial precedent when individual disputes are decided in the courts. These legal precedents are generally relied upon in deciding similar future cases in the same jurisdiction.**
   1. Deference is accorded to decisions made by higher courts within the same jurisdiction; state courts have precedence over local courts, appeal courts over lower courts, and the Supreme Court over appeal courts.
   2. Courts follow past precedents to promote the uniform and predictable application of common law rules based on changing societal values, norms, and cultures; however, courts can reinterpret prior decisions or the application of law to a subject matter in current, future, and past cases.

B *Statutes* **are laws created by state or federal legislatures.**
   1. Statutes may modify existing law or regulate new subject matter.
   2. The legislature may delegate the responsibility for promulgating rules and regulations about a particular matter to an administrative agency.
   3. Statutes may preempt rules and regulations of administrative agencies.
   4. Statutes reflect societal norms and social order; thus laws are enacted or codified as a result of societal changes.

C *Federal law* **is based on the United States Constitution and is the supreme rule of the land; that is, state statutes must be at least as strict as federal law.**

D *State law* **regulates activities within the state's jurisdiction.**
   1. *Civil law* addresses the rights and duties of persons within that state; an example is the Nurse Practice Act.
   2. *Criminal law* is enacted to preserve public order.

3. *Administrative law* is regulated by administrative agencies within each state; for example, the State Board of Nursing is an administrative agency that oversees, monitors, and enforces the Nurse Practice Act within the state.

II Basic Legal Concepts Relevant to Occupational and Environmental Health Nursing Practice

A *Tort* **refers to a private wrong against the person or property of another; examples include assault, battery, and defamation. These wrongs are compensated with money damages.**

B *Negligence* **is the failure to exercise the degree of care in performing one's duties consistent with the standard of care for an occupational and environmental health nurse.**
1. *Standard of care* refers to what the average, reasonable, and prudent occupational and environmental health nurse would do in the same or similar circumstances; the "reasonable occupational health nurse standard."
2. *Exceptional circumstances,* such as emergencies, are taken into consideration when determining negligence.
3. *Duty* refers to the obligation that an occupational and environmental health nurse has to workers to prevent foreseeable harm. For example, if workers are at risk of exposure to a toxin, the occupational and environmental health nurse has a *duty* to ensure that surveillance is conducted to prevent adverse effects from the toxin.
   a. This duty does not apply if there is a reasonable risk of harm to the occupational and environmental health nurse, as in an emergency.
   b. *Breach* of duty occurs when an occupational and environmental health nurse fails to provide care according to the "reasonable occupational health nurse standard."
4. Examples of negligence include the following:
   a. Failure to take action
   b. Failure to communicate danger
   c. Delay in obtaining assistance
   d. Medication errors
   e. Failure to obtain informed consent

C *Informed consent* **means that a worker's decision about a treatment or action plan is made with a clear understanding, including material risks, benefits, and alternative treatments (i.e., complete notice).**
1. To give informed consent, the worker must be advised of the following:
   a. Nature and purpose of proposed treatment
   b. Diagnosis
   c. Material risks of proposed treatment
   d. Alternative treatments
   e. Consequences of lack of treatment
2. The purposes of informed consent include the following:
   a. Allows the worker to make an autonomous decision
   b. Protects the worker from harm
   c. Ensures accountability among health professionals
3. In order to be valid, informed consent must have the following characteristics:
   a. Given freely and without coercion
   b. Given with full understanding

4. The person giving informed consent must be mentally, physically, and legally competent.

D *Malpractice* **is negligence that involves professional misconduct or unreasonable lack of skill.**

1. State statutes will determine the civil action for misconduct by the occupational and environmental health nurse.
2. Malpractice implies that a higher standard of care is owed to the client than the standard implied by simple negligence. Malpractice suits require expert testimony to help the jury understand the standard of care owed to a client by the reasonably prudent occupational and environmental health nurse.

E *Statute of limitation* **is the period of time within which a lawsuit must be filed after a tort occurs.**

1. Typically, the statute of limitation for negligence is 2 years.
2. The statute of limitation for malpractice is typically 1 year.

III Legal Responsibilities of the Occupational and Environmental Health Nurse

A **Occupational and environmental health nurses are responsible for maintaining a current knowledge of the laws affecting occupational health practice in the jurisdiction where they practice, including the following:**

1. Proposed and implemented state and federal administrative rules for nursing, pharmacy, and medicine
2. Proposed and implemented state and federal legislation

B **Because of the dynamic and evolving nature of occupational and environmental health nursing practice, there may be inconsistencies between actual practice and legal guidelines of practice.**

1. Laws, rules, and regulations that are enacted are dynamic; thus they may be challenged as professional practice evolves.
2. The interpretation of laws, rules, and regulations may change as new cases are decided (common law) and legal precedents are established.
3. Laws, rules, and regulations can only be changed by following established procedures and protocols.

IV Occupational Safety and Health Act (Public Law 91-596)

A **The OSH Act was signed into law on December 29, 1970. The purpose of the OSH Act is to "Assure so far as possible every working man and woman in the Nation safe and healthful working conditions and to preserve our human resources . . ." (Appendix V).**

1. The OSH Act applies to employers and employees within the United States and any territory under U.S. jurisdiction.
2. The OSH Act does not apply to self-employed persons, immediate members of family farms that do not employ outside workers, industries regulated by other federal agencies, such as mining, nuclear, and air transportation, or state and local governments.

B **OSHA, a regulatory agency within the U.S. Department of Labor (USDL), was created as a result of the OSH Act.**

1. OSHA, which is responsible for enacting, administering, and enforcing standards to provide workplace health and safety, was the first attempt by

Congress to provide a comprehensive program to protect the health and safety of American workers.

2. States may choose to administer their own occupational health and safety program, with the following provisions:
   a. OSHA approves the state program.
   b. The state's program applies to all employees and includes state, local and private sector employees.
   c. The state's statutes must be at least as restrictive as OSHA statutes; otherwise, OSHA statutes apply.
   (Box 3-1 provides a list of states that have established Occupational Safety and Health Administrations.)

3. General Duty Clause of the OSH Act: Employers are required to furnish all employees "employment and a place of employment which are free from recognized hazards that are causing or are likely to cause death or serious physical harm."
   a. The General Duty Clause can be invoked for hazards not covered by an OSHA standard. For example, citations were issued for ergonomic violations under the General Duty Clause even though an ergonomics standard was not in place.
   b. The general duty obligation is an important means of protecting workers because setting standards is often a slow process.

C **OSHA has the responsibility to promulgate legally enforceable occupational health and safety standards in accordance with Section 6 of the OSH Act.**

1. Standards are developed to eliminate or reduce risks; compliance with standards must occur to the technologic and economic extent possible.
2. OSHA standards must be reasonably necessary or appropriate to provide safe or healthful employment and places of employment.
3. The development of standards is an interdisciplinary process involving individuals from the fields of health care, epidemiology, law, economics,

---

BOX 3-1

States and territories with Occupational Safety and Health Administrations

Alaska	Arizona	California
Connecticut*	Indiana	Iowa
Kentucky	Maryland	Michigan
Minnesota	Nevada	New Mexico
New York*	North Carolina	Oregon
Puerto Rico	South Carolina	Tennessee
Utah	Vermont	Virginia
Virgin Islands	Washington	Wyoming

Source: Levy & Wegman (1999); OSHA 2000 web site

*Plans cover state and local government employees only.

NOTE: Employers should contact their state agency to determine the current status of a state-regulated OSHA

and industrial hygiene; standards are written by OSHA employees and invited consultants.

4. OSHA standards are developed by a public rule-making process that includes the following features:
   a. Public notice: the proposed standard and date of public hearing which are published in the Federal Register
   b. Public hearings: scheduled forums for public input
   c. Public comment: written or offered at public hearings

5. OSHA has enacted many standards, a complete list of which can be found at the OSHA Web site (http://www.osha.gov).

6. OSHA can implement emergency standards as proposed permanent standards effective for 6 months.

7. There are 23 standards that have medical surveillance provisions (Box 3-2).

8. OSHA part 1910 Occupational Safety and Health Standards sub-part Z is a series of Tables, known as the Z *tables,* which list permissible exposure limits for substances for which specific standards are in place and for those for which a standard has not been generated.

D OSHA is authorized to enforce established standards by performing inspections, with or without advance notice to the employer.

1. Inspections may include a review of records, walk-through, and employee interviews.

2. OSHA has established a system of inspection priorities; inspections occur in the following order (USDL, 1993)
   a. Imminent danger situations; that is, when there is reasonable certainty that danger exists that can be expected to cause death or serious physical harm immediately or before the danger can be eliminated through normal enforcement procedures
   b. Fatalities and catastrophes resulting in hospitalization of three or more employees; these situations must be reported to OSHA by the employer within 8 hours of the incident

---

BOX 3-2

OSHA standards requiring medical surveillance

Acrylonitrile	DBCP
Arsenic (Inorganic)	Ethylene Oxide
Asbestos (General Industry)	Formaldehyde
Asbestos (Construction and	HAZWOPER
Shipyards)	Hazardous Chemicals in Labora-
Benzene	tories
Bloodborne Pathogens	Lead
1,3-Butadiene	Methylenedianiline
Cadmium	Methylene Chloride
Carcinogens (Suspect)	Noise
Coke Oven Emissions	Respiratory Protection
Compressed Air Environments	Vinyl Chloride
Cotton Dust	

DBCP, dibromochloropropane; *HAZWOPER,* Hazardous Waste Operations and Emergency Response Standard.

     c. Employee complaints of alleged violation of standards or of unsafe or unhealthful working conditions

     d. Planned inspections aimed at special high hazard industries, occupations, or substances

     e. Random inspections of low hazard and nonmanufacturing work sites

     f. Follow-up inspections to determine if previously cited violations have been corrected

3. Employees or authorized employee representatives may request OSHA to perform an inspection.

     a. If an inspection occurs, the employer has a right to see a copy of the complaint.

     b. The employee's name will be withheld from the complaint if the employee requests.

     c. Inspections can occur without advance notice; however, employers have a right to refuse entry without a court order.

4. OSHA may issue citations identifying violations and specifying the penalty associated with each violation.

E **OSHA consults with business and industry about health and safety issues; these consultation services primarily target small businesses.**

1. The OSHA consultation service is a voluntary program primarily focused on lending assistance to employers to make the workplace free of or safe from recognized hazards.

2. Generally, this service is not punitive; employers who use it are not subject to fines providing efforts are being made to correct deficiencies.

3. Employers can request an OSHA consultation to accomplish the following:

     a. Identify and correct hazards

     b. Provide technical assistance related to work-site hazards

     c. Provide education and training to health and safety personnel

4. Although the consultation service is funded by OSHA, the services are delivered by state governments using well-trained professional staff.

5. OSHA produces a variety of publications designed to provide a basic understanding of occupational health and safety issues and to help with compliance issues.

6. OSHA provides basic to advanced occupational health and safety classes through the OSHA Training Institute.

F **OSHA's Voluntary Protection Program (VPP) was adopted in 1982.**

1. VPP was initiated as a cooperative effort among industry management, labor, and OSHA to recognize excellence in employer-provided programs that go beyond basic regulatory compliance.

2. VPP requirements include the following:

     a. A comprehensive written program demonstrating management commitment and planning

     b. A thorough work-site analysis

     c. Hazard prevention and control systems

     d. Safety and health training

     e. Active employee involvement

     f. A lost workday case rate of below 50% of the national average for the specific industry (based on a review of 3 years of OSHA 200 logs)

     g. Periodic program evaluation with annual report submission

     h. Employee commitment

3. Participating employers are eligible for VPP awards. Award levels are as follows:
   a. STAR: meets all VPP requirements
   b. MERIT: meets some but not all VPP requirements
   c. DEMONSTRATION: special level used to identify use of VPP in industries or employment categories where STAR may not be appropriate, such as when piloting new technology or strategies for health and safety management.
4. Complete information about OSHA's VPP can be found at http://www.osha.gov/oshprogs/vpp/

G In 1988, OSHA instituted measures to ensure nursing representation in policy making.
1. In 1988, the first occupational and environmental health nurse was hired by OSHA.
2. In 1988, an Occupational Health Nurse Intern Program was introduced; this program is available to nurses in graduate school who are specializing in occupational health.
3. In 1993, the Office of Occupational Health Nursing was formally recognized and established.

H NIOSH, an institute within the CDC (under the DHHS), was also created by the OSH Act.
1. NIOSH conducts or funds occupational health and safety research to establish safe levels of toxic materials; this research is the basis for OSHA standards.
2. NIOSH also provides training and education to occupational health and safety professionals.

I The Occupational Safety and Health Review Commission (OSHRC) is an independent regulatory commission authorized by the OSH Act.
1. OSHRC members are appointed by the President with Senate approval.
2. OSHRC is responsible for handling appeals filed by employers who have received OSHA citations.
   a. Employers must file a Notice of Contest within 15 days of receiving an OSHA citation.
   b. OSHRC assigns the appeal to an administrative appeal judge.
   c. Appeal of an OSHRC decision is made to a U.S. Court of Appeals.

V Americans with Disabilities Act (ADA) of 1990

A The ADA is wide-ranging legislation intended to make American society more accessible to people with disabilities (http://www.eeoc.gov/laws.ada.html).
1. Disability is defined as:
   a. A physical or mental impairment that substantially limits one or more major life activities,
   b. A record of such an impairment, or
   c. Regarded as having such an impairment.
2. Title I of the ADA applies to employers (including public and private employers, employment agencies, and labor unions) with more than fifteen employees.

3. Businesses must protect the rights of "qualified individuals with disabilities" in all aspects of employment, including the application process, hiring, firing, compensation and benefits, and training.

B **A qualified person with a disability is one who can perform the essential functions of the job with or without "reasonable accommodation"**

1. Reasonable accommodation is any modification or adjustment to a job or the work environment that will enable a qualified applicant or employee with a disability to participate in the application process or perform essential job functions.
2. Reasonable accommodation may include the following:
   a. Making existing facilities used by employees readily accessible to and usable by persons with disabilities
   b. Restructuring the job, modifying work schedules, or reassigning the employee to a vacant position
   c. Acquiring or modifying equipment or devices; modifying examinations, training materials, or policies; or providing qualified readers or interpreters
3. Considerations related to providing reasonable accommodation include the following (AAOHN, 1994):
   a. Decisions should be made by a multidisciplinary team that includes health and safety professionals, human resources, and management.
   b. The affected employee should be consulted regarding accommodations.
   c. Community resources and national agencies can provide information that can assist with the process of accommodation.
   d. The "reasonableness" of accommodation is based on cost and impact on the business.

C **The ADA affects employment inquiries and medical examinations in the following ways (Equal Employment Opportunity Commission [EEOC], 2000):**

1. Employers may not ask job applicants about the existence, nature, or severity of a disability; however, they may ask about the applicant's ability to perform specific job functions.
2. A medical examination may be performed after a conditional offer of employment has been made, if examinations are required for all entering employees in similar jobs; the post-offer examination does not have to be job related.
3. If an individual is not hired because of the post-offer examination:
   a. The reason for not hiring must be job related and consistent with business need.
   b. The employer must show that no reasonable accommodation was available or that accommodation would impose an undue hardship.
4. Post-offer examinations may disqualify a person if it is determined the individual poses a "direct threat" in the workplace (i.e., a significant risk of substantial harm to the health and safety of the individual or others).
5. After a person is employed, any medical examination or medical inquiry must be job related and consistent with business necessity.
6. Results of medical examinations must be maintained in a confidential manner in medical files that are separate from other employee information and available under limited conditions.

D **The EEOC enforces and regulates Title I of the ADA.**

VI Family and Medical Leave Act (FMLA) of 1993 (29CFR825.118)

A FMLA entitles eligible employees to take up to 12 weeks of unpaid, job-protected leave in a 12-month period for the following reasons: (www.dol.gov/dol/esa/public/regs/statutes/whd/fmla.htm).

1. The birth and care of the employee's newborn child
2. Adoption or foster placement of a child with the employee
3. The care of a parent, spouse, or child with a serious health condition
4. The employee's inability to work because of a serious health condition

B To be eligible for leave under the FMLA, the following conditions must be satisfied:

1. The employee must work for a covered employer in a covered location (at least 50 employees employed within 75 miles)
2. The employee must have worked for the employer for a total of 12 months and worked at least 1,250 hours during the 12 months immediately before the leave.

C Under some circumstances, employees may take FMLA leave on an intermittent basis (e.g., in blocks of time or by reducing a normal work schedule).

D A *serious health condition* means an illness, injury, impairment, or physical or mental condition that involves either of the following:

1. Any period of incapacity or treatment connected with inpatient care (i.e., an overnight stay) in a medical-care facility; and any period of incapacity or subsequent treatment in connection with such inpatient care
2. Continuing treatment by a health care provider that includes any period of incapacity (e.g., inability to work, attend school) because of any of the following:
   a. A health condition lasting 3 or more consecutive days
   b. Pregnancy or prenatal care
   c. A chronic serious health condition (e.g., asthma)
   d. A permanent or long-term condition (e.g., Alzheimer's)
   e. Any absences to receive multiple treatments (e.g., chemotherapy)

E Rights and responsibilities under FMLA (AAOHN, 1995)

1. The employee has the right to return to the same or equivalent position with equivalent benefits, compensation, and conditions of employment.
2. The employee has a responsibility to provide the employer with reasonable notice of the leave (at least 30 days when foreseeable).
3. The employer has the right to require medical certification to support the employee's claim for leave related to health conditions of self or a family member; the Department of Labor has devised a "Certificate of Health Care Provider Form" to obtain medical certification (available on-line at www.dol.gov/dol/esa/fmla).
4. The employer has a responsibility to keep and maintain records regarding compliance with the act; they must also conspicuously post a notice containing information about the FMLA.

F Several states have their own legislation governing family and medical leave.

G The USDL's Employment Standards Administration, Wage and Hour Division administers and enforces FMLA.

VII The Department of Transportation

A The U.S. Department of Transportation (DOT), established by Congress in 1966, is charged with ensuring a fast, safe, efficient, accessible and convenient transportation system to meet the needs of the American people (http://www.dot.gov/about.htm).

1. The DOT has eleven individual operating administrations, including the Federal Motor Carrier Safety Administration (FMCSA), established January 1, 2000 (Public Law No. 106-159, 113 Stat.1748). The FMCSA was formerly part of the Federal Highway Administration.

2. The FMCSA's primary mission is to prevent commercial motor vehicle–related injuries and fatalities.

3. The following provisions from the FMCSA may affect occupational and environmental health nursing practice:

   a. Section 391.41 requires physical examinations for persons who drive commercial motor vehicles (i.e., hold a commercial drivers license).

   b. In general, a motor vehicle is considered a commercial vehicle if it meets any of following guidelines:

   1) Weighs over 26,000 pounds

   2) Is used to transport more than 16 persons

   3) Is used to transport hazardous materials

   c. Guidelines developed by the FMCSA for medical examinations for drivers of commercial motor vehicles are available at http://www.fmsa.dot.gov.rulesregs/fmcsr/medical.htm.

   d. Advanced-practice nurses, in accordance with applicable state laws, may perform the physical examinations for drivers of commercial motor vehicles. (Chapter 10 provides a definition of advanced practice.)

B The DOT administers the Omnibus Transportation Employee Testing Act of 1991 (CFR 49 Part 382.101), which requires alcohol and drug testing of

---

TABLE 3-1

Safety-sensitive employees covered by the Department of Transportation (DOT) Omnibus Transportation Employee Testing Act of 1991

DOT/industry	Covered safety-sensitive employees
Federal Highway Administration (FHWA)/Commercial	Holders of commercial driver's licenses; commercial vehicle drivers
Federal Aviation Administration/Aviation	Flight crews, attendants, instructors, air traffic controllers, aircraft dispatchers, maintenance personnel, screening personnel, ground security
Federal Railroad Administration/ Railroads	Hours of Service Act employees, engine train and signal services, dispatchers, operators
Federal Transit Administration/Mass Transit workers	Vehicle operators, controllers, maintenance workers
Research and Special Programs Administration/Pipelines	Operations, maintenance, emergency response personnel
United States Coast Guard*/Maritime	Crew members operating commercial vessels

Source: DOT, 1994

*Limited rules that require drug testing and postaccident testing

safety-sensitive employees in the aviation, motor carrier, railroad, and mass-transit industries (Table 3-1).

1. Testing is performed under the following circumstances:
   a. Preemployment (for drugs only)
   b. Postaccident
   c. Reasonable suspicion
   d. Return to duty and follow-up testing
2. In 1994, the DOT published rules (49 CFR Part 40) mandating prevention programs for drug and alcohol misuse; they were revised in 1999.
3. The DOT's rules establish procedures for drug testing and breath alcohol testing (Chapter 14).
4. All drug and alcohol testing results and records are maintained under strict confidentiality by the employer, the drug-testing laboratory, and the medical review officer.

C **The FMCSA, through the Office of Hazardous Materials Safety, develops and recommends regulatory changes governing the transportation of hazardous materials, including hazardous waste.**

VIII Documentation

Documentation is the written communication of information that is the basis of the legal occupational and environmental health record.

A **Purposes of documentation and records**
1. Provides information to improve the quality of care and to assist in planning care; for example, the measures that have been implemented and the results of those measures
2. Serves as a means of communication among health professionals
3. Provides a means to audit the quality of care and adherence to established policies and procedures
4. Establishes a baseline by which to gauge improvement or worsening of the client's condition and can be used for comparison should a subsequent injury occur
5. Provides a guide for job placement
6. May be used as the basis for retrospective, current, or prospective research
7. Provides information that can be used for employee education and counseling

B **Characteristics of documentation**
1. Documentation must be complete; if it wasn't written, it wasn't done. Effective, comprehensive record keeping includes the following basics:
   a. The date (including year) must be noted.
   b. The signature of the person who wrote the note must be clearly identified.
   c. Health documentation is legible.
   d. Entries must be permanent; that is, black ink should be used for all handwritten entries in the health records because other colors may not produce legible photocopies.
   e. Entries made via an automated information system must have safeguards so documentation cannot be changed.
   f. Original signatures must be maintained on computer-generated notes or password signatures instituted. (Chapter 7 provides additional information about safeguarding the security of health information.)

g. Each page of the record must be identified with the employee's name and other unique identifier if one is used. Note that special care must be taken when different clients have the same name.

h. Employee questions or comments about instructions given or in response to care must be included.

i. Entries should include normal and abnormal findings.

2. Health documentation should be presented in a concise, descriptive, technical writing style, using accepted health abbreviations and terminology. The SOAP format is recommended (Table 3-2).

3. Errors should be corrected by using the SLIDE rule (Baker, 2000).

a. Draw a **S**ingle **L**ine through the error, leaving the original entry legible.

b. **I**nitial the strike through and write "error" above the notation. White-out and other correction techniques should never be used.

c. **D**ate when the correction was made, including the year.

d. **E**xplain why the correction was made (if correction is other than a spelling or word correction).

4. Corrections should be made as soon as possible after the error is noticed; however, corrections should not be made after there is notice of possible litigation.

5. Stereotypes, generalizations, and judgmental statements should be avoided.

a. Example 1: Rather than "seems uncomfortable" ask the client to identify how much pain they are experiencing using a pain scale from 1 to 10.

b. Example 2: If a client is angry, describe the behavior, such as the words spoken (including obscenities or threats) and whether the client used a loud voice.

6. Health documentation should be contemporaneous with the assessment or done as soon afterwards as possible.

a. Information that was inadvertently omitted should be documented as soon as possible.

b. Late entries should be preceded by the notation "late entry."

c. Late entries should identify the date of each entry and the date of the data being documented.

TABLE 3-2

Example using the SOAP formula for occupational and environmental health documentation

Criteria	Description
Subjective assessment	Reason for visit, why the client is seeing you; location, quality, quantity, timing, setting, aggravating and alleviating factors, associated manifestations
Objective assessment	Physical examination, including inspection, percussion, palpation, auscultation; include any laboratory results; objective description of job demands or monitoring results that may affect the subjective complaint
Assessment or diagnosis	Medical versus nursing
Plan/Treatment	Diagnostic studies to be performed, medications prescribed, oral and written instructions, teaching, counseling, referral, follow-up

Source: Bates, 1995.

IX Types of Records

A OSHA recordkeeping requirements

1. The OSH Act requires most private sector employers with 11 or more employees at any time in a calendar year to prepare and maintain records of work-related injuries and illnesses.

2. Employers and individuals not required to maintain OSHA injury and illness records include the following:

   a. Private employers, such as self-employed individuals, partners with no employees, and employers of domestics in the employers' private residences

   b. Employers engaged in the conduct of religious services or rites

   c. State and local government agencies are usually exempt; however, in certain states, agencies of the state and local governments are required to keep injury and illness records in accordance with state regulations

   d. Low-risk industries such as financial institutions

3. Recordable injuries and illnesses resulting from a work accident or exposure include the following:

   a. Cases that result in a death

   b. Cases that result in an illness

   c. Cases that result in injury that involve any of the following:

      1) Medical treatment other than first aid (Box 3-3)

      2) Loss of consciousness

      3) Restriction of work or body motion

      4) Transfer to another job

      5) Complication requiring medical treatment

4. Occupational and environmental health nurses are often responsible for ensuring that proper records are kept, and thus they must have current knowledge of recordkeeping rules and regulations of OSHA (federal and state) and other regulatory agencies.

5. OSHA has proposed revisions of the Recordkeeping Standard; however, to date, these standards have not been released for implementation.

B Exposure records include the following:

1. All records of environmental (workplace) monitoring or measurement, including toxic agents, air quality, and physical agents (e.g., noise).

BOX 3-3

Comparison of medical treatment and first aid

Medical treatment is any treatment other than first aid (which is defined here) administered to injured employees. Medical treatment involves the provision of medical or surgical care for injuries that are not minor, through the specific application of procedures or systematic therapeutic measures.

First aid is any one-time treatment (it may include a follow-up visit for observation of minor scratches, cuts, burns, splinters, and so forth, which do not ordinarily require medical care).

2. Records reporting the results of any biologic monitoring
3. Material Safety Data Sheets
4. Chemical inventory or any other record that reveals the identity (e.g., chemical, common, or trade name) of a toxic substance or harmful physical agent and where and when the substance is (or was) used

C **The employee health record concerns the health status of an employee and is established and maintained by a physician, nurse, or other health care personnel.**

1. The employee health record may consist of both occupational and nonoccupational health data; the philosophy of the health service determines whether nonoccupational care is provided.
2. It is best to separate nonoccupational data from occupational data. The record may include the following:
   a. Health evaluations, such as preplacement or post-offer examinations and surveillance examinations (e.g., annual audiometric examinations and fitness for duty examinations)
   b. A job hazard requirement analysis or physical demand profile
   c. Work injury/illness and follow-up care, physical assessments, diagnostic procedures, functional capacity examinations, medications administered, consent forms, progress notes, and recommendations
   d. Treatment of injuries and illnesses (occupational and nonoccupational, if indicated)
   e. Other nonoccupational information such as the following:
      1) Health promotion and disease prevention activities, such as cholesterol or blood pressure screening
      2) Primary health care services
      3) Follow-up drug testing related to substance abuse treatment
      4) Monitoring of chronic health care conditions(e.g., blood pressure, glucose monitoring, routine blood work)
3. A written policy for the management, access, and retention of individual health records should be in place; the policy should address the following issues:
   a. Where and how records are stored and secured
   b. Managing records when an employee resigns, transfers, or is terminated
   c. Mechanism for employee access and consent for disclosure
   d. Mechanism for release of information on a need-to-know basis; for example, information on work restrictions
4. Employees' health records should be maintained in a secure place (i.e., locked files) in the exclusive custody and control of company occupational health professionals.

D **Administrative Records**

1. Examples of administrative records that should be retained indefinitely include the following:
   a. All versions of policy and procedure manuals
   b. All versions of approved treatment protocols
   c. Equipment calibration records
2. Examples of administrative records that may be discarded consistent with company policy and prudent practice include the following:
   a. Daily logs
   b. Monthly reports

c. Financial records

d. Staff training records and performance/competency assessments

X Preservation of Employee Health and Exposure Records

A OSHA requires that certain health records must be retained for at least 30 years plus the employee's term of employment.

1. Records of injuries that involve health treatment, loss of consciousness, restriction of work or motion, or transfer to another job are retained.

2. OSHA does not require records of first aid or one-time treatment, or of observation of minor scratches; however, records of cuts, burns, splinters, and the like are to be retained, and the retention of medical documentation demonstrating nursing care is strongly recommended.

3. The health record of an employee who has worked for less than one year need not be retained beyond the term of employment if they are provided to the employee upon termination of employment.

B An employee's exposure records and analyses using the health and exposure records are to be kept for at least 30 years beyond the worker's term of employment.

C Biologic-monitoring records must be kept as specified by OSHA standards.

D Records may be preserved in any manner (including microfilm) as long as the information contained in the record is preserved and retrievable. Note: Chest x-ray films shall be preserved in their original state.

XI Access to Employee Medical and Exposure Records

A OSHA Access to Employee Exposure and Medical Records Standard (29CFR1910.20) requires that the employee or the employee's representative have access to records according the following guidelines:

1. Access will be provided in a reasonable manner and place

2. Records will be provided free of charge, and within 15 working days of the initial request

3. The employer must make provisions for copying of records.

(NOTE: Although this standard uses the term *medical records,* these records may also contain health information that is nonmedical in nature; thus in this publication, these records are called *health records* except when reference is made to published documents that use the term *medical record.*)

B The employee should sign a written consent before health information is released (Fig. 3-1 presents a sample authorization letter); the authorization must include the following information:

1. What records are to be released, including dates of services

2. The purpose of release

3. To whom the records are to be released

4. Period of time for which authorization is valid

5. Date of authorization

6. Authority by which a person is requesting records

7. Identifying data of employee, including date of birth and social security number

8. Signature of the person requesting records

AUTHORIZATION FOR RELEASE OF MEDICAL INFORMATION

I, _____ (full name of employee) _____ hereby authorize

_____ (full name of company/employer) _____ to furnish to:

[name]

[address]

[telephone number]

☐ All information regarding my health conditions, including communicable illnesses, drug use or abuse, drug/alcohol treatment and psychiatric treatment. [*strike through the information that you do not want released.*]

☐ All information regarding any work-related and nonwork-related injuries or disease for which I have consulted you or received your services.

☐ The following information:

_____

_____

You are instructed to release all records from __(date)__ through __(date)__.

I hereby release you from any and all restrictions imposed by law in disclosing or revealing any professional record, observation, or communication in accordance with this release.

A copy of this signed authorization for release of medical records shall be considered as effective and valid as the original. This authorization shall be valid and in force for __(amount of time)__ from the authorization date.

_____   _____

Authorization Date   Signature

_____   _____

Date of Birth   Address

_____   _____

Social Security Number   City, State, Zip Code

FIGURE 3-1 *Sample authorization letter*

C In all cases, the occupational and environmental health nurse should make every attempt to obtain an authorization for release of health records, even when a request for health records is made via subpoena.
1. The authorization for release of medical records must specify whether information obtained from other sources may be released.
2. If there are concerns with such a request, the nurse should consult with legal counsel regarding applicable state law governing access to health records.

D Under no circumstances should the original health record, reports, or x-rays be released to the employee or representative before consulting with corporate legal counsel.

E If it is believed that access to information contained in the records regarding a special diagnosis of a terminal illness or a psychiatric condition could be detrimental to the employee's health, the employer may choose one of the following courses of action:
1. Inform the employee that access will be provided only to a designated representative of the employee having special written consent
2. Deny the employee's request for direct access to this information only

F The occupational and environmental health nurse should notify the designated employer representative whenever there is a nonroutine request for records; for example, when the request references a legal matter or an attorney requests them.

G An employer may withhold trade secret information but must provide information needed to protect employee health; when it is necessary to release a trade secret, the employer may require a written agreement as a condition of release.

H Each employee must be notified of the following information when beginning employment and at least annually thereafter:
1. The existence, location, and availability of any records covered by the OSHA Access to Employee Exposure and Medical Records Standard (29 CFR 1910.20)
2. The person responsible for maintaining and providing access to records
3. Right of access of the employee or a designated representative to these individual health and exposure records

I All health and exposure records subject to 29 CFR 1910.20 must be transferred to the successor employer, to preserve and maintain these same records.

XII Overview of Workers' Compensation

A The workers' compensation system was designed to compensate employees for work-related injuries and illnesses.
1. Workers' compensation benefits generally include the following:
   a. Income replacement (i.e., indemnity benefits) for workers who are unable to work because of injury or illness
   b. Support for dependents in event of occupation-related death
   c. Hospital, medical, and funeral expenses
   d. Incidental expenses such as travel and parking may be covered in some jurisdictions.

2. In general, workers' compensation laws hold that employers must assume costs of work-related injuries and illnesses without regard to fault (e.g., employee or employer negligence).

3. In exchange for providing workers' compensation benefits, the employer is usually immune from further legal action.

4. Each state and the District of Columbia have workers' compensation laws that apply to employees within their respective jurisdictions.

5. Federal civilian employees are covered by federal laws.

6. Courts in each jurisdiction interpret the language of their workers' compensation statute.

7. Workers' compensation laws are generally administered by commissions or boards.

B **Compensable injuries and illnesses are defined by statute in each jurisdiction. In most statutes, workers' compensation benefits are limited to accidents and illnesses "arising out of and in the course of employment." (U.S. Chamber of Commerce, 2000).**

1. Although workers' compensation laws initially had no provision for work-related illnesses, all states recognize responsibility for them.

2. Most statutes do not provide compensation for illnesses that are "ordinary diseases of life," or one that is "not peculiar to or characteristic of the employee's occupation" (U.S. Chamber of Commerce, 2000).

3. Identifying work-related illnesses can be complex and very difficult because of the following factors:
   a. Time elapsed between exposure and onset of illness
   b. Insidious onset of the illness
   c. Multifactorial nature of the illness
   d. Obscurity of exposure because of the inability to detect low levels of toxic substances

XIII Overview of Workers' Compensation Benefits

A **In most jurisdictions, unlimited medical benefits (e.g., hospital care, medications, physician visits, rehabilitative therapy, etc.) are provided by statute.**

1. Many states use managed care concepts to affect workers' compensation benefits and control workers' compensation medical costs.

2. There are jurisdictional differences regarding who can choose the health care provider for the injured or ill employee.
   a. In many states, employees are allowed free choice of treating health care professionals.
   b. In other states, the employer chooses the provider, or employees are limited to choosing from a panel of providers.

3. The employer usually has the right to have the employee examined by a physician of the employer's choice.

4. The employer can generally use an independent medical evaluation, whereby a physician who is not the treating physician evaluates the employee and provides an opinion regarding the following issues:
   a. The employee's health condition in general
   b. Whether the employee can return to work
   c. Recommendation regarding physical limitations
   d. The length of time the employee will be off work

e. Recommendation of current and future treatment

f. The etiology (causation) of the health condition

g. A determination as to whether the person has reached maximum medical improvement

B **Income benefits (i.e., *indemnity benefits*) may not be payable until a waiting period has been met.**

1. If the employee remains off work for days or weeks, most statutes provide payment of income benefits retroactive to the date of injury.

2. Income benefits are generally based on a percentage of the injured or employee's average weekly wage.

3. Many statutes provide income benefits based on a schedule for specific losses (e.g., loss of a limb).

4. Many statutes pay income benefits based on the employee's percent of impairment that results from the injury or illness.

5. Income benefits are generally based on whether the disability is temporary or permanent (i.e., payment for a number of weeks or for life).

6. Definitions of disability are determined by jurisdictional statute. The most common workers' compensation disability classifications* are the following:

a. *Temporary total disability*—a condition in which a worker, because of an occupational injury or illness, is unable to return to any type of continuous gainful employment

b. *Temporary partial disability*—a sub-component of total temporary disability wherein the worker is not medically fixed and stable, but can return to "light" work at a lower wage than before he or she was injured

c. *Permanent total disability*—a condition that permanently and completely incapacitates a worker, preventing the worker from ever performing gainful employment

d. *Permanent partial disability*—condition that results in the permanent loss of a body part or a lasting impairment that has been deemed unlikely to improve

(*These definitions are from Washington State Department of Labor and Industries, 1994. Readers are advised to check the terms and definitions in their respective jurisdictions.)

C **Many statutes include specific provisions for rehabilitation of ill or injured employees (including vocational rehabilitation).**

D **Most jurisdictions require employers to obtain workers' compensation insurance and prove financial ability to assume the risk of worker injury.**

1. States that require workers' compensation insurance through a monopolistic state fund include North Dakota, Ohio, Washington, and West Virginia.

2. Many large corporations prefer to "self-insure" (i.e., assume their own financial liability for workers' compensation).

a. Most states in the United States allow self-insurance in some form (e.g., individual company/group).

b. Companies that self-insure usually use the services of a third party administration (TPA) to manage their workers' compensation benefits.

XIV Professional Position on Ethics

A **AAOHN Standards of Occupational and Environmental Health Nursing, Standard XI, Ethics: The occupational and environmental health nurse**

uses an ethical framework as a guide for decision making in practice. (AAOHN, 1999).

1. Occupational and environmental health nurses are confronted with complex ethical dilemmas that require careful communication with company management and the recipients of care.
2. An ethical framework provides the guidelines within which the nurse makes ethical judgments.
3. The occupational and environmental health nurse is an advocate for clients to receive accessible, equitable, and quality health services, including a safe and healthful work environment.

B The AAOHN Code of Ethics (AAOHN, 1998) provides the ethical framework to guide the conduct of the occupational and environmental health nurse.

XV Ethics: Definitions and Principles

A Definitions

1. *Ethics* is the philosophic study of conduct and moral judgment.
2. *Morals* are principles of right and wrong.
3. *Morality* is society's expectation as to what people should or should not do.
4. *Value* is an expression of worth or goodness.
5. *Moral justification* is the reason for conduct.

B Ethical principles

1. *Autonomy* means self-governance—the ability to make individual decisions and choices, to act, and to think; self-determination.
2. *Nonmaleficence* is the principle of doing no harm to others.
3. *Beneficence* is the principle of doing good for others.
4. *Distributive justice* means that benefits should be equally distributed and equally shared in pursuit of the following three types of equality:
   a. Equality of moral worth
   b. Equality of opportunity
   c. Equality of outcome

C Other principles important to occupational and environmental health nursing practice include the following:

1. *Confidentiality* is the implicit promise that information divulged to another will be respected and not released or repeated (Case Study).
2. *Veracity* is truthfulness.
3. *Honesty* means freedom from deceit.
4. *Promise-keeping* is the act of following through on a pledge.
5. *Integrity* refers to unimpaired moral principles.

XVI Ethical Conflicts

A Confidentiality

1. Employers are charged with the responsibility for maintaining the occupational health and safety records of their employees.
2. The occupational and environmental health nurse, who is an agent of the employer, is charged with providing occupational health services to employees and maintaining health records; the occupational and environmental health nurse has a duty to accomplish the following:
   a. Document care or services provided to a client
   b. Maintain the confidentiality of the client's health records

Case study on confidentiality

N.O. Moore, an occupational and environmental health nurse at E.Z. Con, Ltd., performed spirometry testing and respirator fit testing for Joe Cool. This was Joe's preplacement evaluation at E.Z. Con. During the initial evaluation, Moore noted that Joe smoked two packs of cigarettes for the past 25 years, and that he was an HVAC (heating, ventilation, and air conditioning) specialist. Joe admitted that he used to smoke 2 to 6 joints of marijuana per day, but stopped 10 years earlier. Moore talked with Joe about his smoking, risk factors for disease, and environmental hazards at E.Z. Con.

• Two years later, Moore received several letters in the mail and several phone calls about Joe. The first letter, from an attorney who said that he represented Joe, requested Joe's medical records from E.Z. Con. An authorization signed by the attorney was enclosed.

• The second letter, from Mr. Risk at ABC Company, requested a copy of Joe's medical records at E.Z. Con. An authorization signed by Joe and dated 2 days before Moore received the letter was enclosed.

• The third letter, from Mrs. Cool, stated that Joe had died of a mesothelioma 3 months earlier and requested Joe's medical records from E.Z. Con. An authorization signed by Mrs. Cool was enclosed.

Ms. Snoopy from personnel called Moore and instructed Moore to make a copy of Joe's medical records for the vice president. Snoopy said that she would be down to get the records in 15 minutes. An attorney from H.E.L.P.,

E.Z. Con's corporate counsel, called and demanded a copy of Joe's medical records.

What does N.O. Moore do?

Answer: **No one gets these records.**

1. The authorization must specifically authorize the release of any documentation regarding psychiatric, substance abuse, or communicable illness. Although N.O. Moore did not provide substance abuse treatment, arguably documentation of use of illegal substances may require this specific disclosure.

2. The authorization to release medical records must be signed by the person or a legal representative. Here, because a person who is now deceased signed the form, the signature is not valid. Note: Mrs. Cool stated that Joe died 3 months ago.

3. Mrs. Cool, as Joe's widow, is not his "legal" representative. If the authorization had been signed Charity Cool, Administrator of the Estate of Joe Cool, then Mrs. Cool would legally be able to act in Joe's place.

4. Snoopy has no right to these medical records; neither does the vice president.

5. H.E.L.P. knows better than to request these medical records without a signed authorization.

Moore has no knowledge about why everyone wants these records. If this was the result of a workers' compensation claim filed against E.Z. Con, the employer would arguably have a right to these medical records. However, if E.Z. Con is not a named party in the lawsuit, the medical records must remain confidential.[*]

---

[*]Remember to consult your jurisdictional statutes and case law to determine how you should handle these situations, because every jurisdiction may be different.

3. If asked to divulge information contained in an employee's health record or to provide health records, the occupational and environmental health nurse should consider the following issues:
   a. For what purpose is the information being sought?
   b. Is the requested information work-related?
   c. Who is requesting the information?
   d. Is the requested information aggregate data or individual data?
   e. Why was the information gathered?
   f. Is the information being sought pursuant to an authorization for release of health records signed by the employee?
4. Unauthorized release of health records could result in personal liability, suspension of license to practice nursing by the state agency responsible for regulating the practice of nursing, or termination of employment by the employer.

B **Conflicts of interest and other ethical dilemmas**
   1. The occupational and environmental health nurse has multiple roles in the workplace, including employee, health care provider, client advocate, and coworker; these multiple roles may result in ethical dilemmas that require choosing between two or more compelling ethical or moral values.
   2. The occupational and environmental health nurse may be asked to provide the employer with information about the health needs of employees for use in developing health benefit plans, planning health education programs, and identifying work-site health issues.
      a. The occupational and environmental health nurse may be involved in prioritizing program needs.
      b. The occupational and environmental health nurse may participate in the decision-making process regarding allocation of scarce economic and personnel resources among work-site health programs.
   3. The occupational and environmental health nurse may provide non–work-related health care, such as periodic health assessments and screening programs.
      a. The nurse must document the results of these evaluations and retain such documentation as health records.
      b. The nurse has an ethic and legal duty to maintain the confidentiality of the employee's non–work-related health information.
      c. Release of non–work-related health records requires an authorization for release of health records signed by the client whose records are being released.

BIBLIOGRAPHY

American Association of Occupational Health Nurses (AAOHN). (1994). *The Americans with Disabilities Act* [AAOHN Advisory]. Atlanta, GA: AAOHN Publications.

American Association of Occupational Health Nurses (AAOHN). (1995). The Family Medical Leave Act [AAOHN Advisory]. Atlanta, GA: AAOHN Publications.

American Association of Occupational Health Nurses (AAOHN). (1996). *Employee health records: Requirements, retention, and access* [AAOHN Advisory]. Atlanta, GA: AAOHN Publications.

American Association of Occupational Health Nurses (AAOHN). (1998). *Code of ethics and interpretive statements.* Atlanta, GA: AAOHN Publications.

American Association of Occupational Health Nurses (AAOHN). (1999). *AAOHN standards of occupational and environmental health nursing.* Atlanta, GA: AAOHN Publications.

American Association of Occupational Health Nurses (AAOHN). (2000). Advisory: *Best practices in an occupational health and safety program: Voluntary protection program (VPP) model.* Atlanta, GA: AAOHN Publications.

Americans with Disabilities Act. (1990). P.L. 101-356, 42 U.S.C. §12101 et seq.

Baker, S.K. (2000). Minimizing litigation risk: Documentation strategies in the occupational health setting. AAOHN Journal, 48(2), 100-105.

Bates, B. (1995). *A guide to physical examination and history taking.* Philadelphia: Lippincott.

Commission on Accreditation of Rehabilitation Facilities (CARF). (1992). Standards manual for organizations serving people with disabilities. Tucson, AZ: CARF.

DiBenedetto, D.V. (1995). *OEM occupational health & safety manual* (2nd ed). Boston: OEM Press.

Equal Employment Opportunity Commission. (1992). *A technical assistance manual on the employment provisions (Title I) of the Americans with Disabilities Act.* EEOC-M-1A. Washington, DC: 1192: U.S. Government Printing Office.

Furrow, B.R., Johnson, S.H., Jost, T.S., & Schwartz, R.L. (1991). Liability and quality issues in health care. St. Paul, MN: West.

Haas, T.F. (1987). On reintegrating workers' compensation and employers' liability. *Georgia Law Review, 21,* 843.

Health hazards of the workplace report. Vol. 1 (8). New York: Van Nostrand Reinhold (1990).

Isernhagen, S.J. (1995). The comprehensive guide to work injury management. Gaithersburg, MD: Aspen.

Larson, A. (1991). The law of workmen's compensation. New York:Bender.

Levy, B.S., & Wegman, D.H. (1999). *Occupatio*nal health: recognizing and preventing work-related disease and injuries (4th ed.). Boston: Little, Brown and Company.

Mappes, T.A., & DeGrazia, D. (1996). *Biomedical ethics* (4th ed.). New York: McGraw-Hill.

McCunney, R.J. (1999). Medical center occupational health and safety. Philadelphia: Lippincott, Williams & Wilkins.

Papp, E.M., & Miller, A.S. (2000) .*Screening and surveillance: OSHA's medical surveillance provisions.* AAOHN Journal, 48(2), 59-72.

Pryor, E.S. (1990). Flawed promises: A critical evaluation of the American Medical Association's guides to the evaluation of permanent impairment. *Harvard Law Review, 103,* 964.

Rogers, B. (1994). *Occupational health nursing concepts and practice.* Philadelphia: Saunders.

Shrey, D.E., & Lacerte, M. (1995). *Principles and practices of disability management in industry.* Winter Park, FL: GR Press.

Tate, D. (1992, June). Workers' disability and return to work. *American Journal of Physical Med. & Rehabilitation, 71,* 92-96.

Travers, P.H., & McDougall, C. (1995). *Guidelines for an occupational health and safety service.* Atlanta, GA: AAOHN Publications.

U.S. Chamber of Commerce. (2000). *The 2000 analysis of workers' compensation laws.* Washington DC: U.S. Chamber of Commerce.

U.S. Department of Labor (USDL), Occupational Safety and Health Administration (OSHA). (1993). OSHA safety and health standards [29 CFR 1910.000, et seq]. Washington DC: U.S. Government Printing Office.

U.S. Department of Transportation (DOT). (1994, February 3). *FHWA transportation facts,* Washington, DC: Office of Public Affairs.

Veatch, R. (1986). *The foundations of justice.* Cary, NC: Oxford University Press.

Washington State Department of Labor and Industries. (1994). Industrial insurance: glossary. Olympia, WA: State of Washington Department of Labor and Industries.

CHAPTER

4

Economic, Political, and Business Forces

DEBORAH V. DIBENEDETTO

Economic, political, and business forces (including that of managed care) shape the way business is conducted in national and the global marketplaces. It is essential that occupational and environmental health nurses understand the basics of the economic, political, and business forces and trends that shape the business environment in which they practice. This chapter presents an overview of these trends and discusses how they can affect occupational and environmental health nursing practice.

I Introduction to Economics

A *Economics* **is concerned with the way in which limited resources are allocated; specifically, it involves the following:**
   1. Allocation and management of the income and expenditures of a household, business, community, or government
      a. Production, distribution, and consumption of wealth
      b. Satisfaction of the material needs of people
   2. The study of the world economy (essentially a macroeconomic survey)
   3. Societal establishment of economic systems that serve as a means of achieving the society's economic goals

B **Key economic terms**
   1. *Capitalism:* Allows private ownership of property; income from property or capital accrues to the individual or firms that accumulate it and own it; firms are relatively free to compete with others for their own economic gain; the profit motive is basic to economic life
   2. *Communism:* Production systems are government or state owned, and production decisions are made by official policy and not directed by market action
   3. *Consumer Price Index (CPI):* Measures price changes of goods consumed by an urban family of four on a moderate income.
   4. *Disposable income (DI):* The gross national product (GNP) minus depreciation, business and personal taxes, and transfer payments (such as social security, welfare payments, and so on); "the money in people's pockets" to spend as they want
   5. *Federal Reserve Discount Rate:* The rate at which the Federal Reserve Bank lends funds to its member banks

6. *Gross domestic product:* measures value of all goods and services produced within a nation's borders regardless of the nationality of the producer.
7. *Gross national product:* Monetary value of the total annual flow of goods and services in a nation's economy
   a. GNP is the primary indicator of the national economy.
   b. GNP measures production in the economy by aggregating all goods and services produced by their current prices; for example, bushels of fruits, numbers of automobiles sold.
   c. GNP measures only goods and services that have a market.
   d. International comparisons of GNP are difficult.
   e. GNP does not measure quality of life.
8. *Microeconomics:* Deals with the economic behavior of individual units such as consumers, firms, and resource owners
9. *Macroeconomics:* Concerned with the behaviors of economic aggregates, such as the gross national (domestic) product (national income), consumption, the level of employment, investment, money supply, innovation, and international trade and production relationships
10. *Net national product:* The GNP less capital consumption allowance (allocated costs for depreciation of capital equipment)
11. *Political economy:* A term used to describe the influence of political and social institutions on the aggregate economy
12. *Prime rate:* The rate that banks charge to their commercial customers (those with good credit ratings and lowest risk) for short-term loans
13. *Producer Price Index (PPI):* Measures the wholesale price of goods
14. *Socialism:* An economic system in which government owns or controls many major industries, but may allow markets to set prices in many areas

C Major economic systems include capitalism, socialism, and communism.

D *Economic indicators* measure the relative standing of one economic system (country) versus that of another.
   1. Economic indicators include the gross national (domestic) product (GNP), net national product, and disposable income (DI).
   2. Price indicators that reflect a nation's economic standing include the consumer price index (CPI) and the producer price index (PPI).

E *Labor-force statistics* measure how many noninstitutionalized people are currently working at paid jobs or are willing to work; the *labor force* is the employable population of the economy.
   1. Persons in the military, jails, hospitals/sanitariums (patients), and full-time students are excluded in calculations of the labor force.
   2. Labor-force statistics that include military personnel are also published.
   3. Unemployment statistics indicate the number of people looking for paid work and point to changes in the labor market.

F *Interest rates* are a percentage of a sum of money charged for its use; two important interest rates are the prime rate and federal reserve discount rate.

G *Balance of trade* refers to the net value of a country's imports and exports of merchandise.
   1. The balance of trade consists of transactions in merchandise (automobiles, computers, etc.).
   2. When a country exports more than it imports, it has a surplus, or *favorable,* balance of trade.

3. When a country's imports predominate, the balance of trade is in deficit and is called *unfavorable.*

II Economic State of the Nation

A **During the 1980s, America's economy grew or "expanded" because of the following:**
   1. Decreased taxation (tax cuts) on business and citizens
   2. Deregulation of businesses such as telecommunications, air travel, banking, and many others
   3. Increased consumer spending, investment, and construction
   4. The beginning trend of privatizing government services toward the end of the 1980s

B **The government release of money to the private sector, along with deregulation of business, made the 1980s the longest period of peacetime growth (Bagby, 1995).**

C **Government cuts in spending did not keep pace with the growth of the national economy.**
   1. Tax cuts had a negative impact on government revenue.
   2. Planned spending and reform of national entitlement programs, such as Medicare/Medicaid and Social Security, were not politically supported.
   3. Entitlement program cuts were not large enough to cover the reduction in tax revenue.
   4. American government continued to spend more than it took in; this increased deficit spending by the government, resulting in high deficits.

D **The United States went from the largest creditor nation to the largest debtor nation in the global economy.**

E **Negative effects on Americans living with high national budget deficits include the following (Bagby, 1995):**
   1. Higher interest rates
   2. Less money for investment
   3. Lower economic growth rate
   4. Less revenue to pay interest on debt
   5. Debtor status to foreign countries
   6. Lower sales of exports
   7. Long-term decrease in the standard of living

F **By the end of the 1980s, the American economy was in a recession.**

G **In the 1990s, the inflation rate fell and the U.S. became more competitive in the worldwide marketplace; this resulted in a period of expansion and economic growth.**

H **In the 2000s, the amount and intensity of competition worldwide will increase, augmented by the use of the Internet (Dent, 2000).**

I **In the coming decades, there will be an increase of multinational companies and an expansion of career and investment opportunities around the world.**

III The Impact of Economics on the Individual

A **Unstable, poorly functioning economies produce the following results:**
   1. People have greater difficulty finding jobs that match their abilities and education.

2. Continually rising prices reduce the value of savings, thus affecting the ability of people, especially retirees, to survive.

3. Company managers may have difficulty obtaining a sufficient quantity or quality of materials at a reasonable price.

4. Companies may have difficulty distributing their products and finding buyers able to purchase them.

5. Investment opportunities may be hard to find.

6. Expending accumulated personal assets may be very difficult, because available goods and services may be limited or of poor quality.

B **In a thriving economy, individuals and society as a whole benefit from the efficient production of goods and services.**

1. People are working (society may be at the level of full employment, and unemployment levels are low).

2. Families are receiving income and consuming goods and services that they need or want.

3. Economic progress gives people access to technologically advanced products.

4. A strong market for technologically advanced products stimulates research and investment for further technologic progress.

5. A well-functioning economy is attractive to foreigners for investment of capital or purchasing goods.

6. A stable, advancing economy aids social progress in the following ways:
   a. More students pursue higher levels of education.
   b. Although students are absent from the work force while in school, they enter the work force with a higher level of skill and knowledge.
   c. Well-educated workers function at a higher productivity level and thus benefit the economy.

C **A thriving economy allows managers to accomplish the following:**

1. Plan production and personnel programs with reasonable confidence that they will reap the benefits of the economy and projections for sales, productivity costs, and profits

2. Evaluate company and individual performance factors that have an impact on their "bottom line" without being hindered by an unstable economy

3. Expand businesses or add personnel to payroll

D **A well-run economy facilitates the production and exchange of goods and services.**

E **The low unemployment that results from a thriving economy may result in the following:**

1. A change in the way companies staff their workplaces (U.S. Department of Labor, 1999)
   a. The number of outsourced temporary workers increased 580 percent between 1982 and 1998.
   b. In 1997, 8.5 million workers considered themselves independent contractors.

2. Increasing options available to workers
   a. Businesses may have difficulty hiring and retaining skilled workers.
   b. The hiring of less-skilled workers may diminish the quality of services and products.

IV Changes in the National Economy

The transition in the national economy is from protected markets to international competition.

A Economic competitiveness depends on a nation's financial, industrial, and demographic characteristics, such as its unemployment rate, GNP, per capita income, average hours and conditions of work, and distribution of wealth (Potter & Youngman, 1995).

B The economic competitiveness of a nation also depends on the ability of its individual businesses to sell their goods and services at a profit in domestic (national) and foreign markets.

C America's ability to prosper depends on the ability of U.S. companies to produce and market goods and services that can compete successfully in terms of price, quality, innovation, customization, and serviceability with those of other nations.

V Factors Affecting National and Global Competitiveness

(Potter & Youngman, 1995)

A After World War II, America became the leading economic power, partly because of the destructive impact of the war on the economies of Japan and Europe.

1. Postwar benefits, such as the GI Bill, provided housing and educational opportunities to returning veterans, thus creating a competitive labor force, boosting the construction industry, and encouraging local community development.
2. National and global economies and industrialization surged from 1953 to 1975, increasing world industrial output an average of 6% a year.
3. The postwar economic boom in the United States was facilitated by the deregulation of industry and by industrial developments and manpower planning that occurred during the war.
4. Business, no longer hampered by wartime government constraints, returned to free markets and focused on meeting consumers' (rather than the government's) needs.

B During the immediate postwar decades, the world was divided into domestic and international marketplaces.

1. U.S. companies produced primarily for domestic or regional markets with minimal competition from imports and few multinational companies.
2. American companies led the industrialized markets with increasing technologic advances, mass production, and higher workers' wages through the 1970s.
3. Government regulation and collective bargaining added to costs of American businesses.
4. Europe, Japan, and the Pacific Rim countries, fully rebuilt after World War II, became increasingly competitive with the United States in the world market.

C Customers at home and abroad have become "global shoppers," seeking the best product at the most affordable price without regard to the country in which it was produced.

D Imports to the United States grew 260% between 1975 and 1993, the increase fueled by increased American purchasing power.

E U.S. exports account for the following economic benefits:
1. One out of every six American jobs in manufacturing
2. $115 billion annually in services
3. One-sixth of all U.S. agricultural production
4. Almost 25% of America's gross domestic product (GDP)—over $1 trillion per year.

F The nation's economic status is affected by a multitude of conditions and circumstances.
1. Declining economic competitiveness means potentially fewer jobs, increased unemployment, lower per capita income, and larger budget deficits.
2. The economy entered a recession and business retrenched during the 1970s, affecting manufacturing by decreasing mass production, job creation, wages, and employment levels.
3. The national economy expanded during the 1980s, but American manufacturing lost its competitive edge to foreign competitors who could produce goods at a lower cost than American companies.
4. The United States is no longer a primarily industrialized nation, a producer of manufactured goods; its economy depends more and more on the production of services and technology.

G Since the 1990s, the United States has been the leading provider of services and technology (Dent, 2000).
1. The recent explosion of Internet use has revolutionized communications and has fundamentally altered the way people live, work, and conduct business in the national and global economies
2. The economic competitiveness of the United States has increased through the use of Internet technology, which has resulted in a huge array of customized goods and services at increasingly affordable prices.
3. The vast increase in the use of technology to conduct business and communicate with others in "real time" increases competition and the ability to generate income and wealth.
4. The "information revolution," which began in the 1990s, will continue in the 2000s, with vast changes as business-to-business transactions become electronic and based on Internet technologies.

VI International Trade Status of the Nation

A Presently, the United States has a trade deficit: it imports more than it exports.

B U.S. consumers buy more foreign products than foreigners buy U.S. goods.

C Reasons for this trade imbalance include the following:
1. Some foreign countries have high trade barriers, making it difficult for the United States to sell products there.
2. The U.S. dollar has been high compared to other currencies, making it expensive for foreigners to buy American and inexpensive for Americans to buy foreign.
3. U.S. products are less competitive than foreign products in terms of price and availability.

4. U.S. services (such as architectural, engineering, and consulting) account for billions of dollars in trade, but are not accounted for in calculating the U.S. trade deficit.

D **The United States continues to produce one fourth of the world's gross national product.**

VII The Global Marketplace

A **The global economy is becoming an integrated marketplace and is influenced by a variety of economic and political forces, such as the following:**
1. General Agreement for Trade and Tariffs (GATT)
   a. GATT, which was created after World War II, works to reduce trade barriers and promote free trade among its member nations in the Free World.
   b. In 1994, the member nations of GATT agreed to create the World Trade Organization—a more comprehensive and powerful organization to govern global trade in goods and services.
2. Unification of Europe to form the European Economic Community
3. End of the Cold War and subsequent decline of communism
4. North American Free Trade Act (NAFTA)
   a. Established in 1994, NAFTA lowered trade barriers and opened the borders of Canada, the United States, and Mexico to almost limitless trade.
   b. NAFTA's long-term goal is to remove barriers to trade extending all the way from Alaska to Argentina.
5. Increased economic growth of the Pacific Rim countries

B **The world is moving toward "free trade," that is, trade without taxes or tariffs.**

C **Fewer products are being produced entirely within any single nation; the world is moving toward a single economy—a unified marketplace (Naisbitt & Aburdene, 1990; Dent, 2000).**

D **Economic and political forces are shaping a new world.**

VIII Implications for the Occupational and Environmental Health Nurse

A **The occupational and environmental health nurse is a company's primary resource regarding health care issues and the delivery of occupational health services.**

B **Occupational and environmental health nurses ensure that the work force is fit, healthy, and medically capable of performing work assignments, thus adding to the company's and the nation's productivity and ultimately to the GNP.**

C **With an increasing percentage of temporary and contingent workers, occupational and environmental health nurses will be required to be more creative and innovative in their efforts to ensure that all workers receive appropriate occupational health and safety services.**

D **The role of the occupational and environmental health nurse will expand or contract throughout the business cycle and during periods of economic uncertainty (i.e., business contraction or expansion).**

E Occupational health practice will shift from the manufacturing sector to the service and technology sectors, and will expand to include international issues of health and safety.

F As the work force expands past national borders (i.e., workers transfer to work sites in foreign countries) the occupational and environmental health nurse will be responsible for:
1. Ensuring the health of expatriates and their dependents; occupational and environmental health nursing duties may include the following:
   a. Immunizations for international travel
   b. Access to quality health care abroad
   c. Health education
   d. Psychologic support systems (for example, access to employee assistance programs)
2. Helping identify international health and safety needs of the global work force
3. Identifying national and international regulatory compliance issues that will affect the work force, such as family leave and occupational health laws.

(Chapter 14 presents a sample international travel program.)

IX Business Trends

A Megatrends (large social, economic, and technologic trends) that shaped the 1980s in business include the following (Naisbitt and Aburdene, 1990):
1. Shift from an industrial society to an information society
2. Forced technology to high tech/high touch; for example, interactive technology
3. National economy to a world economy
4. Short-term to long-term planning
5. Centralization to decentralization of company/business lines/units
6. Institutional help to self-help
7. Representative democracy to participatory democracy
8. Hierarchies to networking teams
9. Movement of business from northern states to southern states to save on labor and operating costs
10. Limited options of "either/or" to multiple options

B During the economic expansion in the 1980s, businesses invested, acquired additional product lines, and increased their work forces.
1. Many businesses established operations in southern states, where operating costs were lower.
2. Companies established decentralized business operations wherein operating divisions became dedicated "strategic business units," accountable for their own profits and losses.
3. Businesses merged "horizontally," acquiring companies that enhanced existing product lines.
4. During the latter part of the 1980s, the economy contracted, and business responded by:
   a. Divesting noncore or nonessential business units and product lines
   b. Downsizing work forces through layoffs or reorganizations
   c. Initiating vertical mergers (businesses acquiring similar businesses)

C Trends that affected business and consumers in the 1990s included the following (Naisbitt and Aburdene, 1990):

1. An expanding global economy
2. A renaissance in the arts
3. The emergence of free-market socialism
4. Global lifestyles and cultural nationalism
5. The privatization of the welfare state
6. The rise of the Pacific Rim nations
7. Increasing role of women in leadership
8. Advances in biology and genetics
9. The religious revival
10. Empowerment of the individual

D The technology explosion of the 1990s created eight critical technology trends that will change the way employers and consumers work and live in the 2000s (Dent 2000):

1. Vastly expanded computer power
2. Mass adoption of portable and home personal computers
3. Increased computer literacy among all age groups
4. Evolution of computers so they become simple and affordable appliances and everyday work tools
5. Linkage of microprocessor-embedded home and business products through the Internet
6. Rapid movement of consumers "on line"
7. Expansion of the communication bandwidth
8. Object-oriented programming for customized software

X Major Business Issues

A Increased federalism or regulatory constraints on business include mandatory compliance with regulations set forth by the following:

1. Occupational Safety and Health Administration
2. Department of Transportation
3. Environmental Protection Agency (EPA)
4. Employee Retirement Income Security Act
5. Consolidated Omnibus Budget Reconciliation Act
6. Family Medical Leave Act
7. Americans with Disabilities Act
8. State workers' compensation statutes

B Cost shifting of social insurance programs (Social Security, Medicare, Medicaid) from government to privately funded sources.

C Increasing costs of employee health and welfare benefits, such as workers' compensation and nonoccupational health and disability

D Employers' trends, such as the following:

1. Shift toward managed care for health benefit plans
2. Increased cost sharing of health care expenses and benefits with employees through higher deductibles and coinsurance rates, increasing employees' out-of-pocket expenditures
3. Increased involvement of employees in health care decisions
4. Aggressive negotiation with health providers and packaging of provider services

5. Aggressive management of health care costs through utilization review, second opinions, preadmission certification, concurrent review, case management, and retrospective reviews
6. Increased communication with employees regarding health care costs
7. Encouragement of managed care enrollments
8. Establishment of wellness programs
9. Emphasis on balancing employee work/lifestyle issues *such as elder care, child care, work-life balance*
10. Movement toward a "24-hour" system of health care (i.e., the integration of occupational and nonoccupational medical care)
11. Shift toward integrated benefits and disability management arrangements

E **Issues related to workers' compensation (DiBenedetto, 1999)**
1. Workers' compensation constitutes about 3% of total national medical expenditures; however, 11 million employees suffer work-related injuries resulting in $111 billion in payments for medical care, wage replacement, and disability payments. More than 50% of the $111 billion is associated with the payment of lost wages, and the remainder represents the cost of workers' compensation medical care.
2. *Direct* costs of workers' compensation include medical care and indemnity (wage replacement) payments.
3. *Indirect* costs include lost productivity, required replacements, employee overtime, training, accident investigation, and broken equipment.
4. Identification and correction of the root causes of workers' compensation claims will facilitate a safer workplace and decrease workers' compensation claims, thus increasing work-force productivity.

F **Methods being used by businesses to control the cost of workers' compensation include the following (DiBenedetto, et al., 1996):**
1. Preclaim strategies, such as:
   a. Assignment of responsibilities
   b. Communications
   c. Occupational health and safety programs
   d. Injury prevention programs
   e. Development of job responsibilities (essential functions and physical requirements)
   f. Return-to-work programs
   g. Identification of modified or transitional work assignments
   h. Third party administrator (TPA) performance standards
   i. Medical and case management requirements
   j. Negotiated discounts of fee schedules and managed medical care arrangements
2. At-claim strategies, such as:
   a. Immediate reporting of accidents to management and the carrier or TPA
   b. Timely accident investigation
   c. Claim setup and initiation of medical and case management
   d. Use of disability duration guidelines
   e. Use of treatment guidelines or protocols
   f. Use of independent medical examinations
   g. Fraud investigation
   h. Establishment of appropriate claim reserves

3. Postclaim strategies, such as:
   a. TPA audits
   b. Utilization review
   c. Quality assurance reviews
4. Additional trends include the integration of workers' compensation and nonoccupational disability management to manage costs and facilitate the injured employee's return to work.

G Increasing occurrence of violence in the workplace (Chapter 13)

H Need for advanced information technology and information processing

XI Implications for Occupational and Environmental Health Nursing

(DiBenedetto, 1999)

A The occupational and environmental health nurse plays a primary role in helping the work force attain its maximum level of health and thus adds to work-force productivity.

B The occupational and environmental health nurse performs health care and management functions that vary according to the work setting, the employer's needs and expectations, the company philosophy, and the occupational and environmental health nurse's knowledge of the regulatory requirements that govern occupational health care, safety, and workers' compensation in that particular industry.

C The occupational and environmental health nurse may have the following specific responsibilities:
1. Establish and implement health-related policies and procedures
2. Develop and maintain the company's regulatory compliance programs related to OSHA, EPA, DOT, ADA, FMLA, and workers' compensation requirements
3. Prevent injury and illness through health promotion and health education activities
4. Provide workers' compensation and nonoccupational case management (also referred to as integrated disability management), coordinate independent health examinations, arrange for second-opinion examinations, and perform case management functions to facilitate early return to work of ill and injured workers
5. Identify real and potential hazards in the workplace by conducting facility assessments and report those conditions to appropriate members of management for correction

D The role of the occupational and environmental health nurse and funding for occupational health and safety programs will expand or contract throughout the business cycle.

E Many companies continue to outsource occupational health and safety services; many occupational health providers are now contract providers or vendors.

F As the work force contracts through downsizing and layoffs, employees are more likely to file for workers' compensation; some claims for on-the-job injuries may be fraudulent.

G Occupational and environmental health nurses are increasingly involved in employee benefits; they evaluate plan sponsors and benefit components, arrange for second opinions, educate employees regarding lifestyles and life skills, and integrate health promotion activities to include the needs of families.

H Occupational and environmental health nurses are assuming a greater role in establishing and directing integrated disability management and return-to-work programs to increase the health, safety, and productivity of the work force

XII Health Care Reform and Managed Health Care

A The major arguments for health care reform are the following:
1. The delivery of care is bogged down in administration and insurance underwriting.
2. Health care costs are escalating.
3. At least 44 million Americans lack health insurance or are underinsured.

B Health reform components that have broad support include the following:
1. A standard minimum benefit package
2. Insurance market reform
3. Health plan "report cards"
4. Consumer choice of plans
5. Voluntary purchasing pools

C Major components of health care reform proposals have included insurance market reforms, cost-containment mechanisms, managed care, and subsidies for low-income persons.

D In past proposals, financing of health care reform would have come from employer or individual premium mandates or from voluntary plans that were based upon the then-current health care system.

E Federal efforts to mandate health care reform failed to pass Congress in 1994.

F Currently, market-driven reforms have moved the delivery of health care from "free choice" to managed care.

XIII Overview of Managed Care

A *Managed care* is a broad concept generally applied to "prepayment arrangement, negotiated discounts, and agreements for prior authorization and audits of performance" (Madison & Konrad, 1988, in Wassel, 1995).

B Managed care plans generally provide some restrictions on the traditional unlimited access to providers and payment of reasonable and customary charges for their health care services (Wassel, 1995).

C Managed care plans place responsibilities on consumers and providers in the form of a binding contract (Wassel, 1995).

D A managed care plan is any form of health plan that initiates selective contracting between providers, employers, or insurers to channel employees/clients to a specified set of cost-effective providers (a provider network). These providers have procedures in place to ensure that only medically necessary and appropriate use of health care services occurs.

E Three basic types of health care delivery systems under managed care arrangements are the health maintenance organization, preferred provider organization, and point-of-service plan (Wassel, 1995).

1. A *health maintenance organization (HMO)* provides a specified scope of services or benefits to members for a fixed fee.
   a. There are four types of HMOs: staff, group, network, and independent-practice associations.
   b. HMOs provide 10% to 40% savings over traditional health plans.
2. A *preferred provider organization (PPO)* provides greater consumer choice through use of a limited provider panel, and uses negotiated fee schedules, utilization review, and the physician-as-gatekeeper to hold down costs.
   a. In exchange for reduced rates, providers often receive expedited claim payments or a reasonable market share.
   b. Employees have financial incentives to use PPO providers.
3. A *point-of-service plan (POS)* is a health benefit plan through which several different types of insurance coverage are available. The employee chooses the insurance plan and provider at the time health care services are sought.
   a. POS plans provide incentives for employees to choose cost-effective providers.
   b. If managed care providers are not used by the employee, the extra cost of service is borne by the employee.

F The *24-hour* model of health care incorporates occupational (workers' compensation) and nonoccupational (disability) health care into one health care delivery system to improve continuity of care, manage and reduce claim costs, minimize redundancies in coverage, simplify adjudication, and reduce administrative efforts and costs. Approaches to 24-hour care include the following (Abbott, 1994):

1. 24-hour medical coverage where health benefits for all accidents or injuries fall under an integrated health plan. Disability or lost-time benefits would be paid by workers' compensation.
2. 24-hour disability coverage where disability benefits for both occupational and nonoccupational concerns would be paid from an integrated plan, but health payments would still be divided.
3. Integrated 24-hour medical and disability coverage where medical and indemnity payments would be integrated under one plan.
4. *Accident only* and *sickness only* medical programs may also exist as a subset to these three major categories.

G Managed workers' compensation is characterized by negotiated fee schedules, capitated rates, and the use of PPOs and other provider arrangements.

H *Integrated disability management* is a comprehensive approach to integrating all disability benefits, programs, and services to help control the employer's disability costs while returning the employee to work as soon as possible and maximizing the employee's functional capacity (Mercer, 1995).

XIV Quality Controls in Managed Care

(Employee Benefit Research Institute, 1995)

A Maintaining the quality of health care is Americans' primary concern in the changing health care system.

B Concern over rising health care costs has led private employers and public programs to adopt various strategies to manage health care costs.

C The aim of all these strategies is to purchase the highest quality health care at the lowest cost.

D Defining and measuring health care quality are controversial and costly endeavors.

E *Health care quality* can be viewed narrowly as *clinical effectiveness.*

F Health care quality can be viewed in a broader sense as all the attributes of medical care that clients value.

XV Judging Standards of Care

The following private organizations independently review quality standards in hospitals and other institutions and provide accreditation of those organizations.

A Joint Commission for Accreditation of Healthcare Organizations

B Health Care Financing Administration

C National Committee for Quality Assurance

D Accreditation Association for Ambulatory Health Care

E Utilization Review Accreditation Commission

XVI Defining and Evaluating Quality Outcomes

A Managed care relies on monitoring physicians' treatment patterns (through utilization review, physician profiling, and case management) and changing providers' financial incentives.

B Health Plan Employer Data and Information Set (HEDIS) was established by the private sector (several employers and managed care organizations in 1989) to help large purchasers of health care judge the comparative value of competing health care plans. HEDIS has the following characteristics:

1. Provides a core set of performance measures that can be adapted to serve the needs of other purchasers

2. Provides benchmarks for performance in specific areas such as health plan quality, access and client satisfaction, membership and utilization, finance and management, and activities

3. Relies primarily on structural and process measures of quality; major outcome measures are client satisfaction and readmission rates for major disorders

C Many analysts believe that the future evolution of the health care delivery system will be driven by the development of measures of the quality of care.

D Donabedian (1988) classified attempts to measure quality of care as studies of structure, process, and outcome.

1. *Structure* refers to attributes of care, such as caregiver's qualifications and resources available at the site of care.

2. *Process* examines the caregiver's activities, decisions made at various points in an episode of illness, and appropriateness of care.

3. *Outcome* measures the effects of care on health status and client satisfaction.

XVII Implications for Occupational and Environmental Health Nursing

(DiBenedetto, et al., 1996)

A Occupational and environmental health nurses are providing case management services, return-to-work planning, and management of integrated disability and workers' compensation services.

B As market-driven health care reform continues, the role and scope of occupational and environmental health nursing will expand into the managed care arena as an integrated model that combines both workers' compensation and disability management.

C Occupational and environmental health nurses may be involved in the assessment, evaluation, and implementation of managed health care arrangements and programs.

D Occupational and environmental health nurses will provide value-added knowledge and services as managed care vendors expand services into the occupational health and managed workers' compensation markets.

E Occupational and environmental health nurses will increasingly become involved in managed health care benefits for the following:
1. Employers
2. Employees *and their dependents*
3. Managed health care vendors/organizations

F Occupational and environmental health nurses may become the liaison between employer benefit plans and managed care organizations, thus facilitating lines of communication, professional cooperation, benefit services, and health care delivery.

BIBLIOGRAPHY

Abbott, R.K. (1994, Sept/Oct). 24 hour medical care: A primer. *Innovations in human resources,* 12–14.

Bagby, M.E. (1995). *The first annual report of the United States of America: An account to American citizens of where we stand economically, socially, and internationally.* New York: Harper Business.

Dent, Jr., H.S. (2000) *The roaring 2000s* New York: Simon and Schuster.

DiBenedetto, D.V. (1999, June) Workers' compensation managed care. *OEM report* 13:6, 41-48.

DiBenedetto, D.V., Harris, J.S, & McCunney, R.J. (1996). *Occupational health & safety manual,* (2nd ed.). Beverly Farms,, MA: OEM Press.

Donabadien, A. (1988, Spring). Quality assessment and assurance: Unity of purpose, diversity of means. *Inquiry, 25,* 173–192.

Drucker, P.F. (1989). *The new realities: In government and politics/in economics and business/in society and world view.* New York: Harper and Row.

Drucker, P.F. (1993). *Managing for the future: The 1990s and beyond* [Sections 1C, 9A]. New York: Truman Talley Books/Plume.

Employee Benefit Research Institute (EBRI). (1995, March). *Measuring the quality of health care* [*EBRI Brief No. 159*]: Washington, DC: EBRI.

Epping, R.C. (1995). *A beginner's guide to world economy.* New York: Vintage Books.

Friedman, J.P. (1987). *Dictionary of business terms.* New York: Barron's.

Heilbroner, R., & Thurow, L. (1994). *Economics explained: Everything you need to know about how the economy works and where it's going.* New York: Touchstone.

Katzenbach, J.R, & Smith, D.K. (1994). *The wisdom of teams: Creating the high performance organization.* New York: Harper Business.

Madison, D.L., & Konrad, T.R. (1988). Large medical group-practice organizations and employee physicians: A relationship in transition. *Milbank Memorial Quarterly, 66*(2), 240–282.

Mansfield, E. (1988). *Micro-economics: Theory and applications* (Shorter 6th ed.). New York: W.W. Norton & Company.

McRae, H. (1994). *The world in 2020: Power, culture and prosperity.* Boston: Harvard Business School Press.

Mercer, W. (1995). *The language of managed disability.* New York: Mercer/Met Disability.

Naisbitt, J., & Aburdene, P. (1990). *Megatrends 2000: Ten new directions for the 1990s.* New York: William Morrow & Company.

Peters, T. (1992). *Liberation management: Necessary disorganization for the nanosecond nineties.* New York: Fawcett Columbine.

Potter, E.E., & Youngman, J.A. (1995). *Keeping America competitive: Employment policy for the twenty-first century.* Lakewood, CO: Glenbridge Publishing Ltd.

U.S. Department of Labor Bureau of Labor Statistics (1998). Report on the American Workforce. Washington, D.C.: U.S. Department of Labor.

Thurow, L. (1993). *Head to head: The coming economic battle among Japan, Europe and America.* New York: Warner Books.

Traska, M.R. (1995). *Managed care strategies 1996.* New York: Faulkner and Gray.

Wassel, M.L. (1995). Occupational health nursing and the advent of managed care: Meeting the challenges of the current health care environment. *AAOHN Journal, 43*(1), 23–28.

Webster's new world dictionary of business terms. (1985). New York: Simon & Schuster.

5

Scientific Foundations of Occupational and Environmental Health Nursing Practice

Jacqueline Agnew

The science and practice of occupational and environmental health nursing is based on a synthesis of knowledge gained from multiple disciplines. It is essential that occupational and environmental health nurses understand the principles of the sciences that provide the theoretic, conceptual, and factual framework of the profession. In addition to the nursing and occupational health sciences (e.g., toxicology, industrial hygiene, and ergonomics), effective occupational and environmental health nursing practice requires knowledge and understanding of the public health (e.g., environmental health and epidemiology) and social/behavioral sciences. This chapter provides an introduction and overview of these foundational disciplines.

I History of Nursing Science

A **Florence Nightingale: established public health as an important focus for nursing.**
   1. She emphasized the need for nurses to improve environmental conditions to protect the health of clients, thus laying the foundation for occupational and environmental health nursing.
   2. She provided the initial spark for development of nursing theory and research, although her major influence was on nursing education.

B **Development of nursing research and theory**
   1. Although theorizing has always been a part of nursing practice, the labeling and communication of nursing theories did not occur until the 1950s (Meleis, 1997).
      a. *Nursing Research,* the first journal for nursing science, was established in 1953.
      b. From 1950 to 1965, theories focused on human beings as individuals with a set of needs, and nursing as a set of unique functions to meet those needs.
      c. By 1975, schools of nursing were required to have a theory-based curriculum to be accredited.

d. Most early theories require modification before they can be applied to care delivered in the occupational setting.

2. From 1975 to 1990, the emphasis on using theory to describe and explain nursing phenomena, predict relationships, and guide nursing care resulted in the continued development of theory (Meleis, 1997).

   a. During this period, theory was accepted as a tool that can be used to resolve significant practice problems.

   b. As the commitment of nursing to be a research-based discipline grew, implementing research results into nursing practice became a major goal.

3. From 1990 to the present, clinical outcomes research, and particularly the study of nurse-sensitive outcomes, has become a major focus for nurse researchers; examples of clinical outcomes of occupational and environmental health nursing intervention include the following:

   a. Prevention of work-related illness and injury

   b. The timely return to work of ill or injured workers

   c. Reduction in the cost of health care and disability compensation

   d. Modification of the personal impact of illness and injury on the worker and the family

II Research–Theory–Practice Linkages

A **Relationships between research and practice (Meleis, 1997)**

1. Practice provides a unique context for nursing research.

   a. Problems regularly confronted in occupational and environmental nursing practice should stimulate nursing research studies.

   b. Examples include methods for preventing work-related hearing loss, organizational factors affecting the wearing of personal protective equipment, and the use of modified-duty positions.

2. As a professional discipline, nursing practice should be research-based, and changes in practice should be driven by research findings.

   a. In order to be used in practice, research findings need to be disseminated to appropriate audiences.

   b. Advancements in nursing practice contribute to improvements in worker health and safety.

   c. Examples of such advancements include the institution of latex-safe environments, approaches to the prevention of musculoskeletal injuries, and work-site interventions for violence reduction.

B **Relationships between research and theory (Meleis, 1997)**

1. Qualitative research techniques (e.g., ethnography and grounded theory)

   a. These techniques often lead to the development or refinement of theories about important concepts in nursing practice.

   b. Such research techniques might be used to develop theories and hypotheses about the management of work-related symptoms, workers' self-care, or organizational culture.

2. Quantitative research techniques

   a. These techniques may lead to the development or testing of theories and their associated hypotheses.

   b. Epidemiologic techniques, for example, might be used to test nursing theories about risk factors and risk reduction.

III Early Nursing Theory

Grand theories are more useful as overall frameworks for making decisions in practice than for identifying specific research questions; three categories of grand theories are the following (Meleis, 1997):

A **Needs-based theories**
   1. These theories are based on the idea that nursing care is required to help clients meet specific functional needs (e.g., theories of Virginia Henderson, Dorothea Orem).
   2. Example: Orem's theory might be adapted to promote self-care related to the prevention of work-related symptoms or to modify the work setting for the disabled worker.

B **Interaction-based theories**
   1. These theories are based on the idea that nursing care proceeds through a process of interaction between the nurse and the client (e.g., the theories of Hildegarde Peplau, Ida Jean Orlando, J. Travelbee, Imogene King, J. Paterson, and L. Zderad).
   2. These theories could be adapted to clarify the relationship between the occupational and environmental health nurse and the worker.

C **Outcome-based theories**
   1. These theories are based on the idea that nursing focuses on outcomes of care related to energy conservation, balance, or harmony (e.g., the theories of Dorothy Johnson, Myra Levine, Martha Rogers, and Sister Callista Roy).
   2. For example, Johnson's theory might be adapted to examine physiologic and behavioral outcomes of occupational and environmental health nursing interventions.

IV The Domain of Nursing

Nursing is differentiated from other scientific disciplines by the way it defines the client, or recipient of care; the environment or context of care; the health or illness problems under consideration; and the therapeutic interventions applied. These domains emerged from the grand theories of nursing (Meleis, 1997).

A **Patient/client/recipient of care**
   1. Under what conditions do human beings become recipients of nursing care?
   2. Risks to health, function, equilibrium, or self-care ability tend to define a person or group's need for nursing care.
   3. Occupational and environmental health nurses are concerned primarily with working-age adults and their families.

B **Environment of care**
   1. What are the properties, components, and dimensions of the environment that influence the recipient's health status?
   2. For nursing, the environment includes physical, sociocultural, organizational, economic, political, and interpersonal dimensions.
   3. These dimensions of the environment are all essential considerations for occupational and environmental health nurses, indicating that this is a particularly important domain for occupational and environmental health nursing practice.

C Health/illness problems

1. What are the health or illness conditions that are influenced by nursing care?

2. In nursing, health is considered more than the absence of disease; it includes dimensions of self-actualization as well as illness.

3. Occupational and environmental health nurses focus primarily on work-related illnesses and injuries or potentially disabling conditions that might limit someone's ability to work or that might be worsened by work.

D Nursing therapeutics

1. What are the content and goals of nursing interventions?

2. Nursing interventions are those nursing activities and actions deliberately designed for recipients of nursing care.

3. Occupational and environmental health nurses, for example, perform interventions that are unique to the occupational setting or workers.

V Modern Nursing Theory: Middle-Range Theories

Middle-range theories, in contrast to grand theories, are more amenable to testing through research techniques, and they lend themselves better to testing the interventions used in occupational and environmental health nursing practice.

A Middle-range theories are a compromise between grand theories, which attempt to explain everything about a phenomenon, and narrow-range theories, which address only simple, abstract facts and principles (Meleis, 1997).

B Characteristics of middle-range theories include the following:

1. They evolve from daily practice considerations of nurses and focus on more specific practice problems than grand theories.

2. They are often more amenable than grand theories to testing using research techniques.

3. By contrast, narrow-range theories focus on problems that are unique to individual settings or small groups of clients and are less useful for nursing as a whole.

C Examples of middle-range theories with applicability to occupational and environmental health nursing research

1. Pender's theory of health promotion and health (protection) behaviors
   a. This theory focuses on individual perceptions and the likelihood that an individual will perform a recommended preventive health action
   b. Such a theory has immediate implications for occupational and environmental health nursing research and might be applied to worker perceptions about work-related risks of illness and injury and safe work activities.
   c. For example, a researcher might attempt to identify the factors that influence workers' use of hearing protection.

2. Social support
   a. Multiple theories of social support describe the beneficial effects of support from others, including supervisors and co-workers.
   b. Social support within and among teams of supervisors and co-workers might be studied by occupational and environmental health nurses as a predictor of safer work activities and fewer injuries.

3. Mischel's model of uncertainty
   a. This theory describes the concept of uncertainty and its effects on an individual's choices related to seeking health care and recovering from illness or injury (Mischel, 1988).
   b. An occupational and environmental health nurse researcher might adapt the theory to study recovery from an occupational injury or illness; uncertainty and fear of reinjury, for example, might be a factor in delaying the return to work of clients whose symptoms persist after carpal tunnel syndrome surgery.

VI The Practice of Occupational and Environmental Health Nursing

Occupational and environmental health nursing practice influences and is influenced by nursing science.

A Occupational and environmental health nurses need to actively participate in the development of national activities to ensure that the working population is considered when research priorities are set; examples of these activities are involvement in setting standards and providing input to the development of a research agenda.

B Occupational and environmental health nurses need to participate in determining which outcomes are important for the nursing care of working-age adults and their families and which outcomes are affected by occupational and environmental health nursing interventions.

C The participation of occupational and environmental health nurses in the development of taxonomies (classification systems) is critical to ensure the inclusion of data related to occupations, occupational and environmental health nursing and work-site interventions, prevention programs, worker participation, and work-related injuries and illnesses.

VII The Effects of the Environment on Health

Environmental health is the "freedom from illness or injury related to exposure to toxic agents and other environmental conditions that are potentially detrimental to health" (Institute of Medicine, 1995).

A In 1995, an Institute of Medicine study (Institute of Medicine, 1995) identified three themes related to nursing and the environment:
   1. The environment is a primary determinant of health, and environmental health hazards affect all aspects of life and all areas of nursing practice.
   2. Nurses are well positioned to address environmental health concerns of individuals and communities.
   3. There is a need to enhance the awareness of and emphasis on environmental threats to the health of populations served by all nurses, regardless of their practice arena.

B The expertise and competencies of occupational and environmental health nurses are relevant to the protection of health and safety in community settings and work settings (White, et al., 1999).

C Some of the most significant environmental conditions that are capable of harming the health of humans are experienced at work.

D The following three factors are used to analyze the balance of health (Shortridge & Valanis, 1992):

1. The *causative agent,* which is related to work processes or interactions
2. The *susceptible host,* the worker with the following characteristics
   a. Generally healthy enough to hold a job
   b. Of working age
   c. Often of childbearing age
3. The *environments,* which are highly variable

E Workers are faced with multiple workplace hazards that place them at risk.

1. A *hazard* is defined as a substance capable of causing harm (Chapter 1 describes categories of hazards).
2. *Risk* is the probability that harm will occur.

F A systematic understanding of the agent-host-environment relationship and the principles that govern the association between hazards and health effects can provide the basis for preventing morbidity and mortality and promoting health in a broad range of settings.

1. Workers, work-related exposures, and work environments illustrate one domain in which these principles apply.
2. The influence of industrial conditions on family and community members is another example of health and environment interactions.
   a. Families can be exposed to toxins transported home on workers' bodies or belongings.
   b. Industrial waste or effluent can reach the community.
3. Approaches to risk assessment and principles of health protection similar to those used in the workplace can be used to protect the health of communities faced with natural or manmade hazards in media such as food, air, soil, and water.

G The chief disciplines that guide the occupational and environmental health nurse in an understanding of the agent-host-environment relationship are epidemiology, toxicology, and industrial hygiene; these are described in the following sections.

(Chapter 15 presents more information about environmental health.)

VIII Overview of Epidemiologic Terms and Principles

Epidemiology is the public health science that is fundamental to describing and understanding relationships among agents, hosts, and their environments.

A Definitions

1. The word *epidemiology* is of Greek derivation (from *epi,* meaning *upon; demos,* meaning *people;* and *logos,* meaning *science*).
2. *Epidemiology* is the study of the distribution and determinants of health-related states or events in specified populations, and the application of this study to the control of health problems (Last, 1988).
3. *Incidence rate* is an epidemiologic term that describes the rate of disease development among persons at risk.
   a. The numerator includes only new cases of disease during a given time period; the denominator includes everyone at risk of developing the disease during that period.
   b. Incidence, therefore, measures the probability (or risk) of developing disease.

4. *Prevalence rate* is an epidemiologic term that describes the proportion of the population that has the condition at a given point in time or during a given time period.
   a. The numerator includes new and existing cases; the denominator includes all who are at risk of developing the disease, including those who have it.
   b. Prevalence measures the current burden of disease and is useful for measuring and projecting health care and health resource needs.

B **Examples of applications of epidemiologic research include:**
1. Controlling infectious diseases, such as tuberculosis among migrant farm workers
2. Controlling the effects of chemical hazards, such as asbestosis, mesothelioma, and lung cancers related to exposure to asbestos
3. Understanding genetic susceptibility to disease, such as coronary heart disease, which seems to result from a combination of hereditary and environmental factors
4. Understanding the effects of nutritional status, such as the link between a calcium intake and osteoporosis
5. Linking pathogens to specific disease processes, such as the human immunodeficiency virus (HIV) to acquired immunodeficiency syndrome (AIDS)
6. Identifying risk factors for illness or injury, such as work factors that lead to back injuries in health care workers

C **Epidemiology has great relevance to occupational and environmental health nursing.**
1. It serves as a tool for identifying and preventing hazardous work-site exposures.
2. Findings from epidemiologic studies of worker populations are often reported in the occupational and environmental health literature.
3. Epidemiologic studies of work-related problems help occupational and environmental health nurses provide high-quality health services.

IX Measures of Association

The study of association is central to epidemiology; criteria to evaluate causality of observed association include the following (Mausner & Kramer, 1985):

A **Strength of the association**
1. The strength of the association refers to the magnitude (amount) of risk associated with an exposure.
2. Magnitude of risk is often measured by the ratio of disease rates for those with and without a hypothesized causal factor.

B **Consistency of the association**
1. Similar findings result across several studies of the same association.
2. Conclusions are similar despite the use of different study designs.

C **Temporality of the association**
1. Studies demonstrate that the independent variable (cause) precedes the dependent variable (effect) chronologically.
2. Temporality cannot be evaluated with a cross-sectional study.

D Dose-response relationship
1. As the degree of exposure increases, the risk for developing the outcome increases.
2. Lack of a dose-response relationship does not rule out a causal relationship.

E Plausibility of the association
1. The association is consistent with a plausible biologic explanation.
2. Knowledge of the natural history of the disease and results of animal and other laboratory experiments need to be considered.

X Sources of Epidemiologic Data

A Health outcome data are available through a variety of public and private agencies.
1. Census data (U.S. Census Bureau)
2. Vital statistics (U.S. Census Bureau)
3. National health surveys (National Center for Health Statistics)
   a. Population-based studies such as the National Health and Nutrition Examination Surveys and the National Health Interview Survey are conducted regularly.
   b. Mandatory reporting systems capture data such as OSHA-recordable illnesses and injuries (Bureau of Labor Statistics).
4. Disease and death registries (from state and federal agencies)

B Exposure data are often more difficult to obtain, especially in environmental and occupational settings.
1. Examples of exposure data are air monitoring data and biomarkers of exposure.
2. Data may be obtained from exposure registries such as those maintained for heavy metal exposure, certain pharmaceutics, and needlestick injuries.

XI Comparisons of Rates

A A *rate ratio* (also known as *relative risk*) is a measure of the relationship between two rates, that of the exposed and that of the unexposed population.

B An *odds ratio* is a good estimate of the rate ratio, but is derived from case control or cross-sectional studies.

C A *rate difference* is a measure of the difference between two rates, one for the exposed and one for the unexposed population. Because it describes the increased amount of risk attributed to the exposure, it is known as *attributable risk*.

XII Types of Rates

(Box 5-1 presents examples of the following rates.)

A *Crude rates* are based on the actual number of events for a given time period but do not reflect any important differences in risk among subgroups in the population.

B *Characteristic-specific rates* allow one to compare rates for similar subgroups of two or more populations (e.g., age-specific or gender-specific rates).

BOX 5-1

Using crude, specific, and adjusted rates to describe a health problem

Crude Rates: The crude rates of lung cancer in a population will not reflect the fact that older individuals are at higher risk for lung cancer. To look at the association between smoking and lung cancer, it would not be fair to compare crude rates of lung cancer in groups of smokers and non-smokers who differ in age distribution.

Specific Rates: Rates of lung cancer could be computed for age-specific groups, perhaps by decade of age, to examine differences in lung cancer rates by age.

Adjusted Rates: The age-adjusted rates of lung cancer in the smoking and nonsmoking groups could be compared to examine the question of an association between smoking and cancer.

C *Adjusted* (or *standardized*) *rates* reflect population differences by taking into consideration the distribution of important characteristics that may affect risk (e.g., age-adjusted rates).

XIII Inferential Statistics

Inferential statistics, which are taken from a sample of a population, are used to make inferences about the entire target population (Mausner & Kramer, 1985).

A A *hypothesis* is a supposition, resulting from observation or reflection.
   1. A hypothesis leads to predictions that can be tested.
   2. Hypothesis testing involves conducting a test of statistic significance and quantifying the degree to which sampling variability may account for the observed results.

B Some well-known tests of statistic significance include the t-test and chi-square test.

C A *p-value* is a quantitative statement of the probability that the observed difference (or association) in a particular study could have happened by chance alone.
   1. $p < 0.05$ means that the probability that the observed difference occurred by chance is less than 5%.
   2. $p < 0.05$ is the customary level for accepting an association as statistically significant.

D A *confidence interval* provides an idea of the magnitude of the effect and the inherent variability in an estimated statistic.
   1. A confidence interval is an alternative to a *p*-value.
   2. The calculation of the confidence level is based on the assumption that the distribution of observed rates can be approximated by the standard normal curve.
   3. A 95% confidence level means that there is a 95% probability that the true rate of an observation lies within the calculated interval.

E The *power* of a study is its likelihood of detecting a real association; power is affected by the following four variables:
1. The magnitude of the effect (or association)
2. The variability of the measures of interest
3. The level of statistic significance that has been set (alpha)
4. The size of the sample studied
   a. Larger sample sizes increase the stability of measurements made in an epidemiologic study.
   b. Power calculations based on the above variables suggest the appropriate sample size needed for an epidemiologic study.

XIV Overview of Study Designs

(Chapter 16, Section V.G, presents additional information.)

A *Experimental designs* **are preferred for determining causality**
1. In an experimental study, the investigator assigns the exposure (or putative cause) to the study subjects.
2. *Clinical trials* and *intervention studies* are examples of experimental designs.
3. Experiments are limited by ethical constraints.

B *Nonexperimental designs* **that attempt to simulate the results of an experiment (had one been possible) are primarily** *descriptive studies* **or** *analytic (ex post facto) studies.*
1. *Descriptive studies* are hypothesis generating and therefore are not intended to determine causality.
   a. A *cross-sectional study* examines the relationship between diseases (or other health-related characteristics) and other variables of interest as they exist in a defined population at one point in time.

TABLE 5-1

Advantages and disadvantages of various designs of nonexperimental epidemiologic studies

Study design	Advantages	Disadvantages
Cohort or Prospective	Good for study of rare exposures Allows classification of exposure before disease develops Can determine incidence of disease Can determine true relative risk Can follow multiple outcomes	Lengthy Large sample size required Generally expensive
Case-Control	Good for study of rare outcomes Can estimate relative risk by odds ratio Takes less time Less expensive Requires smaller sample size Can look at multiple risk factors	Exposure histories may be difficult to construct Potential for subject loss to follow-up Recall bias can be a problem Must select appropriate control group
Cross-Sectional	Generates hypotheses Useful in study of exposures that do not change (e.g., blood type)	Cannot determine causality Current exposure does not represent relevant past exposure

Source: Mausner & Kramer, 1985.

b. An *ecologic study* involves the group rather than the individual as the unit of analysis, usually because information is not available at the individual level.

2. *Analytic studies:* the investigator systematically determines whether risk of disease is different for exposed and nonexposed individuals.

a. A *cohort study* (also called a *prospective study* or *follow-up study*) is an analytic study in which persons who are initially free of the disease (or outcome) but vary in one or more factors (such as exposure or potentially protective factors) are followed over a period of time for the occurrence of the disease (or outcome).

b. In a *case-control study*, a group of persons with a disease (cases) are compared with a group without the disease (controls) to study the characteristics (such as exposure) that might predict, cause, or protect against the disease.

3. Table 5-1 lists advantages and disadvantages of cohort, case-control, and cross-sectional study designs.

XV Bias and Confounding in Epidemiologic Studies

Detection of associations that are not real is usually the result of biased study methods or the presence of confounding variables (Mausner and Kramer, 1985).

A *Bias* **refers to systematic error in an epidemiologic study that results in an incorrect estimate of the association between exposure and risk of disease.**

1. Selection bias
a. This type of bias occurs when the identification of subjects for inclusion in the study, on the basis of either exposure (cohort study) or disease (case-control study) status, depends in some way on the other axis of interest.
b. Selection bias can result from differential surveillance, diagnosis, referral, or participation of individuals in the study.

2. Information (or observation) bias
a. This type of bias results from systematic differences in the way data on exposure or outcomes are obtained from various study groups.
b. Examples of information bias are recall bias, interviewer bias, loss of subjects to follow-up over time, and misclassification (Table 5-2).

3. Study results may be biased either toward or away from the null hypothesis—or in both directions.

B *Confounding* **results when the estimate of the effect of the exposure of interest is distorted because it is mixed with the effect of an extraneous factor; in occupational epidemiology studies, age and smoking status are usually important confounding variables.**

C **Methods to avoid and manage study biases and confounding include the following:**

1. A strict study protocol with attention to how subjects are selected for study is a means of avoiding study bias in the design phase of the study.

2. Systematic, standardized data collection techniques that are consistent for all study participants will help avoid bias in the data collection phase.

3. Confounding can be avoided by making comparisons only among individuals with the same level of the confounding variable; this is also known as *controlling for the effect of the confounding variable.*
a. Confounding is usually avoided by stratifying or adjusting during data analysis.

TABLE 5-2	

Types of bias in epidemiologic studies

Type of bias	Description
Information	Exposure and outcome data are ascertained differently from study groups.
Recall	Individuals with negative outcomes are more likely to remember and report exposure.
Interviewer	Interviewers' prior knowledge of outcome status affects ascertainment of exposure information in interview.
Lost to follow-up	Prospectively, those with negative outcomes may be lost to follow-up at greater rate than controls.
Misclassification	Ascertainment of either exposure or outcome status is incorrect for some subjects.
Selection	Entry into study or control group is affected by factors related to exposure (case-control) or outcome (cohort).
Self-selection	Individuals' participation is affected by their knowledge of disease or exposure status.

    b. Matching subjects is another way to control for confounding.

    c. In an experimental study, confounding is avoided by randomization of treatment between cases and controls.

    d. Subjects who are lost to follow-up should be evaluated to assess whether they differ in important characteristics from those who have remained in the study.

XVI Screening

Screening is the practice of testing people who are as yet asymptomatic; its purpose is to classify them with respect to their likelihood of having a disease.

A **An implicit assumption of screening is that early detection will help prevent death or disability; criteria for screening include the following:**

    1. A recognizable presymptomatic stage of disease must exist.

    2. An effective treatment must be available.

    3. The screening test should have sufficient validity.

B **A sufficiently valid screening test is one that is highly sensitive and specific.**

    1. *Sensitivity* is the ability of a test to identify correctly those who have the disease; a sensitive test yields few false negatives.

    2. *Specificity* is the ability of a test to identify correctly those who do not have the disease; a specific test yields few false positives.

    3. Sensitivity and specificity do not change when the prevalence of the disease in the population changes.

C **The *predictive value* of screening tests is the ability to predict disease status from test results.**

    1. *Positive predictive value* is the likelihood that an individual with a positive test truly has the disease.

2. *Negative predictive value* is the likelihood that an individual with a negative test does not have the disease.
3. Levels of predictive value change when the prevalence of a disease in a population changes.
   a. As the prevalence of a disease in a population increases, the positive predictive value of the test will increase.
   b. However, as the prevalence increases, the negative predictive value will decrease.

D **Screening may be done for disorders related to work-site exposures or to nonoccupational causes.**
1. OSHA standards require periodic screening of some employees (Papp and Miller, 2000).
   a. Examples are workers exposed to asbestos, cadmium, or cotton dust.
   b. This type of screening is generally called *medical surveillance* in OSHA standards.
2. Screening for early detection is done for diseases such as breast cancer, prostate cancer, and colon cancer.

XVII Overview of Toxicologic Terms and Principles

Toxicology is the study of the adverse effects of chemicals on biologic systems (Doull & Bruce, 1986).

A A *target organ* **is the organ that is selectively affected by a harmful agent.**

B **A chemical is toxic—that is, it can cause harm—if all of the following five conditions are met:**
1. Its properties make it capable of producing harm
2. It is present in sufficient amount
3. It is present for sufficient time
4. It is delivered by an exposure route that allows it to be absorbed
5. It reaches a susceptible body organ, also known as the target organ.

C *Toxic agents* **can be classified by their form of action on biologic systems.**
1. *Asphyxiants* deprive the body tissue of oxygen.
   a. Simple asphyxiants displace oxygen and cause suffocation; examples are carbon dioxide, nitrogen, and argon.
   b. Chemical asphyxiants prevent oxygen use by the cell, even when enough oxygen may be present; examples are carbon monoxide and cyanide.
2. *Corrosives* cause irreversible tissue death; ozone and acids are examples of corrosives.
3. *Irritants* cause temporary, but sometimes severe, inflammation of the eyes, skin, or respiratory tract; an example is ammonia.
4. *Sensitizers* cause allergic reactions after repeated exposure; examples are nickel and toluene diisocyanate.
5. *Carcinogens* are capable of causing cancer; examples are asbestos, coal tar, and vinyl chloride monomer.
6. *Mutagens* are toxins that cause changes to the genetic material of cells that can be passed on to future generations; known human mutagens include ethylene oxide and ionizing radiation.
7. *Teratogens* cause malformations in an unborn child; some teratogenic agents are organic mercury compounds, ionizing radiation, and some pharmaceutics.

8. Toxins may have more than one form of action and may act at more than one site. For example, formaldehyde is irritating to the eyes and respiratory tract, can irritate and sensitize the skin, and is suspected of being a carcinogen.

D **Characteristics of exposure**
1. The *dose* of an agent is the amount that reaches the target organ.
   a. The dose is usually impossible to determine accurately.
   b. The dose is usually estimated by measuring the amount administered (as with drugs) or the amount to which a person has been exposed (as with work-related exposures).
   c. Vapors or gases are expressed as parts per million (ppm).
   d. Solids (dusts or fumes) are expressed according to their weight per volume of air, usually as milligrams per cubic meter (mg/m^3).
   e. Higher concentrations of substances are generally absorbed in greater amounts.
   f. Longer or more-frequent periods of exposure also lead to greater absorbed doses.
2. Acute and chronic exposures
   a. *Acute exposure* occurs when exposure is short-term and absorption is fairly rapid.
   b. *Chronic exposure* refers to longer duration or repeated periods of contact.
   c. In general, acute toxic exposures tend to be at higher levels, and chronic exposures occur at lower concentrations.
3. *Guidelines and standards* serve to evaluate the seriousness of an exposure.
   a. Examples of workplace guidelines are *threshold limit values;* examples of workplace standards are *permissible exposure limits* (described in detail in Section XXVII).
   b. Guidelines and standards indicate upper limits of exposure concentrations that are not felt to pose a danger to workers who are exposed over normal work hours.
   c. Published limits cannot be viewed as definitely "safe" levels.
   d. Guidelines and standards may be controversial because of a lack of scientific data, lack of agreement over the levels associated with health effects, and the reality that levels that protect most individuals may yet affect susceptible subgroups.

XVIII Major Exposure Routes

A *Inhalation:* **This is the most important route of exposure in the occupational environment because it is the most common route by which occupational exposures are absorbed.**
1. Most absorption takes place in the alveoli, where blood flow is high and close to the inhaled air; to reach the alveoli, the substance must be a gas or a particulate ranging in size from approximately 1 to 10 microns in diameter.
2. Absorption by inhalation is influenced by the rate and depth of respirations; thus workers performing heavy physical labor may absorb substances at a higher rate.
3. Although the lung may serve as the target organ of some inhaled toxins, other substances gain entry through the lungs but exert their effect

elsewhere in the body; examples are solvents and carbon monoxide, which have systemic effects.

B *Cutaneous:* **The skin does provide a barrier to most substances, but its effectiveness as a barrier varies according to its condition, site, and the properties of the chemical agent.**

1. Some substances cross the epidermal layer or enter through hair follicles.
2. Some substances may enter by the trauma of injection or impalement; this entry method is less common.
3. In general, gases penetrate most freely, liquids less freely, and solids that are insoluble in water or fats do not penetrate the skin.
4. Longer contact promotes higher levels of absorption.
5. Damage to the epidermal cells by a chemical may promote its further absorption.

C *Ingestion:* **In the occupational setting, ingestion is the least common route of entry.**

1. Caustic or irritant chemicals, if ingested, may have a direct adverse effect on the gastrointestinal tract.
2. Some toxins act systemically following their absorption.
3. Smoking or eating at work sites can lead to consumption of toxins by way of contaminated hands, food, or smoking materials.

XIX The Dose-Response Relationship

This is the relationship between the level of exposure and the resulting toxic effects in a susceptible population of humans or experimental animals (Klaassen, 1986b).

A **Higher doses are generally associated with effects in a greater proportion of individuals.**

B **Identification of a dose-response relationship lends support to a theory that a substance causes a given effect.**

C **Dose-response curves provide a basis for evaluating a chemical's relative toxicity; an agent is considered more toxic when a smaller dose is needed to produce effects comparable with those produced by a greater dose of a less toxic substance.**

1. Terms that describe toxicity of a substance are *lethal dose, 50%* (LD_{50}) and *lethal concentration, 50%* (LC_{50}).
2. These terms refer to the dose (LD_{50}) or concentration (LC_{50}) that produce death in 50% of a group of experimental animals.
3. These indices are smaller for more-toxic agents. For example, the LD_{50} of acetone is 5,340 mg/kg, whereas hydrogen cyanide, a much more toxic compound, has an LD_{50} of 0.5 mg/kg (Dreisbach and Robertson, 1987).
4. Animal studies are useful because they provide information about potential toxic effects or target organs in humans; however, they must be interpreted cautiously because of the many differences in response that exist among species.

XX Nature of Effects

A **The effects of toxins with long latency periods may not be apparent until years after the exposure period.**

B **Work-related exposures commonly consist of chemical mixtures (McCauley, 1998); this is a concern because interactive effects may occur with two or more concurrent exposures (Klaassen, 1986b).**

1. *Synergistic effects* are effects caused by exposure to more than one toxin that surpass the sum of the separate effects of those toxins.
2. *Antagonism* between toxins results in an overall effect that is less than the sum of their separate effects.
3. *Potentiation* means that a chemical has no adverse effect on its own, but its presence increases the effect of another substance or makes that substance capable of exerting an effect.

XXI The Fate of Toxins in the Body

Once absorbed, the fate of toxins in the body varies (Klaassen, 1986b).

A Excretion
1. Some chemicals are excreted unchanged into expired air, urine, feces, bile, or perspiration.
2. Other avenues of excretion include milk, spinal fluid, saliva, and hair.
3. Most chemicals and their metabolic products are excreted through the kidney/urine pathway.

B Transformation
1. Chemicals may be transformed into substances that can be excreted by a process called *biotransformation.*
2. Products of biotransformation may be either less toxic or more toxic than their parent chemical.
3. This is an important concept when individuals differ in the rate at which they metabolize substances, because this rate can affect individual susceptibility to a toxin.

C Factors affecting excretion
1. Many agents are not metabolized or excreted immediately, but instead are deposited in body tissue and slowly released and excreted over time.
2. *Half-life* is the term that describes the time it takes for one half of the total absorbed amount to be eliminated from the body.
3. The length of the half-life depends on the agent and the tissue in which it is stored; for example, the half-life of lead is more than 20 years in bone, compared with about 25 to 30 days in blood.

XXII Endogenous and Exogenous Host Factors

These factors can influence susceptibility and the magnitude of the toxic response.

A *Endogenous* **factors are inherent to the individual and are beyond the control of that individual.**
1. *Gender* may influence susceptibility to some toxins, although the cause of this difference is not well understood in all cases.
   a. Some cancers and other diseases are associated with gender.
   b. Women have a greater proportion of body fat and therefore may accumulate more lipid-soluble toxins than men.
   c. Other differences in metabolism, anthropometry, and genetic types may account for varying susceptibility to toxins.
2. *Genetic differences* may cause variation in metabolism, detoxification, excretion, and cellular response to toxins.

3. *Aging* is related to rate and efficiency of metabolism, levels of organ function, and patterns of excretion.
   a. Age-related factors may increase toxic responses among older adults.
   b. Similarly, children may experience increased susceptibility because of their higher respiratory and metabolic rates, less mature nervous systems, and immature livers, which lack the detoxification mechanisms of adults.
   c. Children are also more susceptible than adults to some cancers because they are growing and their cells are dividing more rapidly.
   d. Pregnant mothers may be exposed to work-site agents that have the potential to cause perinatal malignancies.
4. *Health conditions* can increase individual susceptibility to toxins; for example, heart disease can influence effects of exposure to asphyxiants that affect oxygen availability or utilization.

B **Individuals may be able to exert some control over *exogenous* factors, because those factors are related to behavior or environmental conditions.**
   1. *Nutrition* factors can enhance or inhibit absorption or toxic responses.
   2. *Obesity* may promote more storage of lipid-soluble substances.
   3. *Lifestyle* factors such as smoking or alcohol consumption increase overall chemical exposures that must be handled by the body.
   4. *Stress* may have an effect on the function of some organs, such as those of the cardiovascular, immune, and gastrointestinal systems.
   5. Some adverse health conditions are temporary and manageable but may affect an individual's vulnerability to toxins.

Note: Table 5-3 presents some major effects seen in various body systems and gives examples of work-site exposures that cause them.

TABLE 5-3

Potential toxic effects by system, with examples of toxins

System	Effects	Sources of exposure
Respiratory	Irritation	Hydrogen chloride, ammonia
	Sensitization	Isocyanates
	Fibrosis	Silica, asbestos, beryllium
	Carcinogens	Asbestos, arsenic, chromium VI
Dermatologic	Irritation	Acetone, carbon disulfide
	Corrosive burns	Alkali, hydrogen fluoride
	Sensitization	Chromate, nickel
	Carcinogenesis	Ultraviolet light, arsenic
Nervous System	Depression/altered consciousness	Carbon monoxide, solvents
	Behavior and mood disturbance	Lead, mercury, manganese
	Cognitive disturbance	Lead, solvent
	Cerebellar impairment	Toluene, mercury
	Parkinson-like effects	Carbon monoxide, manganese, pesticides
	Peripheral neuropathy	Acrylamide, *n*-hexane, methyl *n*-butyl ketone

Continued

TABLE 5-3

Potential toxic effects by system, with examples of toxins—cont'd

System	Effects	Sources of exposure
Hearing and Vision	Acid burns of eyes	Hydrochloric and tannic acid
	Alkali burns of eyes	Sodium hydroxide, calcium oxide
	Blindness	Methanol
	Deafness	Noise
Hematopoietic	Bone marrow suppression	Ionizing radiation, benzene
	Red cell lysis	Arsine, trinitrotoluene (TNT), naphthalene
Hepatic	Necrosis	Carbon tetrachloride, chloroform, tetrachloroethane
	Cirrhosis	Carbon tetrachloride
	Malignancy	Vinyl chloride monomer
Renal and Bladder	Nephrotoxicity	Heavy metals, carbon tetrachloride, chloroform
	Renal cancer	Coke oven emissions
	Bladder cancer	Benzidine, B-naphthylamine
Reproductive	Decreased sperm production	Ionizing radiation, heat
	Decreased female fertility	Ionizing radiation, carbon disulfide
	Spontaneous abortions	Ethylene oxide
	Congenital defects	Rubella, varicella

XXIII Examples of Work-Related Exposures and Their Effects

Exposures may be classified in many ways, such as by their chemical properties (e.g., metals) or by their action (e.g., asphyxiants). This section presents some of the major groups of work-site toxins with information about selected examples (Sullivan and Kreiger, 1992).

A Metals

1. Arsenic, in the inorganic form, is found in operations such as mining, smelting, and electronics manufacturing and in products such as pesticides, paints, and wood preservatives.
   a. It is important to distinguish inorganic arsenic, which is toxic, from organic arsenic, which is not toxic but is found in foods such as seafood; dietary seafood can lead to high total arsenic levels in urine without any threat to health.
   b. Acute arsenic exposure leads to gastrointestinal symptoms, abdominal pain, and a garlic odor on the breath. This may progress to renal failure, shock, encephalopathy, and death.
   c. Chronic arsenic toxicity can lead to hyperpigmentation of the skin, hyperkeratosis, dermatitis, and skin cancer. A sign of arsenic exposure is the presence of Mee's lines, which are transverse white lines on the fingernails.
   d. Multiple systems can be affected by arsenic.
      1) Arsenic can cause a sensorimotor polyneuropathy, often noted in the hands and feet.

2) Vascular effects can simulate Raynaud's syndrome or lead to gangrene of the extremities.

3) Liver effects include cirrhosis and angiosarcoma.

4) Respiratory effects include lung cancer.

5) Anemia or leukopenia may result from bone marrow suppression.

  e. The treatment for arsenic toxicity is chelation.

  f. The OSHA standard for inorganic arsenic requires medical surveillance for exposed workers.

2. Beryllium is currently found in metal alloys, tools, and instruments, particularly in the aerospace industry, but was once used in manufacturing fluorescent lights and nuclear weapons.

  a. Acute toxicity to beryllium is a result of hypersensitivity of the lungs or mucous membranes.

  b. Allergic and irritant contact dermatitis with skin ulceration may also occur.

  c. Chronic beryllium disease, berylliosis, is marked by granulomas of the skin, lungs, and other organs. Other signs are dyspnea, cough, anorexia, fatigue, weight loss, and arthralgias.

3. Cadmium is found in battery manufacturing, electroplating, welding, and zinc and lead smelting. Cadmium is also present in cigarettes.

  a. The primary route of cadmium exposure is inhalation.

  b. Acute cadmium exposure can lead to metal fume fever or pulmonary edema.

  c. Cadmium causes renal failure resulting from proximal renal tubular damage.

  d. Cadmium also causes osteomalacia, emphysema, and possibly lung and prostate cancer.

  e. The OSHA standard for cadmium-exposed workers requires, among other tests, medical surveillance for blood and urinary cadmium levels and urinary Beta$_2$- microglobulin.

4. Chromium is found in metal alloys, tanning and dye operations, and chromium plating; welding can also be a source of exposure.

  a. The principle forms that cause toxicity are trivalent and hexavalent chromium.

  b. Chromium exposure occurs through inhalation and absorption through cracks in the skin.

  c. Skin and mucous membrane exposure can lead to deep, painful ulcers and perforation of the nasal septum.

  d. Chronic exposure can lead to asthma or allergic contact dermatitis.

  e. The hexavalent form of chromium can cause lung cancer.

5. Lead exposure can arise from a number of occupational sources. Examples include the manufacture or use of paint, alloys, and ceramics, and smelting, demolition, and radiator repair operations. The more common form of lead encountered today is inorganic lead; the organoleads were formerly used as gasoline additives.

  a. Lead is also a significant environmental toxicant found in residential paint and soil, and is used in hobbies such as stained glass work and soldering.

  b. Routes of exposure to lead are inhalation and ingestion.

  c. Most lead is stored in the bone, but the toxicity of lead is related to the amount that reaches target organs.

    d. Gastrointestinal effects of lead such as constipation and abdominal colic are sometimes mistaken for other problems like appendicitis.

    e. Lead causes central nervous system effects, such as memory deficits, and mood disturbances, such as irritability and depression.

    f. Lead toxicity results in peripheral neuropathy that primarily affects motor nerves.

    g. Lead exposure can result in renal failure, gout, and possibly hypertension.

    h. Reproductive effects of lead include sperm abnormalities and effects on the fetus that may lead to spontaneous abortion or developmental delays in childhood.

    i. The OSHA standard for lead-exposed workers specifies medical surveillance requirements and medical removal criteria.

    j. The treatment for lead toxicity, in addition to removal from exposure, consists of chelation.

6. Mercury is found in many products and processes, including the manufacture and repair of medical instruments, pesticides, and the preparation of dental amalgams. Organic mercury accumulates in fish.

    a. The three forms of mercury differ by mode of exposure and effect. Exposure to elemental mercury, the form used in thermometers, is through inhalation; inorganic mercury compounds are absorbed through the gastrointestinal tract and lungs; organic mercury is ingested.

    b. The classic triad seen with elemental and inorganic mercury toxicity are tremor, gingivitis, and personality changes that include shyness, paranoia, and labile mood.

    c. Stomatitis and dermatitis may also be present.

    d. Mercury exposure can cause renal dysfunction.

    e. A distal peripheral neuropathy can also result from mercury exposure.

    f. Organic mercury toxicity has been associated with ingestion of fish contaminated with methyl mercury.

    g. Organic mercury toxicity in adults has been associated with neurobehavioral changes, ataxia, tremor, and constriction of the visual field and has caused severe central nervous system defects in unborn children.

    h. Chelation is sometimes used to treat elemental and inorganic mercury toxicity.

B **Respirable dusts**

1. Asbestos has been used for pipe and furnace insulation, tiles, automobile and train brakes, and other heat-resistant products; health risks occur when asbestos fibers become airborne.

    a. Different types of asbestos are associated with differently shaped fibers; the most common type in the United States is chrysotile.

    b. Pleural effusions and pleural plaques are seen with chronic asbestos exposure.

    c. Asbestosis is characterized by interstitial fibrosis.

    d. Mesothelioma occurs only with asbestos exposure and can affect the pleura or peritoneum; the latency period is 30 to 40 years.

    e. Bronchogenic carcinoma also can be caused by asbestos; the risk is much greater if a person exposed to asbestos also smokes.

    f. Asbestosis is possibly associated with cancers of the gastrointestinal tract.

    g. There is an OSHA standard for asbestos-exposed workers that requires medical surveillance.

2. Coal-dust exposure occurs primarily in coal mining.
   a. Coal-dust exposure causes coal workers' pneumoconiosis, also known as *black lung*.
   b. Changes are first noted on chest x-ray, starting in the upper lobes and resulting in progressive massive fibrosis.
   c. Coal-dust exposure is also associated with bronchitis and emphysema (chronic obstructive pulmonary disease).
   d. Coal dust may be associated with gastric cancers.
   e. Medical surveillance for underground coal miners consists of chest x-ray and spirometry evaluations, administered as part of the Coal Worker's X-Ray Surveillance Program.
3. Silica exposure occurs in sandblasting, manufacturing of glass and pottery, mining of stone, and foundries.
   a. Acute, high level exposure to silica leads to a severe alveolar consolidation process known as *acute silicoproteinosis*.
   b. Silicosis is characterized by nodules in the upper lung lobes.
   c. Silicosis can be slowly progressive or can lead to progressive massive fibrosis.
   d. Silicosis puts a worker at increased risk for tuberculosis.
   e. Those with silicosis should be screened annually for tuberculosis.

C Solvents
1. Solvents are a diverse category of chemicals, defined by their ability to dissolve other substances; some are chemical reactants.
2. Many solvents are lipid soluble and can cross cell membranes easily.
3. Solvents generally have short half-lives in the body; they are metabolized in the liver and excreted through exhalation or in the urine.
4. Acute health effects of solvent exposure include central nervous system effects such as dizziness, confusion, convulsions, coma, and death.
5. Aspiration of solvents can sometimes lead to chemical pneumonitis, which can be fatal; this is the main risk when petroleum distillates are ingested.
6. Chronic health effects associated with solvents can include neurobehavioral dysfunction, peripheral neuropathy, liver disease, renal disease, dermatitis, and reproductive disorders.
7. Benzene is an aromatic hydrocarbon found in the petrochemical industry and as a component of gasoline.
   a. Chronic exposure causes acute myeloblastic leukemia, aplastic anemia, and cytopenia.
   b. The OSHA standard for benzene exposed workers includes requirements for periodic complete blood counts with criteria for follow-up and referral.
8. Carbon disulfide is sometimes used as a grain fumigant; exposure also occurs in the manufacture of rayon and rubber.
   a. Skin or eye contact with carbon disulfide can cause severe chemical burns.
   b. Chronic exposure to carbon disulfide can lead to nervous system effects of peripheral neuropathy, Parkinson's-like effects, cranial neuropathies, and optic neuritis.
   c. Vascular effects of carbon disulfide include accelerated atherosclerosis with hypertension, elevated cholesterol, and changes in retinal blood vessels.
   d. Carbon disulfide is a reproductive toxin that causes decreased and abnormal sperm and increased risk of spontaneous abortions.

9. Ethylene oxide is used as a sterilant in hospitals; other exposures occur in industry.
   a. Acute toxic effects of ethylene oxide exposure include irritation of the eyes, respiratory tract and burns.
   b. Chronic exposure leads to neurotoxic and reproductive effects and possibly chromosomal changes and leukemia.
   c. The OSHA standard for ethylene oxide includes medical surveillance requirements.
   d. Exposure-prevention efforts have included improvements in sterilization equipment and ventilation.
10. Formaldehyde exposure occurs in laboratories, when using formaldehyde resins in particle board, and in paper, rubber, and dye manufacturing.
   a. Acute exposure to formaldehyde leads to irritation of the upper and lower respiratory tract.
   b. Chronic formaldehyde exposure is linked to asthma and allergic dermatitis.
   c. Formaldehyde causes nasal cancer in animal models and is a possible human carcinogen.
   d. The OSHA standard for formaldehyde has medical evaluation requirements that include periodic administration of a questionnaire.
11. n-Hexane is used in thinners, glues, and the manufacture of rubber.
   a. n-Hexane causes a sensorimotor polyneuropathy.
   b. The toxic metabolite of n-hexane is 2,5-hexanedione.
   c. The distal portions of long nerves, such as those of the extremities, are most susceptible.
   d. The pattern of sensory loss is that of stocking-glove (feet/ankles and hands/wrists), and motor function is also impaired.
   e. After exposure ceases, the neuropathy often continues to worsen before improving; residual signs and symptoms may persist.
12. Methylene chloride is used as a degreaser and is the active agent in furniture strippers.
   a. Acute exposure to methylene chloride leads to central nervous system depression.
   b. Methylene chloride is metabolized to carbon monoxide; toxic effects are associated with this asphyxiant.
   c. The OSHA standard for methylene chloride requires medical surveillance.
13. Toluene has been used as a substitute for benzene and is used in many household products, including inks, aerosol paints, and dyes.
   a. Toluene is an irritant of the respiratory tract, causes central nervous system depression, and is toxic to the fetus.
   b. Toluene products, such as spray paint, are favored by solvent abusers. Long-term, high doses of toluene, such as those experienced by chronic abusers, are associated with severe neurobehavioral dysfunction, and cerebellar signs such as ataxia and poor coordination; abusers also commonly die from cardiac arrythmias.
   c. A major metabolite of toluene is hippuric acid; medical surveillance is based on urinary hippuric acid levels.
14. Trichloroethylene is commonly used in degreasing operations.
   a. High exposure levels cause liver and kidney toxicity.
   b. The metabolite dichloracetylene causes trigeminal neuropathy with facial numbness and masseter muscle weakness.

    c. Trichloroethylene may also cause optic neuropathy and may be linked to ventricular arrythmias.

    d. Symptoms are worse in the presence of ethanol; the combination of ethanol and trichloroethylene may cause what is known as the *degreaser's flush.*

D **Pesticides**

1. Pesticides are a potential toxic exposure for agricultural workers, home pesticide users, and workers manufacturing these agents.
2. Organophosphates are one class of pesticide that includes parathion and mevinphos.
   a. These pesticides inhibit acetylcholinesterase, allowing the accumulation of acetylcholine at synapses.
   b. Parasympathetic responses include diarrhea, urination, miosis, bronchospasm, emesis, lacrimation, and salivation ("DUMBELS") and bradycardia.
   c. Nicotinic responses include weakness, paralysis, muscle twitching, and tachycardia; central nervous system effects range from excitation to depression to seizures.
   d. Death is caused by respiratory failure.
   e. Treatment for organophosphate toxicity is atropine and 2-PAM (pralidoxime).
   f. Medical surveillance includes plasma and red blood cell cholinesterase levels.
3. Carbamates are a class of pesticide that includes aldicarb and carbaryl.
   a. Their action is similar to that of organophosphates, but symptoms are less severe and of shorter duration.
   b. The treatment is atropine, but not 2-PAM.
4. Organochlorines include the well-known examples of chlordane and DDT (dichlorodiphenyl-trichloroethane).
   a. Organochlorines are very persistent in the environment.
   b. In humans, this type of pesticide is stored in fat; consequently, they have a long half-life in the body.
   c. Because of their toxicity and persistence, carbamates are not commonly used at this time.
   d. Acute toxic effects are related to the nervous system and include weakness, paresthesias, mental status changes, and seizures.
   e. Chronic toxic effects include liver, kidney, and possibly carcinogenic outcomes.

E **Asphyxiants**

1. Asphyxiants are inhaled and result in hypoxia or anoxia; angina and adverse effects to a fetus are other potential consequences.
2. Simple asphyxiants displace oxygen in the atmosphere; oxygen is then unavailable to the body.
   a. Examples are carbon dioxide, argon, methane, and nitrogen.
   b. Treatment for exposure to simple asphyxiants is oxygen.
3. Chemical asphyxiants interfere with the body's ability to transport or use oxygen.
4. Carbon monoxide (CO) is an example of a chemical asphyxiant; sources are incomplete combustion and methylene chloride metabolism.
   a. CO binds to hemoglobin; the affinity of hemoglobin for CO is much greater than it is for oxygen.
   b. The transport of oxygen is therefore prevented.

    c. Long-term central and peripheral nervous system effects can result from acute exposure to CO.

    d. The treatment is oxygen, sometimes under hyperbaric conditions.

5. Hydrogen cyanide is another example of a chemical asphyxiant.

    a. Sources of hydrogen cyanide exposure are pesticides, gold and silver purification, combustion of some synthetic materials, and chemical processes.

    b. Hydrogen cyanide is characterized by an odor of almonds that many people cannot detect.

    c. Hydrogen cyanide inhibits cellular enzymes, preventing the use of oxygen for energy production.

    d. Treatment includes the administration of oxygen and the use of cyanide kits that include nitrites and thiosulfate; these help to bind and detoxify cyanide.

XXIV Overview of Industrial Hygiene

Industrial hygiene refers to the "the anticipation, recognition, evaluation, and control of environmental factors or stresses arising in or from the workplace, which can cause injury, sickness, impaired health and well-being, or significant discomfort among workers or among citizens (Niland, 1994).

A The field of industrial hygiene draws upon knowledge from many scientific disciplines, including engineering, physics, chemistry, and biology.

B Industrial hygiene "involves evaluation of the extent of exposure and development of corrective measures to control health hazards by reducing or eliminating hazards" (Plog, 1996).

C Professional organizations for industrial hygienists include the American Industrial Hygiene Association and the American Conference of Governmental Industrial Hygienists (Appendix I).

XXV Sources of Information to Facilitate Hazard Recognition

A *Qualitative assessment* of the work site, which requires the following:

    1. Communication with key personnel, such as plant management representatives and supervisors, to learn about materials and processes

    2. Communication with other occupational and environmental health professionals to learn about health problems that may be related to exposure

    3. Communication with workers to learn about their perceptions of exposure

B *Observational assessments,* which are achieved through strategies such as walk-through surveys, focused inspections, and job-hazard analyses. (Chapter 9 describes these and other strategies in detail.)

C Material safety data sheets (MSDSs)

    1. MSDSs provide the following information (Hathaway, 1994):

        a. Identification of the material and its manufacturer

        b. Hazardous ingredients and regulatory and advisory levels

        c. Physical and chemical properties

        d. Fire and explosion hazard data

        e. Reactivity data

        f. Health hazard data

        g. Precautions for safe handling and use

h. Control measures

i. Special precautions and comments

2. Some caveats are in order when using information provided in MSDSs (Fowler, 1990).

a. The quality of MSDSs is variable; the information is sometimes outdated and unclear, and may be inconsistent for the same materials from different manufacturers.

b. Recommended protective measures need to be considered in the context of the specific material's actual use and the control measures in effect.

XXVI Sampling Methods

Approaches for estimating the dose of an exposure received by workers include personal and environmental *sampling* and *biologic* and *medical monitoring* (Plog, 1996). (Chapter 9 provides additional details regarding sampling and monitoring methods.)

A Sampling techniques may measure exposure before absorption has occurred.

1. Approaches to sampling depend on the type of agent and the route by which it is absorbed by workers (Smith, 1988).

a. *Skin wipes* measure amounts of materials that has come in contact with the skin.

b. *Noise dosimeters,* worn near the worker's ear, record work-site noise levels.

c. *Airborne contaminants* can be assessed by means of personal monitoring at the worker's breathing zone or environmental monitoring in the work area.

2. Several important factors govern whether the sampling results truly represent worker exposure (Gross and Morse, 1996).

a. The location of the sampling device with regard to the worker and source of contaminant should be based on worker location and movements.

b. The workers to be sampled usually are those who are most highly exposed.

c. Timing of sampling should take into account seasonal changes, shifts, and other sources of variation.

d. Length of sampling time generally represents a full shift.

e. The number of samples depends on the type of instrumentation, concentration of the contaminant, and purpose of sampling.

B Biologic and medical monitoring identify the presence of a chemical in the body following exposure.

C Exposure records are extremely important and must be maintained for at least 30 years.

XXVII Airborne Contaminants

Levels of airborne contaminants can be compared with the following guidelines and standards.

A Permissible exposure limit (PEL)

1. PELs are promulgated by OSHA and are legally enforceable.

2. PELs are 8-hour, time-weighted averages of airborne exposure.

B Threshold limit value (TLV)

1. TLVs are guidelines developed by the American Conference of Governmental Industrial Hygienists and are published annually by that organization (Appendix I).
2. TLVs are 8-hour, time-weighted averages, with the following exceptions:
   a. *Ceiling levels,* or uppermost TLV levels, cannot be exceeded.
   b. *Short-term exposure levels* are the maximum, 15-minute, time-weighted averages permitted over a workday, with at least 60 minutes between successive exposures.

C Recommended exposure level (REL)

1. RELs are developed by NIOSH.
2. These levels are the exposures that, in the judgment of NIOSH, will not cause adverse health effects in most workers.

XXVIII Control Strategies for Occupational Exposures

Approaches to eliminating or reducing exposure to hazardous substances at the work site are ordered into a *hierarchy* based, in general, on their degree of overall effectiveness.

A *Engineering controls* to enclose or isolate operations, improve ventilation, or change the process to reduce or eliminate exposure; include elimination and substitution.

B *Administrative controls* (such as worker rotation) to minimize exposure, including the development of monitoring or surveillance programs and worker training, including work practices.

C *Personal protective equipment* such as ear plugs and muffs, safety goggles, gloves, coveralls, and respirators—the least preferred control strategy

XXIX Overview of Ergonomic Terms and Principles

The term *ergonomics* (sometimes known as *human factors*) refers to the study of the interaction between humans and their work.

A The term literally means the *laws* (from the Greek word *nomos*) *of work* (*ergos*).

B The field of ergonomics is concerned with the design of the work-site, equipment, and physical environment and the organization of work.

C The field is multidisciplinary, involving health professionals, engineers, behavioral scientists, physiologists, and others.

D Its purpose is to prevent acute and chronic injuries, make work sites comfortable, enhance productivity, reduce fatigue and errors, and promote job satisfaction.

E Proper job design can make jobs appropriate for workers of both sexes and all ages; considerations are given to size, strength, visual capacity, hearing, capabilities, and limitations.

F Ergonomics seeks to fit the job to the person rather than the person to the job.

XXX Musculoskeletal Disorders

Several *musculoskeletal health problems* can be caused or aggravated by work-site factors.

A Affected tissue structures include muscles, tendons, ligaments, peripheral nerves, blood vessels, joints, cartilage, and bones.

B Problems occur in the upper and sometimes lower extremities, cervical spine, and lower back; symptoms of musculoskeletal disorders include pain, swelling, erythema, numbness, and paresthesia.

C Examples of work-related musculoskeletal disorders are tendinitis, tenosynovitis, epicondylitis, DeQuervain's syndrome, synovitis, ganglion cysts, and rotator cuff tendinitis.

D Nerve entrapment syndromes include carpal tunnel syndrome (median nerve entrapment at the wrist), tarsal tunnel syndrome (tibial nerve entrapment at the ankle), and ulnar nerve entrapment at the elbow or wrist.

E Another form of peripheral nerve impairment has been termed hand-arm vibration syndrome; this is thought to result from vibration such as that experienced with the use of power tools (Galszechy, 1999).

XXXI Risk Factors for Musculoskeletal Problems

The major work-site risk factors for musculoskeletal problems of the upper extremities are repetition, force, mechanic stresses, awkward postures, low temperatures, and vibration.

A The goal in task and tool design is to avoid or minimize these risk factors.

B *Repetition* refers to the performance of the same or similar tasks again and again; for example, if one work cycle (a series of motions that is then repeated) lasts less than 30 seconds, or if, in the case of cycles lasting several minutes, there are subcycles that constitute more than 50% of the overall cycle, the job is generally considered repetitive (NIOSH, 1988).

C *Force* is exerted in tasks that require lifting weights, handling heavy tools, pinching with the fingers, or applying other grips while working.

D Repetition seems to be a stronger risk factor than force for carpal tunnel syndrome (Silverstein, et al., 1987).

E *Mechanical stress* refers to the forces that result from a worker's direct contact with work surfaces or tools.

F The *compressive forces* that result from striking objects with hand-held tools or from leaning against hard surfaces or corners on work tables can lead to nerve compression disorders.

G Work frequently requires workers to assume awkward positions for prolonged periods or repetitive shorter periods; deviation from neutral posture has been identified as a risk factor for injury, as illustrated by the following:
  1. Cervical spine injury—caused by extreme neck flexion and twisting
  2. Back injury—caused by twisting at the waist; lifting with legs straight; bending and reaching repetitively; maintaining awkward postures for long periods; carrying, pulling, pushing, or lifting heavy objects from below the

knees or above the shoulders; or lifting weight beyond one's capabilities (Garg, 1995)

3. Shoulder injury—caused by raising the arm or elbow above midtorso without support, reaching behind one's body

4. Forearm/elbow injury—caused by repeated rotation (i.e., supination and pronation)

5. Wrist/hand injury—caused by repeated wrist flexion and extension, holding the hand in ulnar deviation

H *Vibration* **caused by power tools or other work equipment can adversely affect the upper extremities.**

I **Whole-body vibration, such as that experienced by drivers of trucks and heavy equipment, can affect the back, lower extremities, and possibly shoulder and neck.**

J *Cold environmental conditions* **have an effect on manual dexterity and muscle strength and may directly or indirectly cause hand disorders.**

XXXII High-Risk Jobs

Types of jobs that are considered particularly high risk in terms of ergonomic exposures include the following:

A **Office work**

1. Work with technology such as computers may require individuals to assume static or awkward positions for typing if workstations are not properly adjusted.

2. Other conditions in the office environment that may introduce hazards include poor lighting, obstructions in walkways, slippery floors, and heavy objects.

B **Manual materials handling—a part of many jobs, from loading trucks and moving heavy goods to working in grocery stores**

1. In addition to repeated bending, lifting, and twisting, this work sometimes involves exposure to vibration.

2. The risks of back injury are high for these types of jobs.

C **Assembly work, which is often machine-paced, giving the worker little control over the speed at which he or she works**

1. Repetitive motions tend to be characteristic of assembly work.

2. Sometimes work is performed in static or awkward postures or with poorly designed tools.

XXXIII Evaluating Risk Factors

Various methods can be used to evaluate work sites for ergonomic risk factors; each approach has its advantages and disadvantages.

A *Interviews or questionnaires* **that ask workers about their work**

1. Advantages: Workers have the most complete view of their tasks throughout all work periods. This method may reveal factors that might not otherwise be noted.

2. Disadvantages: There may be high variability in the way workers report their perception of work performance; reports may be incomplete or biased.

B *Observation and use of checklists*—observing workers while they work and noting any risk factors
  1. Advantages: Observers using the same methods will look at all workers in the same way and thus introduce less variability; this method is fairly efficient—that is, one observer evaluates many workers in their work setting.
  2. Disadvantages: People may change the way they behave when they are under observation; the limited time period for observation may cause some things to be missed; and observers must be trained to be accurate and consistent.

C *Videotaping and analysis*—taping the worker on the job and later conducting a detailed analysis of motions and other risk factors
  1. Advantages: Analysis is recorded and does not rely on one person's assessment; tape can be repeated, slowed, or frozen to evaluate details of work tasks; measurement of time and motion can be highly accurate.
  2. Disadvantages: Videotaping requires expensive equipment and experienced personnel; behavior may change when being taped; only a small window of worker's time is recorded, and therefore it is not useful for evaluating highly variable tasks.

XXXIV Ergonomic Improvements

Some considerations and guidelines for analyzing or designing jobs are as follows (Ross, 1994; U.S.D.L., 1990):

A General environment: Provide adequate illumination, comfortable levels of temperature and humidity; good visibility of labels and signs; and clear, audible auditory signals.

B Workstations and chairs: These should be adjustable to accommodate workers of different sizes.

C Layout: Place tools, controls, and materials in front of the worker to prevent twisting, reaching, and bending; keep work space free of obstacles.

D Postures: Avoid static postures; locate and orient work to promote neutral positions.

E Repetition: Engineer the product or process to reduce repetition; vary tasks; rotate workers to different jobs; allow rest time.

F Forces: Reduce the size and weight of objects held; use power grips rather than pinch grips; balance tools; provide correctly fitting gloves (not tight or bulky); sharpen tools often.

G Mechanic stresses: Ensure that handles on equipment fit the worker's hands; pad or eliminate sharp edges.

H Vibration: Eliminate vibrating tools if possible; isolate sources of vibration; keep tools and equipment properly maintained; maintain even floor surfaces to reduce vibration from driving; reduce driving speeds.

I Lifting: Reduce size and weight of tools and objects that are lifted often; use mechanic lifting devices; use gravity to move work; raise the work (or lower the operator); provide grips and handles; reduce friction where objects are slid from one point to another; increase friction when objects are held; evaluate lifting tasks according to NIOSH lifting guidelines (Garg, 1995).

TABLE 5-4

Example of occupational injury occurrence: a fracture

Host	Injury	Agent	Vector	Exposure event	Physical environment	Sociocultural environment
Employee • Age • Sex • Health status • Physical condition	Fracture	Kinetic energy	Cement floor	Slip and fall	Oil, grease, dirt, and water on floor; painted cement floor; equipment and supplies on floor; lighting; integrity of floor	Attitude toward housekeeping; costs associated with injuries and lost time not accounted for under department budget

J Work organization: Alternate physically demanding and mentally demanding tasks; vary the rate and nature of tasks as much as possible; provide breaks (more-frequent short breaks are generally better than less-frequent long breaks).

Chapter 14 provides a sample ergonomics program.

XXXV Occupational Injury Epidemiology

The study of the natural history of injuries helps to define the host, agent, vector, and environmental (psychosocial and physical) factors that contribute to injury.

A Characteristics of occupational injury

1. Occupational injuries are not random events.
2. Injuries are predictable and preventable.
3. Injuries result when energy is exchanged in a manner and dose sufficient to overcome the host's threshold of resistance in the presence or absence of certain environmental conditions (Table 5-4).

B Examples of sources of injuries

1. *Mechanic or kinetic energy:* impact of an object, dashboard, floor, knife, noise, extreme air pressure (explosion)
2. *Thermal energy:* steam, flame, hot substances, and lasers
3. *Electric energy:* man-made sources, such as high-tension wires, and natural sources, such as lightning
4. *Radiation:* both ionizing and nonionizing, including sunlight, radioactive minerals, and radiotherapeutic devices, implants, and pharmaceutics
5. *Chemical energy:* effects of acids, bases, poisons/toxins, and irritants
6. Absence of energy-producing mechanisms necessary to sustain life, such as absence of respiration secondary to drowning

C The energy-exchanging event causing an injury can be studied as a sequence of interactions viewed in pre-event, event, and post-event phases.

TABLE 5-5

Haddon matrix: case example of control countermeasures—slips and falls on the same level in a maintenance area

Phase	Human factors	Environmental and engineering factors	Social, legal, and political factors
Preevent	• Shoes—nonskid soles • Safety training—increase awareness • Establish work practices, including housekeeping	• Nonskid floor (paint, strips) • Oil/grease absorbing material for spills • Good lighting • Proper storage of equipment and supplies	• OSHA inspections and regulation compliance • Safety audit • Risk management—insurance losses and litigation
Event	• Padded clothing • Optimal physical condition of employees	• Energy absorbing floors (with non-skid surface) • Emergency notification system	• Injury investigation, reporting, and tracking • Coordination of medical care
Postevent	• Effective first-aid response • Interaction with ambulance and hospital emergency services	• Prompt access to work location • Access to first-aid equipment and supplies	• Emergency response system—triage, first aid, evacuation, and definitive medical care

Source: Haddon, 1963 and 1979. In Hayes, 1990.

XXXVI Countermeasures

Strategies that are effective in preventing or reducing the extent of injuries were identified and categorized by William Haddon as control *countermeasures* (Table 5-5).

A Pre-event countermeasures include:
1. Preventing the creation of the workplace hazard
2. Reducing the severity of the hazard
3. Preventing the release of the hazard
4. Modifying the rate of release of the hazard
5. Separating the hazard from the employee

B Event countermeasures include:
1. Placing a physical barrier between the hazard and the person
2. Modifying the basic qualities of the hazard
3. Increasing the individual's resistance to injury

C Post-event countermeasures include:
1. Rapidly evaluating the injury that has occurred or is occurring, preventing continuation of the injury, and mitigating or halting the extension of its effects
2. After stabilizing the injured party, providing definitive medical and surgical treatment and rehabilitative and reconstructive care, with a goal of restoring the employee to an optimal level of functioning.

XXXVII Implications for Occupational and Environmental Health Nurses

A An understanding of occupational injury epidemiology will enable occupational and environmental health nurses to analyze and characterize the potential for injury in their work setting.

B The occupational and environmental health nurse can use injury prevention and control principles to study, prevent, and control the occurrence of injury-producing events and the extent of injury.

XXXVIII Effects of Social Conditions and Behavior on Health

Social and behavioral sciences examine the influences of workers' social milieus and lifestyles on their health.

A Modern approaches to health services have been influenced by a variety of factors.

1. Life expectancy has substantially increased.
2. Patterns of disease have changed; the leading causes of death have shifted from infectious diseases to chronic diseases related to behaviors and environmental factors.
3. Traditional approaches such as the medical paradigm are not responsive to many modern-day health problems.

B Research in the behavioral sciences has examined the relationship between human behavior and the occurrence of illness and injury.

1. The behavior of individuals and groups is complex, and understanding behavior is a complicated process.
   a. People often make choices that they know are not good for their health (e.g., not wearing hearing protection).
   b. The key to effecting behavioral change is understanding the human thought processes that affect behavior (e.g., ear plugs are not comfortable).
   c. Focusing on behavioral strategies may result in workers' making healthier behavioral choices (e.g., allowing worker participation in selection of hearing protection devices).
   d. Behavioral approaches to research may also facilitate a better understanding of the neurologic and behavioral effects of certain exposures (to lead, for example).
2. Many theories and models have been developed to help us understand behavior. (Chapter 12 presents examples of behavioral theories and models.)
   a. These theories and models explain why people behave as they do.
   b. They provide a rich source of ideas that can be used to further our understanding of behavior.
   c. They enable health care providers to develop more effective interventions.

C Research in the social sciences has examined the contribution of social environments to the occurrence of illness and injury.

1. There is increased recognition of the relationship of social phenomena to health and illness outcomes.

2. Examples of social indices that may affect occupational health include rates of violence, divorce, and unemployment and the degree to which workers have care-giving responsibilities or hold multiple jobs.
3. The provision of appropriate health services depends on complete understanding and appreciation of the nature of work and the social context of the workplace.

D Unique attributes of social and behavioral sciences include the following:
1. Qualitative techniques, which are more likely to be used for collecting data
2. Quality of life, which is an important outcome for the social and behavioral sciences; quality of life considers emotional, social, intellectual, physical, and spiritual health

XXXIX Health Promotion and Risk Reduction

Health promotion and risk reduction require an understanding of the psychosocial determinants of health.

A There is a need to develop organizational "healthy policy" as a strategy to improve workers' health.
1. Healthy policy facilitates and supports healthy behaviors.
2. Health-promoting and health-damaging policies of organizations are likely to receive increased scrutiny in the coming years (Pender, 1996).
3. Organizational change is a critical factor in achieving a healthy occupational environment.

B An important area that would benefit from the attention of the social and behavioral sciences is health promotion that focuses on lifestyle and stress reduction.

C Social and behavioral sciences can identify and examine factors that threaten the health of workers.
1. The psychosocial environment of the workplace plays a critical role in the occurrence of occupational injury and illness.
2. The organization of work is influenced by the ideologies, values, and beliefs of people within the organization (managers and workers) and outside of it (scientists and government); these ideologies affect the social dimensions of the workplace.
3. The organization of work has been identified as a research priority by NIOSH (NIOSH, 1996).
4. Implementing strategies based on findings from social and behavioral investigations is likely to result in cost savings to employers and a better quality of life for employees.

BIBLIOGRAPHY

Cowan, M., Heinrich, J., Lucas, M., Sigmon H., & Hinshaw, A. (1993). Integration of biological and nursing sciences: A 10-year plan to enhance research and training. *Research in Nursing and Health, 16*, 3–9.

Doull, J., & Bruce, M.C. (1986). Origin and scope of toxicology. In C.D. Klaassen, M.O. Amdur, & J. Doull (Eds.), *Casarett and Doull's toxicology: The science of poisons* (3rd ed.) (pp. 3–10). New York: Macmillan Publishing Co.

Dreisbach, R.H., & Robertson, W.O. (1987). *Handbook of poisoning: Prevention, diagnosis, and treatment* (12th ed.). Norwalk, CT: Appleton & Lange.

Eastman Kodak Company. (1983). *Ergonomic design for people at work* (Vol. 1). New York: Van Nostrand Reinhold.

Eastman Kodak Company. (1986). *Ergonomic design for people at work* (Vol. 2). New York: Van Nostrand Reinhold.

Ewart, C.K., & Fitzgerald, S.T. (1994). Changing behaviour and promoting well-being after heart attack: A social action theory approach. *Irish Journal of Psychology, 15,* 219–241.

Fitzgerald, S. (1991). Self-efficacy theory: Implications for the occupational and environmental nurse. *AAOHN Journal, 39(12),* 552–557.

Fowler, D.P. (1990). Industrial hygiene. In J. LaDou (Ed.), *Occupational medicine* (pp. 499–513). Norwalk, CT: Appleton & Lange.

Galszechy, T. (1999). The effects of vibration on hands and arms: Clinical brief. *AAOHN Journal, 47(3),* 117–119.

Garg, A. (1995). Revised NIOSH equation for manual lifting: A method for job evaluation. *AAOHN Journal, 43,* 211–216.

Gross, E.R., & Morse, E.P. (1996). Overview of industrial hygiene. In B.A. Plog, J. Niland, & P.J. Quinlan (Eds.), *Fundamentals of industrial hygiene* (4th ed.) (pp. 453–483). Itasca, IL: National Safety Council.

Hathaway, B.K. (1994). Understanding the material safety data sheet. *AAOHN Journal, 42,* 291–295.

Hayes, W. (1990). Nursing advances in occupational injury prevention and control. In J.M. Radford (Ed.), *Recent advances in nursing (26). Occupational health nursing,* Edinburgh, Scotland: Churchill, Livingstone.

Henry, S. (1995). Informatics: Essential infrastructure for quality assessment and improvement in nursing. *Journal of the American Medical Informatics Association, 2,* 169–182.

Institute of Medicine. (1995). *Nursing, health, and the environment.* A.M. Pope, M.A. Snyder, & L.H. Mood (Eds.). Washington, DC: National Academy Press.

Klaassen, C.D. (1986a). Principles of toxicology. In C.D. Klaassen, M.O. Amdur, & J. Doull (Eds), *Casarett and Doull's toxicology: The science of poisons* (3rd ed.) (pp. 11–32). New York: Macmillan Publishing Co.

Klaassen, C.D. (1986b). Distribution, excretion, and absorption of toxicants. In C.D. Klaassen, M.O. Amdur, & J. Doull (Eds), *Casarett and Doull's toxicology: The science of poisons* (3rd ed.) (pp. 33–63). New York: Macmillan Publishing Co.

Landrigan, P.J. (1992). Commentary: Environmental disease—a preventable epidemic. *American Journal of Public Health, 82,* 941–943.

Last, J.M. (1988). *A dictionary of epidemiology* (2nd ed.). New York: Oxford University Press.

Mausner, J.S., & Kramer, S. (1985). *Mausner & Bahn epidemiology—An introductory text* (2nd ed.). Philadelphia: W.B. Saunders Company.

McCauley, L.A. (1998). Chemical mixtures in the workplace: Research and practice. *AAOHN Journal, 46(1),* 29–40.

Meleis, A.I. (1997). *Theoretical nursing: Development and progress.* (3rd ed.). St. Louis, MO: Lippincott.

Mischel, M.H. (1988). Uncertainty in illness. *Image–The Journal of Nursing Scholarship, 20,* 225–232.

National Institute for Occupational Safety and Health (NIOSH). (1988). *Cumulative trauma disorders: A manual for musculoskeletal diseases of the upper limbs.* V. Putz-Anderson (Ed.). New York: Taylor & Frances.

National Institute for Occupational Safety and Health (NIOSH). (1996). *National occupational research agenda.* Atlanta: U.S. Department of Health and Human Services.

Niland, J. (1999). Industrial hygeine. In C. Zenz, O.B. Dickinson, & E.P. Horvath (Eds.). *Occupational Medicine* (3rd ed., pp. 1012–1127). St Louis: Mosby.

Papp, E.M., & Miller, A.S. (2000). Screening and surveillance: OSHA's medical surveillance provisions. *AAOHN Journal, 48(2),* 59-72.

Pender, N. (1996). *Health promotion in nursing practice.* (3rd ed.). Los Altos, CA: Appleton & Lange.

Plog, B.A. (1996). Overview of industrial hygiene. In B.A. Plog, J. Niland, and P.J. Quinlan, (Eds.), *Fundamentals of industrial hygiene* (4th ed.) (pp. 3–32.). Itasca, IL: National Safety Council.

Ross, P. (1994). Ergonomic hazards in the workplace: Assessment and prevention. *AAOHN Journal, 42(4),* 171–176.

Salazar, M.K. (1991). Comparison of four behavioral theories: A literature review. *AAOHN Journal, 39(3),* 128–135.

Shortridge, L., & Valanis, B. (1992). *The epidemiological model applied in community health nursing.* Baltimore: Mosby Year Book.

Silverstein, B.A., Fine, L.J., & Armstrong, T.J. (1987). Occupational factors and carpal tunnel syndrome. *American Journal of Industrial Medicine, 11,* 343–358.

Smith, T .J. (1988). Industrial hygiene. In B.S. Levy and D.H. Wegman (Eds.), *Occupational health: recognizing and preventing work-related disease* (2nd ed.) (pp. 87–103). Boston: Little, Brown & Co.

Sullivan, J.B., & Kreiger, G.R. (1992*). Hazardous materials toxicology: Clinical principles of environmental health.* Baltimore: Williams & Wilkins.

U.S. Department of Labor, Occupational Safety and Health Administration (USDL OSHA). (1990). *Ergonomics program management guidelines* for meatpacking plants [OSHA publication No. 3123]. Washington DC.

Weinstein, N.D. (1988). The precaution adoption process. *Health Psychology, 7(4),* 355–386.

Weinstein, N.D., and Sandman, P.M. (1992). A model of the precaution adoption process: Evidence from home radon testing. *Health Psychology, 11(3),* 170–180.

White, K., Cox, A.R., and Williamson, G.C. (1999). Competencies in occupational and environmental health nursing: Practice in the new millennium. *AAOHN Journal, 47(12),* 552-568.

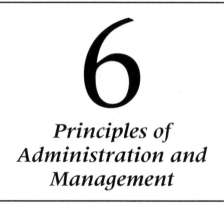

CHAPTER

6

Principles of Administration and Management

Joy Wachs

Occupational and environmental health nurses must have leadership, management, and administrative skills to give the direction, provide the services, manage the resources, and document the outcomes related to employee health. As business and industry in America seek new solutions to the high cost of health care, these abilities will enable occupational and environmental health nurse managers to promote, maintain, and restore the health of workers and positively affect corporate profits.

I Leadership

Leadership is the "desire and ability to influence others to set and achieve goals that represent the values and the motivations of both leader and followers" (Perra, 1999).

A **Various leadership approaches are used in American business and industry.**

1. *Tactical leadership* is demonstrated when a leader "clarifies the goal, convinces us that it is absolutely essential to achieve that goal, explains the plan and strategies, organizes and coordinates our activities, and deals aggressively with individual performance issues" (Crislip & Larson, 1994).

2. *Transactional leadership* occurs "when one person takes the initiative in making contact with others for the purpose of an exchange of valued things" (Burns, 1978).

3. *Collaborative leadership* involves a leader who can mobilize a diverse group to work with ambiguous issues and make sure the process is constructive and outcome-driven (Crislip & Larson, 1994).

4. *Transformational leadership* is exemplified when "one or more persons engage with others in such a way that leaders and followers raise one another to higher levels of motivation and morality . . . " (Burns, 1978).

5. *Servant leadership* occurs when the leader is servant first, "to make sure other's highest priority needs are being served" (Greenleaf, 1970).

B **Leaders and followers have distinct but related responsibilities.**

1. Leaders are responsible for the following (Depree, 1989):
   a. Defining what is (reality) and what could be (vision)

      b. Serving by enabling others to reach their potential

      c. Saying thank you for the opportunity to lead

   2. Leaders need followers who demonstrate the following behaviors (Chaleff, 1998):

      a. Assume responsibility through personal growth, passion, and risk-taking

      b. Serve both the leader and the cause

      c. Challenge themselves, the leader, and the group

      d. Participate in transformation by being a catalyst, resource, and role model

      e. If necessary, leave the organization to allow the organization and the follower to grow

C **Characteristics of today's leaders include the following (Depree, 1992):**

   1. Integrity

   2. Vulnerability

   3. Discernment

   4. Awareness of the human spirit

   5. Courage in relationships

   6. Sense of humor

   7. Presence

   8. Intellectual energy and curiosity

   9. Respect for the future, regard for the present, and an understanding of the past

  10. Predictability

  11. Breadth

  12. Comfort with ambiguity

D **Leadership tasks include the following (Kouzes & Posner, 1987):**

   1. Challenging the process

   2. Inspiring others to share a vision and see its exciting possibilities

   3. Enabling others to act by building teams based on trust and respect

   4. Modeling the way for others

   5. Recognizing individual and team achievements

II Strategic Planning

Strategic (long-range) planning sets the course for the organization.

A **A clearly articulated vision results in the development of purpose, mission, and goals.**

   1. The vision, philosophy, mission statement, goals, and objectives of occupational health services should reflect those of the greater organization (Yoder-Wise, 1999).

   2. Vision statements describe the future of the organization and provide a context for the philosophy and mission statements (Yoder-Wise, 1999).

   3. The philosophy in an occupational health unit should articulate the following:

      a. The inherent worth of individual workers to the company

      b. A commitment to quality care based on standards of nursing practice

      c. An expectation that nursing practice be research-based

      d. An emphasis on health-promotion and risk-reduction services

      e. An emphasis on continuing education and appropriate certifications

4. The mission aims to promote, protect, and restore the health of workers.
5. Goals and objectives clarify the essential actions necessary to achieving the philosophy and mission (Yoder-Wise, 1999), such as services provided and resources used.
6. The philosophy, mission, goals, and objectives need to be developed by management and staff of the health unit, approved by upper management, and revised periodically to fit the ever-changing business environment.

B **The strategic planning process must accomplish the following (Yoder-Wise, 1999):**
1. Assess the internal and external environments
2. Identify strengths and weaknesses as well as threats and opportunities
3. Identify strategies
4. Implement prioritized strategies
5. Evaluate activities and outcomes

C **The goals of strategic planning include the following (Yoder-Wise, 1999):**
1. Improved likelihood of success in achieving goals and outcomes
2. Effective and efficient use of resources
3. Creative vision for the future direction of the occupational health unit

D **Planned change can be approached from a linear or nonlinear frame of reference (Yoder-Wise, 1999) (Box 6-1).**
1. *Linear change* is a systematic process used in organizations to facilitate needed, semipermanent change through mutual goal-setting between worker and the change agent (Lewin, 1951).
   a. The role of the occupational and environmental health nurse as an agent for change includes the following:
      1) Identifying problems
      2) Assessing the forces that will drive or restrain the change
      3) Determining costs and benefits of the change
      4) Establishing a helping relationship with management and workers
      5) Ensuring that the change will last until it is time to change again
   b. Planned change may relate to programs, services, staffing, facilities, cost containment, or health outcomes of workers (Case Study).

BOX 6-1

Stages of planned change

- **Unfreezing:** when workers become aware of the need for change and realize that change could be positive
- **Moving:** when the change is actually being implemented and problems related to the change are resolved

- **Refreezing:** when the change is accepted as part of the organization's culture and workers are no longer tempted to revert to "prechange" ways

Source: Lewin, 1951.

Case study using Lewin's stages of planned change

Unfreezing: The occupational health nurse manager of Company X was displeased with the quality of service provided by three contract physicians. They were often late for appointments with workers, tended to keep workers off the job for extended periods, and often missed critical details in assessing workers during preplacement and occupational injury examinations.

Moving: It was determined by occupational health unit staff, line management, safety staff, and human resource staff that the occupational health unit needed a full-time provider with prescriptive authority at a cost less than or equal to current costs. After much research and discussion, it was decided to hire an occupational health nurse practitioner and retain one physician as a consultant to the occupational health unit staff and a preceptor to the occupational health nurse practitioner.

Refreezing: The change was made, and within a few months, feedback from managers and workers was positive regarding the occupational health nurse practitioner's competence, availability, professionalism, and attitude. Within a year, the occupational health nurse practitioner left for personal reasons, but the company immediately hired another occupational health nurse practitioner to replace her.

2. Chaos theory and learning organization theory are examples of nonlinear change models (Wheatley, 1992; Senge, 2000)
   a. Organizations are analogous to living organisms, not to machines that can be controlled linearly (Senge, 2000).
   b. People in organizations "seek to create a world in which (they) can thrive" by working from the inside, identifying needs, applying experience and perceptions, enlisting support, and creating their own solutions (Wheatley, 1999).

III The Management Process

The *management process* "consists of achieving organizational objectives through planning, organizing, directing, and controlling human and physical resources and technology" (Douglass, 1992, p. 7).

A **Management differs from leadership in that managers do things right whereas leaders do the right things.**
   1. Managers "meet their goals by organizing, staffing, controlling, and problem-solving (Yoder-Wise, 1999).
   2. Leaders "set direction, develop a vision and communicate the new direction" (Yoder-Wise, 1999).

B **Management theories can be used to guide the occupational and environmental health nurse manager's activities (Box 6-2).**

C **Management styles include the following:**
   1. Authoritarian/autocratic style or "do as I say" approach
      a. Most effective in emergency situations
      b. Used when followers have little experience or limited motivation

---

BOX 6-2

Overview of management theories

Classical Theory (Taylor, 1911)
- Focuses on efficiency through design.
- Work is reduced to specific tasks, and workers are trained to do those tasks (division of labor).
- A hierarchy of supervisors and managers provide direction to workers (chain of command) and workers are expected to obey supervisors, be loyal to the organization, and be rewarded for production (Sullivan & Decker, 1997).

Neoclassical Theory
- Begins with the principles of classical theory
- Adds the human-relations approach, the desire for social relationships in the workplace, group pressure, and personal fulfillment (Sullivan & Decker, 1997)
- Assumes workers can create a rational structure through participation, cooperation, and motivation

Theory X and Y (McGregor, 1960, 1966)
- Theory X managers believe people intensely dislike working and must be "coerced, controlled, and directed" by management in doing the work required (Grohar-Murray & DiCroce, 1992).

- Theory Y managers believe that people enjoy work and are "self-directed, responsible, and capable of solving their own problems" (Grohar-Murray & DiCroce, 1992).

Theory Z (Ouchi)
- Derived from studies of Japanese organization
- Uses the concepts of "collective decision making, long-term employment, slower promotions, indirect supervision, and holistic concern for employees" as the centerpiece of the theory (Tappen, 1989)

Contingency Theory (Fiedler, 1964)
- Situational theory
- Argues that workers, managers, and the environment are a unique blend, and the effectiveness of a particular management approach is *contingent* on the blend (Tappen, 1989)
- Argues that the most successful managers are those who adapt their approach to the situation

Other Theorists
- Herzberg (1959) focused on motivation.
- Argyris (1960) centered on organizational and individual goals.
- Likert (1967) developed a continuum of management systems from autocratic to participatory.

---

2. Democratic/participatory style
   a. Most effective in long-term situations when followers are motivated and possess interpersonal and organizational skills
   b. Empowers followers through collaborative teamwork; focuses on communication and constructive relationships.
3. Bureaucratic style, or "the book says so" approach
   a. Often used by managers who do not tolerate creative problem-solving but rather want order and consistency in the way situations are handled day to day
   b. Tends to be impersonal

BOX 6-3

Sources of power

- **Legitimate power** or authority arises from one's position within the organization.
- **Referent power** or charisma comes from one's personality and other personal characteristics; confidence, controlling emotions, and dress may all contribute to referent power.
- **Reward power** is based on one's ability to reward others, for example, with merit pay increases and employee recognition.
- **Expert power** allows the occupational and environmental health nurse manager to make health care decisions because others recognize a nurse's special knowledge, skills, and abilities.

- **Connection power** is created when individuals work together, as when health and safety professionals collaborate with human resources staff (Ellis & Hartley, 1991).
- **Information power** is held by those who control and possess information; they are often more powerful than those who need the information but are barred from access to it (Ellis & Hartley, 1991).
- **Coercive power** is often used by authoritarian managers to control the behavior of others through fear, threats, and punishment.

---

  4. Laissez-faire, or permissive, style, sometimes called "anything goes"
      a. Allows full utilization of talents; may work well with highly motivated employees
      b. Requires an awareness of the level of competence and personal integrity of employees; may fail because of lack of direction

D Occupational and environmental nurse managers must develop power bases in order to implement decisions regarding the health and safety of workers (Box 6-3).

IV The Organization: Its Culture, Climate, and Structure

A Organizational culture
  1. *Organizational culture* is a set of assumptions about the organization, outside the conscious awareness of, but nonetheless "known" by the workers, that guide the collective organization in dealing with internal and external situations and challenges (Moran & Volkwein, 1992).
  2. An organization's culture is rooted in the founding, history, and leadership of that organization.
  3. Paradigms explaining the origin of organizational culture include the following (Zamanou & Glaser, 1994):
      a. Fundamentalist: "Organizations *produce* culture."
      b. Interpretive: "Organizations *are* culture" because they are the product of interaction among people.

B **Organizational climate**
1. The *organizational climate* is a set of employee perceptions, environmental properties, or relatively enduring characteristics of an organization that describe how an organization operates, what is important to an organization, and what ultimately influences worker behavior (Butcher, 1994; Al-Shammari, 1992; Moran & Volkwein, 1992).
2. Organizational climate both influences and is influenced by communication patterns within the organization and with the greater community.
3. Organizational climates form as a result of the following (Moran & Volkwein, 1992):
   a. Workers' perceptions of the organization's structure
   b. Individual "descriptions of organization conditions"
   c. Worker interaction
   d. A shared culture
4. Comparison of organizational culture and climate
   a. *Organizational culture* is an anthropologic concept, is highly enduring, emerges from a historical context, is often held in workers' unconscious, and influences the organization's climate (Moran & Volkwein, 1992).
   b. *Organizational climate* is a concept of social psychology, is relatively enduring, is mediated by the organization's internal and external environments, is held in the awareness of workers, and is a manifestation of the organization's culture (Moran & Volkwein, 1992).

C **The *organizational structure* includes positions, job responsibilities, and relationships among the positions (Ellis & Hartley, 1991; Marriner-Tomey, 1992).**
1. *Vertical structures* are associated with clear lines of authority; power is held by a few.
   a. Also called hierarchical, centralized, or bureaucratic
   b. Characterized by role clarity, specialization, delegation of authority
   c. Advantages include efficiency and clarity
   d. Disadvantages include an inclination to autocratic leadership, lack of cooperation among workers, and a loss of worker creativity and commitment
2. *Horizontal structures* are associated with few layers of management.
   a. Also known as decentralized or organic culture
   b. Characterized by worker self-reliance, tolerance for ambiguity, open communication, acceptance of change, and risk-taking
   c. Advantages include speed in responding to challenges, job satisfaction, opportunities for staff development, and less need for higher-paid supervisory personnel
   d. Disadvantages include training costs, costs of poor decisions by inexperienced workers, time spent to reach consensus
3. Mixed structures:
   a. Use a more centralized approach for routine, day-to-day functions
   b. Use a decentralized approach for managing change and innovation

V Policies and Procedures

Policies and procedures provide uniform ways of responding to situations and meeting organizational challenges.

A Policies and procedures, which are often developed as a result of problems in the workplace or regulatory mandates, should be handled as follows:

1. They must be developed through collaborative efforts requiring the participation of all affected parties and the approval and support of management.
2. They must be reviewed and revised regularly.
3. They should be deleted once they have outlived their usefulness (after careful consideration).

B *Policies,* which serve as guidelines for decision-making and action (Ebaugh, 1998), should accomplish the following:

1. Provide direction for goal attainment
2. Define the scope of the occupational health unit's activities and to whom they apply
3. Must be clear, flexible, and consistent

C *Procedures* are the specific chronological steps necessary to implement policy.

1. Procedures include a purpose, responsibilities, resources, expected results, documentation precautions, and other considerations (Ebaugh, 1998).
2. Not all tasks performed in the occupational health unit require a procedure; if the task is a common one that staff members are all familiar with, writing a procedure is not necessary.

D Once the policy and procedures are developed and approved, they should be disseminated to affected workers through an employee handbook, newsletters, payroll stuffers, closed-circuit television, or in-house computer networks when available.

VI Fiscal Issues: Budgeting and Resource Management

A *Budgeting* is the process of planning and managing financial resources for a given time period.

1. Budgets usually fall within two categories: operating and capital expenditure.
   a. *Operating budgets* itemize the following:
      1) Expected revenues to be generated by the occupational health unit (i.e., cost avoidance or actual income from providing services to another organization)
      2) Expected expenses to be incurred, including personnel salaries, benefits, and contract payment; facility expenses (rent, utilities, maintenance, repairs, and depreciation); supplies; travel; and staff development
   b. *Capital expenditure budgets* include major investments (equipment or facility renovation).
2. Methods of budgeting include the following:
   a. The *incremental budget method* begins with the previous year's budget and adds or subtracts from each line item to fund programs and services.
      1) Advantages: the historical foundation requires little need to justify continuing services and programs.
      2) Disadvantages: resources may be lost if not used in a given year; thus there may be an incentive to overspend the budget to justify the need for increases the next year.

b. The *zero-based budget method* requires annual justification for each program and service in terms of outcome and cost.
   1) Advantages: it requires annual analyses of all occupational health programs and services to evaluate their productivity and cost.
   2) Disadvantage: extra time is required to produce the analyses and provide prioritized alternatives for each program and service.
3. The budgeting process includes the following steps (Yoder-Wise, 1999):
   a. Gathering information and planning programs and services based on mission, goals and objectives
   b. Developing individual program and service budgets
   c. Negotiating and revising the budget
   d. Evaluating via variance analysis and critical performance reports
4. The occupational health unit manager has the primary responsibility for controlling the occupational health unit budget.
5. In order to demonstrate the cost savings of services, the manager must accomplish the following (Table 6-1):
   a. Use zero-based budgeting to determine which program and services are cost effective and which need to be modified or eliminated.

TABLE 6-1

Sample of format for demonstrating cost savings

Service category	Number of visits	Outsource costs	In-house costs	Net costs or savings
Clinical				
Preplacement Exams				
Clinical Follow-Up (Occupational)				
Clinical Follow-Up (Nonoccupational)				
Screening (vision, hearing)				
Health Risk Appraisals				
Health Surveillance				
Diagnostic				
Blood Pressure				
Blood Work, Urinalysis				
Pregnancy Test				
Strep Screen				
Electrocardiogram				
Drug/Alcohol Screen				
Treatment				
Immunization				
Physical Therapy Modalities				
Wound Care				
Health Education				
Counseling				
Miscellaneous & Administration				
Special Projects				
Health Promotion Programs				
Disability Management				
Case Management				
Professional Consultation				
Reports				

Source: Childre, 1995.

   b. Compare costs of providing services in-house with the price of outsourcing to community providers.

B *Resource management* **refers to the timely monitoring of fiscal resources. Managing resources involves the following:**
   1. Determining the costs of resources
   2. Identifying methods to reduce waste
   3. Maintaining appropriate inventory (sufficient supplies without excess)

C **Quarterly and annual reports can be used to document productivity, quality of services, and progress toward goal attainment.**
   1. Quarterly or monthly reports should include the following (Marrelli, 1993; Travers & McDougall, 1995):
      a. Budget projections versus actual expenditures
      b. Update on quality activities and measures
      c. Human resource summary (e.g., hires, vacancies)
      d. Staff-development activities
      e. Outcomes, such as participation in particular programs and services
      f. Staff participation in interdepartmental and interdisciplinary activities
      g. Trends related to injuries and illnesses
   2. Annual reports provide an overview of accomplishments during the past year.

VII Human Resource Issues

A *Assessments* **of job functions serve the following purposes:**
   1. Are often a prerequisite to writing position descriptions (Zwanenberg & Wilkinson, 1993)
   2. May serve as the basis for hiring and developing staff
   3. Also serves as the foundation for performance appraisals (i.e., the measurement of employees' job performance quality and productivity)

B *Position descriptions* **delineate requirements of the job.**
   1. Position titles should be clearly described in terms of "knowledge and skills required, levels of complexity and responsibility, actual work effort, and work conditions" (Forsey, Cleland, & Miller, 1993).
   2. Descriptions should include line authority and responsibility, roles, functions, obligations, and qualifications and should reflect current practice standards (Yoder-Wise, 1999)
   3. Occupational and environmental health nurses can refer to AAOHN's guidelines for job descriptions (AAOHN, 1998) and other AAOHN resources for guidance in developing job descriptions.

C **Strategies for** *recruiting* **applicants, especially in a limited labor market, may include the following:**
   1. Increasing the diversity of the applicant pool through the following methods:
      a. Committing to hiring racial and ethnic minority candidates and supporting these employees with aggressive retention programs (Adams, 1998)
      b. Developing accommodating retirement policies that encourage older workers to remain in or rejoin the work force (Powell, 1998; Steinhauser, 1998)
      c. Providing family-centered benefits that allow employees to balance home and work obligations

2. Innovative recruitment processes may occur through the Internet (Thaler-Carter, 1998)
    a. Strengths
        1) Reaches millions of people around the world in a timely manner
        2) Results in cost savings because of efficiency
    b. Limitations
        1) Overwhelming to applicants as the number of Internet sites expands
        2) Potential breach of confidentiality when resumes are shared among recruiters via the Internet
        3) Only those with Internet access join the applicant pool, resulting in a more homogenous work force.
        4) Increased number of applicants, many of whom are unqualified or uninterested

D The *screening* of applicants can take many forms, including background checks, psychological profiling, handwriting analysis, and interviews (Yarborough, 1994).
    1. Screening techniques must have the following characteristics:
        a. They must be linked to actual job requirements
        b. They must be reliable and valid, meaning that the results would be the same if the screening were administered multiple times and are indeed predictive of worker success in a particular job
    2. Resumes provide a summary of the applicant qualifications.
        a. The resume may be organized chronologically or functionally, or it may be targeted toward a particular position (Amann, 1997).
        b. A cover letter should tie the accomplishments documented in the resume to the opportunities detailed in the position announcement.
    3. Interviews are a common type of selection screening used in business and industry today.
        a. Questions asked must be limited to job functions and performance requirements; acceptable questions relate to the applicant's ability to complete the job tasks with or without accommodation (Alfus, 1994; Lissy, 1995).
        b. Interviewers often ask how the applicant dealt with a situation in a prior position or provide hypothetical situations and ask how the applicant might respond in the future (Pulakos & Schmitt, 1995).
        c. Managers want to assess the applicant's abilities to work within the organization but also are interested in what the applicant can bring to the organization that will further organizational goals (Alderman, 1995).

E *Staff development activities* include mentoring, training. and coaching (Wachs, 1992c).
    1. *Mentoring* is a process whereby a seasoned, skilled, and influential worker (mentor) commits to a long-term relationship with a novice worker (mentee) for the purpose of enhancing the career of the mentee (Carey & Campbell, 1994; Hensler, 1994; Ondeck & Gingerich, 1994).
        a. The mentoring process can be either formal (managed by the organization) or informal (spontaneous relationship) and is marked by four stages: initiation, cultivation, separation, and redefinition (Shaffer, Tallarica, & Walsh, 2000; Bartlett, 1995; Burgess, 1995; Hernandez-Piloto Brito, 1992).
        b. Mentoring is directed at ensuring professional competency.

     c. Mentoring is used to prepare occupational and environmental health nurses to effectively apply nursing and occupational health and safety principles in an occupational setting.

2. *Training* is a more structured process of preparing staff to meet the needs of the organization.
   a. Training begins with orientation to the department and the position.
   b. Training activities may include on-site, in-house presentations; on-site, vendor-generated seminars; off-site offerings; or independent study.
   c. Training activities are initiated based on the individual needs of staff members, annual performance appraisals, and organizational needs.
   d. Training priorities may result from legislative mandates, such as the ADA and the Drug Free Workplace Act.
   e. Staff development activities must be evaluated by workers and managers in terms of the following:
      1) The desired behavior change as a result of the training
      2) The desired improvement in knowledge, skills, or attitudes
      3) The usefulness to the organization of the knowledge, skills, or attitudes to be taught

3. *Coaching* is "a system that *grows* people by enabling them to learn through guided discovery and hands-on experience" (Renke, 1999). Coaches facilitate self-discovery via the following methods:
   a. Listening for meaning rather than words
   b. Encouraging critical thinking
   c. Sharing relevant experiences

4. The key to mentoring, training, and coaching is motivation.
   a. *Motivation* is an "intrinsic drive" resulting from an individual's instincts, needs, and actual or expected rewards; it determines an individual's behavior (Tappen, 1989; Sullivan & Decker, 1997).
   b. Motivation is stimulated by others, including managers, mentors, or a work team.
   c. Motivation is an important concept in management and leadership theories.
   d. Motivating others requires effective communication skills, credibility, caring, praise, constructive criticism, and inclusion of others in the decision-making process (Ellis & Hartley, 1991).

5. *Team building*
   a. *Team building* is important when tasks are complex and work requires a collaborative effort.
   b. Team building results in mutual respect and appreciation of each member's contributions.
   c. One goal of team building is the creation of *empowered teams* whose members demonstrate the following qualities (Renke, 1999):
      1) They focus on results.
      2) They are risk-takers who make mistakes and learn from them.
      3) They communicate effectively to build coalitions and networks.
      4) They lead.
      5) They are creative and visionary.
   d. Because teams take a long time to develop into efficiently functioning entities, the stability of team membership and frequent opportunities for team members to collaborate are important.
   e. Interdependent teamwork is required when multiple workers playing

a variety of unique roles must interact in order to achieve the desired outcome (Drexler & Forrester, 1998).

    f. Interdependent interactions require trust, an affinity for working with other people, a balance of inner strength and other-directedness, and a tolerance for conflict (Drexler & Forrester, 1998).

6. Interdisciplinary occupational health and safety teams

    a. An effective interdisciplinary occupational health and safety team is more than a collection of individuals; the team has a vision and accomplishes goals that none of the members could formulate or implement in isolation.

    b. The interdisciplinary team may include an occupational and environmental health nurse, occupational physician, industrial hygienist, safety manager, ergonomist, toxicologist, and others.

    c. The coordination of the interdisciplinary team is often the responsibility of the occupational and environmental health nurse manager.

    d. The mission and goal of each discipline's contribution to the interdisciplinary team must be clearly articulated.

F *Performance appraisals* **are based on position descriptions, particularly job responsibilities, and standards of performance.**

1. The purpose of performance appraisals is to develop the individual employee and to strengthen the organization through improved productivity and quality outcomes (Webb & Cantone, 1993).

2. Methods of appraisal include verbal feedback, corrective demonstration, conferences, memos, and other forms of communication.

3. Standards of performance "specify for the employee the conditions that will exist when the job is done to the manager's satisfaction" (Webb & Cantone, 1993).

    a. Each job responsibility should have a companion performance standard.

    b. Examples of performance standards are as follows:

        1) Provides professional nursing care appropriate to worker needs

        2) Identifies worker health needs accurately using health history and physical assessment skills for 95% of the workers who present in the occupational health unit

        3) Following signed protocols, prescribes appropriate treatment to meet identified health needs for 100% of workers who present in the occupational health unit

4. Documenting progress toward standards of performance is important; it serves to justify salary increases and promotions.

    a. Begin with annual self-appraisal of accomplishments and contributions.

    b. Write an objective assessment of employee performance based on data collected throughout the year.

    c. Provide time for discussion with a core message of strengths, needs for immediate improvement, and opportunities for development.

    d. Tell the truth (Falcone, 1999; Grote, 1998; Amann, 1996).

    e. Evaluate the efficacy of computer-assisted performance appraisal systems in providing objective, timely assessments and stimulating employee behavioral change (Flowers, Tudor, & Trumble, 1997).

G **Other sources of information that can be used to evaluate occupational health services include surveys of workers who use health services, upper**

management, community resources, vendors, professional colleagues, and occupational health unit staff (Wells, 1999; Eckes, 1994; Weber, 1995).

VIII Communication

A *Listening* is hearing plus the thought processes that allow an "accurate perception of what is being communicated" (Meiss, 1991 [Tape 1]; Wachs, 1995b).
  1. Obstacles to effective listening include the following:
     a. Multiple demands on occupational and environmental health nurses
     b. Biases and beliefs, especially among diverse groups (Tannen, 1994)
     c. Misunderstanding the meaning or tenor of words
     d. Differences in the rates of speech and listening
     e. The need to solve the problem rather than listen to the person
  2. Effective listening requires the following:
     a. Encouraging the speaker to continue the interaction through the use of verbal and nonverbal communication
     b. Listening for others' observations, feelings, needs, and requests (Rosenberg, 1999)
  3. The listening role is a powerful one, often making the difference in whether or not agreements can be reached and work can be accomplished.

B Negotiation and conflict resolution
  1. These skills are most effective when both parties listen and aim for a win-win solution (Badawy, 1994).
  2. "The most common sources of conflict are personal differences, lack of information, role incompatibility, and environmental stress" (Lemieux-Charles, 1994).
  3. Approaches to conflict resolution include the following (Orchard, 1998):
     a. *Competition:* The manager "overpowers the opposition" to meet his or her needs or goals.
     b. *Accommodation:* The manager is more concerned with working relationships than with outcomes and thus will allow others to achieve their goals.
     c. *Avoidance:* The manager refuses to address the issue.
     d. *Compromise:* The manager attempts to find a "middle ground"—a mutually acceptable solution that partially satisfies both parties.
     e. *Collaboration:* All parties work together to find the most satisfying solution for everyone involved.
  4. *Negotiation* is "working side by side with another party to achieve mutually satisfactory results" (Dolan, 1990). *Principled negotiation* is a method designed to decide issues on their merits rather than on a process of haggling (Fisher & Ury, 1991).
     a. A *distributive* approach tends to be competitive; each party is attempting both to resolve the issue and to gain something.
     b. An *integrative* approach focuses on problem solving, seeking a win-win situation for all (Lemieux-Charles, 1994).
  5. Successful negotiation requires the following (Fisher & Ury, 1991; Fisher & Ertel, 1995):
     a. Clarifying each party's interests and searching for underlying interests
     b. Creating alternative ways to meet needs
     c. Developing a best alternative if negotiations fail
     d. Using effective communication and building relationships
     e. Identifying issues to be included in an agreement and defining steps to reach that agreement

C *Networking* **is a process of establishing connections through introductions, promoting and supporting others, and helping others connect (Wachs, 1991).**
  1. Methods of networking include the following:
     a. Identifying essential contacts in the organization and in the community
     b. Being involved in community activities, such as serving on health-related advisory boards or attending community events
     c. Serving as a mentor
  2. Networking is beneficial not only for the occupational and environmental health nurse manager, but also for the organization.
     a. It helps to recruit and retain employees.
     b. It increases visibility within the community and is excellent publicity for the organization.

D **Day-to-day communication is handled with meetings and in writing.**
  1. Meetings are a means of disseminating information, brainstorming, planning, problem solving, or motivating (Wachs, 1992b).
  2. Keys to an effective meeting include the following:
     a. Drawing up an agenda that describes the who, what, when, where, and why of the meeting
     b. Reviewing the purpose of the meeting and establishing the ground rules
     c. Reserving sufficient time for the meeting
     d. Using audiovisuals as needed to help convey information
     e. Distributing the minutes or a written summary of the meeting to all participants and other interested parties
  3. Business writing conveys information, presents facts and conclusions, and motivates or persuades.
  4. The primary audience of the written document makes decisions and acts; the secondary audience "needs to know" but will not act.
  5. An effective document is clear, concise, grammatically correct, and requests action within a time frame (Crowe, 1999).

IX Project Management

Project management is "getting the job done on time, within budget, and according to specifications" (Eichenberger, 1997).

A **A project is "a set of activities planned for the purpose of achieving a specific outcome" (Eichenberger, 1997).**

B **Projects should be goal directed, consist of interrelated activities, be of finite duration, and be unique.**

C **Project scheduling can be accomplished through a work breakdown structure (WBS), Gantt chart, and schedule networks that help accomplish the following:**
  1. Defining tasks, subtasks, responsible parties, and time frame
  2. Alerting participants regarding time delays and devising methods to modify the schedule to keep the project moving toward completion (Eichenberger, 1998a)

D **Budgets are numerical plans and control devices.**
  1. Budget components may include direct labor, overhead, fringe benefits, and auxiliary costs.
  2. Project costs can be estimated using one of the following strategies:
     a. *Bottom up* strategy, in which dollar amounts are assigned to each WBS activity

b. *Parameteric* strategy, in which all costs are estimated based on total labor costs

3. Control devices include variance analysis and cumulative cost curves (Eichenberger, 1998b).

X Time Management

A The principal benefits of managing time are the following:

1. Feelings of accomplishment and control over work, resulting in job satisfaction
2. Long-term commitment to the profession and the organization (Wachs, 1993)

B To manage time effectively, it is important to adhere to the following guidelines:

1. Set realistic, prioritized goals for the occupational health unit and allow staff adequate time to achieve them.
2. Limit additional programs and services the occupational health unit may be asked to provide (Wachs, 1993).
3. Develop a "to do" list, avoid time wasters and paper shuffling, use technologies such as computers, create a supportive work environment, and reward oneself for a job well done (Wachs, 1993).

C Delegating responsibility and commensurate authority to occupational health unit staff is not only effective time management but also effective nursing management (Pollock, 1994; Klock, 1995).

XI Critical Thinking

A *Critical thinking* is the "intellectually disciplined process of actively and skillfully conceptualizing, applying, analyzing, synthesizing, or evaluating information gathered from, or generated by, observation, experience, reflection, reasoning, or communication, as a guide to belief and action (Paul, 1995).

B *Decision-making* is "a purposeful and goal directed effort using a systematic process to choose among options" (Yoder-Wise, 1999).

1. Decision-making styles range from solving problems and making decisions independently to facilitating group discussion and group decision-making processes.
2. The continuum of decision-making styles parallels management styles; the style used in any given situation should be matched to the problem, time frame, and the level of group commitment.
3. The hallmark of decision-making is "the identification and selection of options" (Yoder-Wise, 1999).

C *Problem solving* is "focused on trying to solve an immediate problem; a gap between "what is" and "what should be" (Yoder-Wise, 1999).

1. The problem-solving process includes the following steps:
   a. Defining the problem
   b. Gathering and analyzing data
   c. Developing solutions
   d. Selecting a solution
   e. Implementing the solution
   f. Evaluating the outcome

2. Common methods of problem solving include trial and error, experimentation, and purposeful inaction (Yoder-Wise, 1999).

D *Creativity* **is the "ability to conceptualize new and innovative approaches to a problem or issue by being more flexible and independent in thinking" (Yoder-Wise, 1999).**
   1. Critical thinking links creativity to decision making and problem solving.
   2. Foster creative problem solving by pursuing the following practices:
      a. Establish a safe environment for trying innovative practices without fear of failure
      b. Promote interaction between occupational health unit staff and others (both within and outside the organization)
      c. Reward staff for unique approaches to occupational health unit problems

XII The Image of the Occupational and Environmental Health Nurse

The occupational and environmental health nurse should be seen as a competent business person who has particular expertise in health and safety.

A *Image* **is created through the display of personal characteristics and interpersonal skills.**
   1. Personal appearance plays a major role in the occupational and environmental health nurse's image.
   2. Professionalism displayed through interactions with workers, managers, and community members attests to the positive image of nurses.
      a. A nurse's caring and competence are often evaluated by workers and managers.
      b. Dealings with community providers, vendors, and other business people will color the community's perception of not only an individual occupational and environmental health nurse but of nurses in general.
   3. The occupational and environmental health nurse can also positively affect the image of nurses by engaging in the following activities:
      a. Publishing articles in the organization's newsletter and the community newspaper
      b. Belonging to professional organizations such as AAOHN
      c. Recognizing and publicizing excellence among staff members (Brown, 1995)

B **The image of the occupational and environmental health nurse relates directly to the nurse's influence and ability to promote health and safety in the organization.**

XIII Application of Ethics to Decision-Making

Ethics is the "science of using moral criteria to guide human conduct and morals as accepted values and standards of human behavior" (Key & Popkin, 1998).

A **"The incorporation of ethics into decision-making can improve the functioning of an organization and ultimately can maximize corporate profits (Key & Popkin, 1998).**
   1. Identify the interests the organization intends to serve
      a. Private interests (e.g., providing a healthy and safe work environment for all employees)

      b. Public interests (e.g., proper disposal of hazardous waste for the entire community)

2. Analyze these identified interests in terms of moral, social, and legal responsibilities
3. Create processes whereby an understanding of various interests and responsibilities becomes part of any decision-making within the organization (Key & Popkin, 1998)

B **Organizations are often very adept at after-profit ethical decision-making (philanthropy).**

1. Philanthropy is an essential part of corporate life but will not guarantee corporate success.
2. The occupational and environmental health nurse manager has daily opportunities to incorporate ethics into decisions made regarding the health and safety of workers; these opportunities include the following:
   a. Confidentiality of health-related documents and interactions
   b. Recommendations regarding malingering
   c. Return to work policies
   d. Employee assistance program evaluation

XIV Outcomes Management

Outcomes management is "the systematic approach to evaluate, through process, all steps leading to a result (outcome) and proactively use the information at the front end to design and implement best practices" (Kosinski, 1998).

A **Outcomes management is used to measure the following:**

1. The cost versus benefit of programs and services
2. The effect of programs and services on organizational profit margin

B **To design an effective outcomes management program, execute the following steps:**

1. Determine what outcomes can be measured or evaluated
2. Compare possible measures with the needs of the organization
3. Assess current resources and additional needs to determine the feasible scope of the program
4. Describe expected results based on appropriate benchmarks (past performance or goals for future performance) (Kosinski, 1998)

C **Collect data from more than one source if possible**

D **Focus the program by avoiding too broad an evaluation, lost variables, or global outcomes (Kosinski, 1998)**

E **Use results to modify best practices to better approximate the benchmark**

XV Benchmarking

Benchmarking is the "continuous process of measuring a company's products, services, and practices against industry leading competitors" (Collins, 1995) and "against industry's best practice" (Landwehr, 1995).

A **The purposes of benchmarking include the following (Beasley & Cook, 1995):**

1. Modifying organizational culture or climate
2. Fostering competition

3. Creating an awareness of the quality standard within the industry
4. Measuring productivity and performance quality
5. Setting performance standards
6. Managing the organization to achieve the best results

B **The benchmarking process includes the following steps (Brown, 1995; Collins, 1995; Murray & Murray, 1992; Landwehr, 1995; Bergman, 1994):**

1. Planning: decide which processes will be benchmarked and what the assessment activities will be; develop measurement tools; and assess internal functioning
2. Data collection: identify best-practice companies and sharing information
3. Data analysis: identify performance gaps between the study company and the benchmark companies
4. Change: use the data to unfreeze workers to accept the need for modification in the work process under review and then implement the change based on the benchmark criteria
5. Monitoring: oversee the change process, of course, but also recalibrate benchmarks at regular intervals

C **Benchmarking has some potential problems, such as the following (McWilliams, 1995):**

1. Choosing the wrong benchmark organizations for comparison
2. Failure to appreciate that although organizations may be comparable, they will also be unique in ways that may affect the legitimacy of the comparison
3. The need for common definitions of processes and criteria
4. The need to be the best no matter what the cost
5. Reluctance to use quality interventions other than benchmarking

D **The occupational and environmental health nurse must understand benchmarking sufficiently to communicate with others in the organization about the opportunities and challenges of quality management.**

XVI Total Quality Management

A *Total quality management* **(TQM) and** *continuous quality improvement* **(CQI) are processes used to put customers' needs and quality products first.**

1. TQM is a business strategy that focuses on work processes and outcomes.
2. In health care, a similar strategy is known as continuous quality improvement (CQI).
3. Quality improvement is defined as conformance to customer requirements and specifications, fitness for use, buyer satisfaction, and value at an affordable price (Harrington, 1987).
4. The quality improvement process is a disciplined, ongoing process for producing outputs and preventing errors in products and services.

B Approaches to total quality management

1. W. Edwards Deming's TQM program, called the *Deming Cycle,* includes the following steps (Deming, 1986):
   a. Plan a work process
   b. Do or implement a work process
   c. Check or measure a work process
   d. Act on results to continuously improve the process
2. Joseph Juran's program focuses on quality planning, quality control, and quality improvement of processes (Juran, 1988).

3. Philip B. Crosby's program is based on organizational development, with the following absolutes for quality management (Crosby, 1979):
   a. Conformance to organizational requirements
   b. Prevention of potential problems
   c. Zero defects in products or services
   d. Determination of the cost of quality

C Interpersonal behaviors are at the center of total quality management or continuous quality improvement.

D Task behaviors that get work done include the following:
1. Proposing a new idea or making a suggestion
2. Building on others' ideas or suggestions
3. Seeking information by soliciting facts, data, experiences, or clarifications from others
4. Giving information by offering facts, data, experiences, or clarifications to others
5. Seeking opinion by soliciting values, beliefs, or sentiments from others
6. Giving opinions by offering values, beliefs, or sentiments to others
7. Disagreeing by opposing or raising doubts about an issue, not a person
8. Summarizing by restating the content of previously shared dialogue in condensed form
9. Testing comprehension by asking questions for one's own understanding of previous communication
10. Checking to find out if consensus has been reached or if more discussion is needed

E Group maintenance and facilitation behaviors are important elements of TQM.
1. Encourage others by supporting or recognizing their contributions
2. Resolve disagreements and conflict by searching for alternatives and/or agreements
3. Check performance by temporarily suspending task operations to facilitate the internal group process
4. Set standards to improve the quality of the group's process
5. Relieve tension and increase enjoyment by suggesting breaks or proposing fun approaches to work

F Beyond TQM
1. Business process reengineering (BPR) focuses on redesigning work processes in an effort to reduce specific resource needs and the work force with an ultimate reduction in overhead costs (DeCock & Hipkin, 1997).
   a. BPR led to the "right sizing" of the work force typical in the 1990s.
   b. Organizations expected more output from fewer workers.
   c. BPR has not necessarily resulted in improved products or services or increased profitability.
2. To improve quality and profitability, an organization can use techniques such as TQM or BPR; but most importantly the entire organization must have a commitment to improve structure and processes to positively affect outcomes.

BIBLIOGRAPHY

Adams, M. (1998). Building a rainbow, one stripe at a time. *HRMagazine, 43,* 72-79.

Alderman, L. (1995). What you need to ace today's rough-and-tough job interviews. *Money, 24(4),* 35.

Alfus, P. (1994). Know new interview guidelines—or risk legal trouble. *Hotel and Motel Management, 209(19)*, 16-17.

Al-Shammari, M.M. (1992). Organizational climate. *Leadership & Organization Development, 13(6)*, 30-32.

Amann, M. (1996). Performance management. Part 2: Performance review and appraisal. *AAOHN Journal, 44*, 421-422.

Amann, M. (1997). Business skills for occupational health nurses: Preparing the perfect resume. *AAOHN Journal, 45*, 107-108.

American Association of Occupational Health Nurses (AAOHN). (1998*). Guidelines for developing job descriptions in occupational & environmental health nursing.* Atlanta, GA: AAOHN Publications.

American Association of Occupational Health Nurses (AAOHN). (1999). *Success tools: Developing business expertise—strategies for thriving & surviving in business.* Atlanta, GA: AAOHN Publications.

Argyris, C. (1960). *Understanding organizational behavior.* Homewood, IL: Dorsey

Badawy, M.K. (1994). Listening is an art in negotiation. *Electronic Business Buyer, 20(12)*, 19.

Bartlett, R.C. (1995). The mentoring message. *Chief Executive, 101*, 48-49.

Beasley, G., & Cook, J. (1995). The "what," "why," and "how" of benchmarking. *Agency Sales, 25(6)*, 52-56.

Bergman, R. (1994). Hitting the mark. *Hospitals and Health Networks, 68(8)*, 48-51.

Brown, S. (1995). Measures of perfection. *Sales & Marketing Management, 147(5)*, 104-105.

Burgess, L. (1995). Mentoring with the blindfold. *Employment Relations Today, 21(4)*, 439-444.

Burns, J.M. (1978). *Leadership.* New York: Harper & Row.

Butcher, A.H. (1994). Supervisors matter more than you think: components of a mission-centered organizational climate. *Hospital & Health Services Administration, 39(4)*, 505-521.

Carey, S.J., & Campbell, S.T. (1994). Preceptor, mentor and sponsor roles: Creative strategies for nurse retention. *Journal of Nursing Administration, 24(12)*, 39-48.

Chaleff, I. (1998). *The courageous follower.* San Francisco: Berrett-Koehler Publishers.

Collins, M.J. (1995). Benchmarking with simulation: How it can help your production operations. *Production, 107(7)*, 51-52.

Crislip, D.D., & Larson, C.E. (1994). *Collaborative leadership.* San Francisco: Jossey-Bass Publishers.

Crosby, P.B. (1979). *Quality is free.* New York: New American Library.

Crowe, R. (1999). Business writing: A necessary skill for occupational and environmental health nurses. *AAOHN Journal, 47*, 383-385.

DeCock, C., & Hipkin, I. (1997). TQM and BPR: Beyond the beyond myth. *Journal of Management Studies, 34*, 661-675.

Deming, W.E. (1986). *Out of the crisis.* Cambridge, MA: MIT-CAES.

Depree, M. (1989). *Leadership is an art.* New York: Dell Publishing.

Depree, M. (1992). *Leadership jazz.* New York: Dell Publishing.

Dolan, J.P. (1990). *Negotiate like the pros* (audiotape). Boulder, CO: CareerTrack.

Douglass, L.M. (1992). *The effective nurse: Leader and manager.* St. Louis, MO: C.V. Mosby.

Drexler, A.B., & Forrester, R. (1998). Interdependence: The crux of teamwork. *HRMagazine, 43*, 52-62.

Ebaugh, H. (1998). Defining the scope of occupational health services: Effective policy and procedure development. *AAOHN Journal, 46*, 547-553.

Eckes, G. (1994). Practical alternatives to performance appraisals. *Quality Progress, 27(11)*, 57-60.

Eichenberger, J. (1997). Project management for occupational health nurses. *AAOHN Journal, 45*, 607-608.

Eichenberger, J. (1998a). Project management, Part II. AAOHN Journal, 46, 96-98.

Eichenberger, J. (1998b). Project management, Part III. Budgets for projects. *AAOHN Journal, 46,* 268-270.

Ellis, J.R., & Hartley, C.L. (1991). *Managing and coordinating nursing care.* Philadelphia: J.B. Lippincott Company.

Falcone, P. (1999). Rejuvenate your performance evaluation writing skills. *HRMagazine, 44,* 126-136.

Fiedler, F.E. (1964). A contingency model of leadership effectiveness. In L. Burkowitz (Ed.), *Advances in experimental social psychology.* New York: Academic Press.

Fisher, R., & Ertel, D. (1995). *Getting ready to negotiate.* New York: Penguin Books.

Fisher, R., & Ury, W. (1991). *Getting to yes.* New York: Penguin Books.

Flowers, L.A., Tudor, T.R., & Trumble, R.R. (1997). Computer assisted performance appraisal systems. *Journal of Compensation and Benefits, 12,* 34-35.

Forsey, L.M., Cleland, V.S., & Miller, B. (1993). Job descriptions for differentiated nursing practice and differentiated pay. *Journal of Nursing Administration, 23(5),* 33-40.

Greenleaf, R.K. (1970). *The servant as leader.* Indianapolis, IN: Robert K. Greenleaf Center for Servant Leadership.

Grohar-Murray, M.E., & DiCroce, H.R. (1992). *Leadership and management in nursing.* Norwalk, CT: Appleton & Lange.

Grote, D. (1998). Painless performance appraisals focus on results, behaviors. *HRMagazine, 43,* 52-58.

Harrington, H.J. (1987). *The improvement process: How America's leading companies improve quality.* New York: McGraw-Hill.

Hensler, D.J. (1994). Mentoring at the management level. *Industrial Management, 36(6),* 20-21.

Hernandez-Piloto Brito, H. (1992). Nurses in action: An innovative approach to mentoring. *Journal of Nursing Administration, 22(5),* 23-28.

Herzberg, F., Mausner, B. & Snydermann, E.E. *The motivation to work.* New York: Wiley.

Honeywell Solid State Electronics Center. (1990). *Quality improvement tools.* Minneapolis, MN: Honeywell Solid State Electronics Center.

Juran, J.M. (Ed.). (1988). *Juran's quality control handbook* (4th ed). New York: Random House.

Key, S. & Popkin, S.J. (1998). Integrating ethics into the strategic management process: doing well by doing good. *Management Decision, 36,* 331-338.

Klock, J.P. (1995). Learn to be a master delegator! *Real Estate Today, 28(3),* 50-53.

Kosinski, M. (1998). Effective outcomes management in occupational and environmental health. *AAOHN Journal, 46,* 500-510.

Kouzes, J.M., & Posner, B.Z. (1987). *Leadership challenge.* Palo Alto, CA: TPG/Learning Systems.

Landwehr, W.R. (1995). Focus on benchmarking: Achieving world-class maintenance and superior competitive performance. *Plant Engineering, 49(7),* 120-121.

Lemieux-Charles, L. (1994). Physicians in health care management: Managing conflict through negotiation. *Canadian Medical Association Journal, 151(8),* 1129-1132.

Lewin, K. (1951). *Field theory in social sciences.* New York: Harper & Row.

Likert, R. (1967). *The human organization.* New York: McGraw-Hill.

Lissy, W.E. (1995). Interviewing job applicants under the ADA. *Supervision, 56(3),* 17.

Marrelli, T.M. (1993). *The nurse manager's survival guide.* St. Louis, MO: C.V. Mosby.

Marriner-Tomey, A. (1992). *Guide to nursing management.* St. Louis, MO: Mosby YearBook.

McGregor, D. (1960). *The human side of enterprise.* New York: McGraw-Hill.

McGregor, D. (1966). *Leadership and motivation.* Cambridge, MA: MIT Press.

McWilliams, B. (1995). What's wrong with benchmarking? *CFO, 11(5),* 105-106.

Meiss, R. (1991). *Effective listening* (audiotape). Boulder, CO: CareerTrack Publications.

Moran, E.T., & Volkwein, J.F. (1992). The cultural approach to the formation of organizational climate. *Human Relations, 45(1),* 19-47.

Murray, J.A., & Murray, M.H. (1992). Benchmarking: A tool for excellence in palliative care. *Journal of Palliative Care, 8(4),* 41-45.

Ondeck, D.A., & Gingerich, B.S. (1994). The mentoring relationship. *Journal of Home Health Care Practice, 6(4),* 1-7.

Orchard, B. (1998). Creating constructive outcomes in conflict. *AAOHN Journal, 46,* 302-313.

Paul, R.W. (1995). *Critical thinking: How to prepare students for a rapidly changing world.* Santa Rose, CA: Foundations for Critical Thinking.

Perra, B.M. (1999). The leader in you. *Nursing Management, 30,* 35-38.

Pollock, T. (1994). Secrets of successful delegation. *Production, 106(12),* 10-11.

Powell, D.H. (1998). Aging baby boomers: Stretching your workforce options. *HRMagazine, 43,* 82-85.

Pulakos, E.D., & Schmitt, N. (1995). Experience-based and situational interview questions: Studies of validity. Personnel Psychology, 48(2), 289.

Renke, W.J. (1999). Manage like a coach not a cop. *Balance, 3,* 24-26.

Rosenberg, M.B. (1999). *Nonviolent communication.* Del Mar, CA: PuddleDancer Press.

Senge, P.M. (1990). *The fifth discipline.* New York: Doubleday.

Senge, P.M. (2000). Leadership in living organizations. In F. Hesselbein, M. Goldsmith, & I. Somerville, (Eds.), *Leading beyond the walls* (pp. 73-90) San Francisco: Jossey-Bass Publishers.

Shaffer, B., Tallarica, B., & Walsh, J. (2000). Win-win mentoring. *Nursing Management, 31,* 32-34.

Steinhauser, S. (1998). Age bias: Is your corporate culture in need of an overhaul? *HRMagazine, 43,* 86-91.

Sullivan, E.J., & Decker, P.J. (1997). *Effective leadership and management in nursing.* Menlo Park, CA: Addison-Wesley.

Tannen, D. (1994). *Talking from 9 to 5.* New York: Avon Books.

Tappen, R.M. (1989). *Nursing leadership and management: Concepts and practice.* Philadelphia: F.A. Davis.

Taylor, F.W. (1911). *The principles of scientific management.* New York: Harper & Brothers.

Thaler-Carter, R.E. (1998). Recruiting through the web: Better or just bigger? *HRMagazine, 43,* 61-68.

Travers, P.H., & McDougall, C. (1995). *Guidelines for an occupational health and safety service.* Atlanta, GA: AAOHN.

Wachs, J.E. (1991). Strategies to develop "interconnectedness." Part I: Connections within the organization. *AAOHN Journal, 39(12),* 578-579.

Wachs, J.E. (1992b). Facilitating an effective meeting. *AAOHN Journal, 40(6),* 294-296.

Wachs, J.E. (1992c). Developing health service staff. *AAOHN Journal, 40(9),* 448-450.

Wachs, J.E. (1993). Managing time. *AAOHN Journal, 41(6),* 300-302.

Wachs, J.E. (1995b). Listening. *AAOHN Journal, 43(11),* 590-592.

Wachs, J.E., & Price, M. (1995). Asking questions: A management tool. *AAOHN Journal, 43(5),* 285-287.

Webb, P.R., & Cantone, J.M. (1993). Performance evaluation: Triumph or torture? *Journal of Home Health Care Practice, 5(2),* 14-19.

Weber, A.J. (1995). Making performance appraisals consistent with a quality environment. *Quality Progress, 28(6),* 65-69.

Wells, S.J. (1999). A new road: Traveling beyond 360-degree evaluation. *HRMagazine, 44,* 82-91.

Wheatley, M.J. (1992). *Leadership and the new science.* San Francisco: Berrett-Koehler.

Wheatley, M.J. (1999). Good-bye, command and control. In F. Hesselbein & P.M. Cohen (Eds.), *Leader to leader* (pp. 151-162). San Francisco: Jossey-Bass Publishers.

Wywialowski, E. (1993). *Managing client care.* St. Louis, MO: C.V. Mosby.

Yarborough, M.H. (1994). New variations on recruitment prescreening. *HR Focus, 71(10),* 1-5.

Yoder-Wise, P.S. (1999). *Leading and managing in nursing.* St. Louis, MO: Mosby

Zamanou, S., & Glaser, S.R. (1994). Moving toward participation and involvement. *Group & Organization Management, 19(4),* 475-502.

Zwanenberg, N.V., & Wilkinson, L.J. (1993). The person specification—A problem masquerading as a solution? *Personnel Review, 22(7),* 54-65.

7

Information Management in the Occupational Health Setting

Mary Amann

The ability to manage information efficiently is critical to the successful delivery of health services. An increase in the volume and complexity of information that must be managed in the modern day workplace requires new organizational skills and the use of advanced technological tools. This chapter provides an overview of the multiple systems and techniques that can help the occupational and environmental health nurse effectively manage information, and describes how these systems can be used to optimize service delivery.

I Introduction to Nursing Informatics

A ***Nursing informatics* is a "combination of computer science, information science and nursing science designed to assist in the management and processing of nursing data, information and knowledge to support the practice of nursing and the delivery of nursing care" (Graves & Corcoran, 1989, p. 227).**

1. Nursing informatics consists of management and processing components.
    a. The *management* component of informatics is the functional ability to collect, aggregate, organize, move, and represent information in an economical, efficient way that is useful to the users of the system.
    b. The *processing* component of informatics refers to the transformation of data into information and of information into knowledge.
2. Factors that necessitate more efficient management of information include the following:
    a. An increase in health-related legislation with requirements for extensive recordkeeping, reporting, and documentation
    b. The rapid emergence of new health issues requiring immediate action
    c. The changing demographics of client populations that may include employees who are older, more mobile, working from home, caring for family members, working multiple jobs, sharing jobs, or engaging in activities that may compound the effects of work on health
    d. An expectation that the occupational and environmental health nurse will work collaboratively as part of multidisciplinary teams to address complex health issues in the workplace

e. A need to justify occupational health services as a worthwhile expenditure in a competitive market

f. The need to operate occupational health services as a "business"

B **The occupational and environmental health nurse applies the principles of nursing informatics in the following activities:**

1. Assessing the needs of employees for services, education, and surveillance programs
2. Developing interventions that are appropriate for the client audience
3. Evaluating services to ensure desired outcomes
4. Disseminating information to employees, peers, managers, and others in a timely, efficient manner
5. Ensuring compliance with all regulations and legislation that affects the occupational health service and the corporation
6. Conducting research by accessing and using information from expert sources to support decision making

C **Information management systems can be applied to all aspects of the occupational health service, including the following:**

1. Developing and managing budgets
2. Selecting, training, and managing the performance and professional development of staff members
3. Overseeing the physical plant from which services are delivered
4. Anticipating, acquiring, and managing the resources required to deliver effective services
5. Producing and presenting reports that help business leaders make informed decisions
6. Developing and implementing policies that protect the health of employees
7. Developing and implementing protocols and standards of practice that ensure consistent delivery of goal-oriented services

II Tools Available to the Occupational and Environmental Health Nurse

A *Occupational health information management systems* **are computerized programs that provide a mechanism to collect, access, and use large amounts of information from many different sources in a single repository. They may be designed to be client-centered or site-management systems, or a combination of both.**

1. *Client-centered systems* facilitate the development of an electronic medical record that tracks health experiences of an individual from placement through the period of employment and for the period of retention as required by the Occupational Safety and Health Administration (OSHA) (AAOHN, 1996); information maintained in a client-centered system includes the following:

   a. Preplacement health evaluations
   b. On-the-job injury treatment documentation
   c. Clinic visit notes
   d. Work restriction management records
   e. Disability case management notes
   f. Exposure documentation
   g. Participation in workplace surveillance programs
   h. Assignment and fitting of personal protective equipment
   i. Examination and test results

2. *Site-management systems* enable the occupational health professional to document activities related to a physical work environment, a corporation, or some geographical region; examples of the type of data captured by a site-management system include the following:
    a. Industrial hygiene sampling activities and results over time
    b. Exposures and actions taken
    c. OSHA recordkeeping
    d. Equipment calibration and maintenance records
    e. Vendor, supplier, and community provider lists
    f. Motor vehicle accident records

B *Combination systems* **are usually modular in design, and thus can be tailored to the specific needs of the organization.**
    1. These systems enable occupational health professionals to select, purchase, and implement those functions that are most applicable to their specific needs.
    2. Because of the expanding role of the occupational and environmental health nurse and the need to manage many different types of data, combination systems are increasingly preferred.

III Selecting and Implementing Information Management Systems

A **The American Nurses Association Taskforce on Nursing Information Systems (1993) has described the essential characteristics of effective health information systems; they must have the following characteristics:**
    1. Be flexible to meet changing requirements, such as incorporating new functionality to help track employees in a new exposure group
    2. Be compatible and able to integrate with other internal and external systems, such as Personnel or Human Resources
    3. Have a simple, logical approach to language and codes, including minimal technical jargon
    4. Support the work of the nurse without increasing effort, including eliminating double entry of the same data
    5. Provide useful outputs, such as reports, letters, and notices that the nurse develops
    6. Be cost efficient and cost beneficial to the organization and the user
    7. Ensure sustained performance with minimal downtime and ensure that data are easily recovered in the event of system failure
    8. Ensure system security that prevents unauthorized entry or access to health information
    9. Ensure data integrity that prevents loss, changes, or corruption to information captured in the system
    10. Ensure confidentiality of sensitive information recorded by a health professional regarding the health status of a client

B *Selection* **of an occupational health information system must be a well-organized, thoughtful process that involves the input of any individual or group who will be using, interfacing with, or supporting the system.**
    1. Typical team members participating in the selection process include the following:
        a. Occupational and environmental health nurses
        b. Safety/industrial hygienist

    c. A management representative

    d. A person assigned from the corporate information systems department

    e. Representatives from Human Resources or Personnel

2. The following steps will provide a framework for the team:

    a. Identify and define the information needs of users, other departments, and the company

        1) List all services and functions to be supported by the system

        2) Develop workflow diagrams for each process (Fig. 7-1)

        3) Identify the data needs for each step in the diagram (e.g., forms, questionnaires, notices, reports) (Fig. 7-2)

        4) Specify all interfaces and information exchanges required for each work process

        5) Specify the methods of communication required for each interface (e.g., automatic fax, e-mail, hard-copy mail)

        6) Develop a list of all requirements and assign priorities for each function (Table 7-1)

    b. Determine whether to develop the system internally or purchase a commercial product

    c. If the decision is made to purchase a commercial product, initiate the following activities to research suppliers and products:

        1) Attend trade shows and vendor exhibits at conferences such as the American Occupational Health Conference

        2) Secure lists such as the Technology Resource List available from AAOHN

        3) Network with occupational and environmental health nurses who are users of automated systems

        4) Review the literature on specific products in journals, newsletters, and web sites

        5) Invite vendors to demonstrate software products using the list of functionality and specifications generated by the selection team

        6) Interview customers of specific software programs regarding functionality and support provided by the vendor

    d. Prepare and submit a business case justifying the purchase or development of an electronic health information system

C *Implementation* **of an occupational and environmental health information system may be facilitated by using project management techniques and tools (Chapter 6 describes the principals of project management). The following strategies will help ensure that the process of implementation is well organized and that all possible barriers have been anticipated.**

1. Widely publicize the purchase and planned implementation

2. Secure the commitment of top-level management, unions, and other authority figures

3. Develop policies and procedures for appropriate use of the system

4. Appoint a lead representative to work directly with the system vendor/developer

5. Secure a designated representative from company information systems department

6. Establish evaluation criteria, including the following:

    a. Cost savings versus expenditures

    b. Time savings

    c. Improved communication between departments

Text continued on p. 181

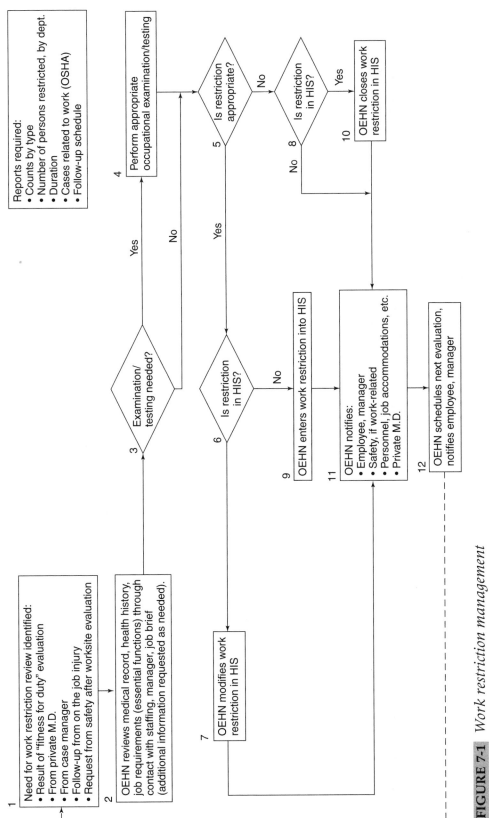

FIGURE 7-1 *Work restriction management*

OEHN, Occupational and environmental health nurse; *HIS*, health information system.

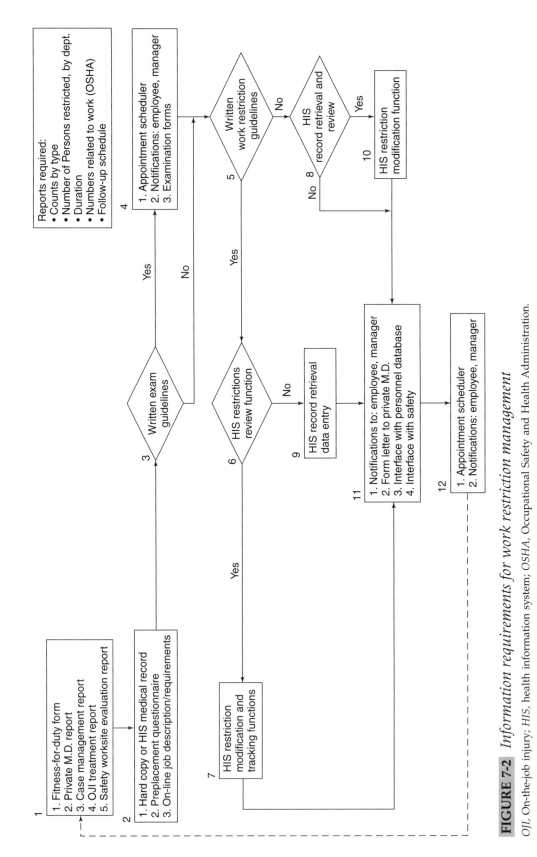

FIGURE 7-2 *Information requirements for work restriction management*

OJI, On-the-job injury; *HIS*, health information system; *OSHA*, Occupational Safety and Health Administration.

TABLE 7-1

Occupational health system review grid*

Function	Priority	System 1 Score/ weighted score		System 2 Score/ weighted score		System 3 Score/ weighted score	
Windows based, 32 bit							
Interfaces with other departments							
Imports demographics from HR							
Ad hoc reporting							
User-defined standardized reports							
User-defined lists							
User-generated letters, notices							
Schedules appointments							
Maintains activity log by site, staff, etc.							
Contains standards lists, ICD, MSDS							
Tracks costs/savings							
Archives records							
On-line help for users							
Maintains vendor/provider lists							
Internet enabled							
E-mail connected							
Produces charts/graphics							
Interfaces with laboratory							
Instrument interfaces (audio, PFT)							
Word processing editing							
Search engine							
Preplacement							
Questionnaire/form							
Notices							
Establishes evaluation by job title							
Total weighted score for page 1							

*Using a scale of 1 (least) to 5 (greatest), indicate the *priority* of each function to you. Give each system a *score* accrding to its ability to perform each function; then multiply the score by the priority to arrive at a *weighted score* for each function.

HR, Human resources; *ICD,* international classification of diseases; *MSDS,* material safety data sheets; *PFT,* pulmonary function testing.   *Continued*

TABLE 7-1

Occupational health system review grid—cont'd

Function	Priority	System 1 Score/ weighted score		System 2 Score/ weighted score		System 3 Score/ weighted score	
Employee health record							
Encounters							
Clinical notes							
Procedures							
Allergies/serious health problems							
Medical Surveillance							
Target groups by risk							
Exam protocols/test panels							
Tracks exam/test results							
Imports environmental monitoring							
Imports job description, phys. req.							
Track equipment calibration records							
Hearing conservation program							
Respiratory protection program							
Immunization/vaccination records							
BBP required forms							
Titer results							
Prophylaxis records							
Notification of boosters/doses							
Captures serum information							
Motor vehicle accidents							
Accident details							
Claim details							
Costs to the company							
Employee training							
Documents course, attendance, hrs.							
Schedules							
Notifies							
Generates rosters							
Total weighted score for page 2							

TABLE 7-1

Occupational health system review grid*—cont'd

Function	Priority	System 1 Score/ weighted score		System 2 Score/ weighted score		System 3 Score/ weighted score	
Case management							
Case profile							
Duration guidelines							
PVT MD/IME reports							
Workers compensation history							
Rehab record							
Tracks costs							
Tracks days lost/restricted days							
Records FMLA criteria							
Drug testing							
Produces random selection							
Notifies employee/supervisor							
Records results							
Produces DOT reports							
Work restrictions							
Automatic re-evaluation notification							
Lists essential functions by job							
Transmits info to HR database							
Notifies employee/supervisor							
Industrial hygiene							
Tracks sampling by area, employee							
Calculates exposure levels, TWA							
Security							
Multi-level password protected							
Audit trails for all files and records							
Encryption/coding capability							
Time lock for changes to records							
Total weighted score for page 3							

PVT MD, Private medical doctor; *IME,* independent medical examiner; *FMLA,* Family and Medical Leave Act; *DOT,* Department of Transportation; *HR,* human resources; *TWA,* time-weighted average.

Continued

TABLE 7-1

Occupational health system review grid—cont'd

Function	Priority	System 1 Score/ weighted score		System 2 Score/ weighted score		System 3 Score/ weighted score	
Audits							
Standard forms							
Schedule of locations/areas							
Produces randomized site selection							
Generates supervisor report							
System management							
System cost							
Module/feature costs							
Cost of required hardware							
Cost of on-going support							
User training							
User groups							
Loss of customizations with upgrades							
Designated customer rep							
Response to change requests							
Health promotion							
Lists programs							
Captures roster/attendance							
Distributes notices							
Captures costs							
Information technology							
Compatibility							
Networking capability							
Firewall issues							
Expandability							
Total weighted score for page 4							
Total of weighted scores for pages 1-4							

      d. Improved access to critical information for professional decision making
      e. More-useful reports
      f. Increased satisfaction of users

7. Determine and institute measures to ensure security(e.g., passwords for users, etc.)
8. Provide ways to obtain and maintain appropriate hardware and software
9. Ensure that users have basic computer skills; if not, institute tutorials or workshops
10. Train one or more users to be "super users" who can support others during implementation and troubleshoot problems
11. Establish a pilot program at a single location and document the experience thoroughly
12. Implement the system on a limited basis (e.g., one function or one location at a time)
13. Have users keep a log of their progress, issues, and problems
14. Have regular meetings to debrief employees and resolve issues as they occur
15. Monitor direct and indirect costs associated with implementation

IV The Internet

A **The *Internet* is a worldwide network of computers and users who are able to communicate using standardized protocols.**

1. Many forms of media, including voice, graphics, sound, video, and data, may be transmitted among different users, user sites, machines, and networks of machines.
    a. The Internet (originally called the ARPANET or Advanced Research Project Agency Network) was created in 1969 for the purpose of communicating research data among four universities.
    b. The World Wide Web (WWW) is a widely used protocol developed much later that allows users to move freely from one site to another.
2. *Protocols* are sets of rules or common directions for accomplishing a task; the following protocols are commonly used on the Internet:
    a. TCP/IP (Transmission Control Protocol/Internet Protocol) is the suite of protocols that are required for Internet use.
    b. SMTP (Simple Mail Transfer Protocol) is the protocol used to send electronic mail via the Internet.
    c. POP has the following two meanings:
       1) *Point of presence* refers to a location where a user connects to a network, usually a city and often with dial-up phone lines. Internet customers should clarify with their Internet service provider if connecting using the assigned POP will require a long distance phone call.
       2) *Post Office Protocol* refers to the way e-mail software retrieves mail from a mail server.
    d. FTP (File Transfer Protocol) is a very common method of moving files from one site to another (e.g., accessing material from a library or catalog).
    e. HTTP (Hypertext Transfer Protocol) is the most important protocol used on the WWW because it allows files to be moved across the

Internet using hypertext, or the language that makes it possible to call up and display another site simply by selecting it.

3. There are other important terms that one needs to know to understand and use the Internet to its fullest potential, including the following:

a. *HTML* (Hypertext Markup Language) is a coding language.
   1) *Hypertext* enables words, symbols, graphics, sound and video files, and other items to be linked to other sites or items within a site.
   2) Selecting hypertext items allows users to "navigate" or "surf" from site to site in a nonlinear way.

b. *Bandwidth* is the amount of data that can be transmitted at once.

c. *Bits* are the smallest unit of computerized data (bandwidth is measured in bits-per-second).

d. *Bytes* are a set of bits (usually 8).
   1) A *kilobyte* is 1000 bytes, and a *megabyte* is a million bytes.
   2) This metric is most often used to describe the space available on a drive or in memory.

e. *Baud* is the speed at which a computer can send or receive bits of data.

f. A *bookmark* (sometimes called a *favorite*) is a direct link created by the user to a site that was once visited and is likely to be visited again.
   1) Creating bookmarks is a fast, efficient way to use the browser to navigate directly to a site without searching.
   2) Occupational and environmental health nurses can use bookmarks to create directories of sites that contain commonly used information, such as the sites maintained by the Centers for Disease Control and Prevention (CDC), OSHA, AAOHN, American Board for Occupational Health Nurses, and National Institute for Occupational Safety and Health (NIOSH) (Appendix IV provides the addresses for these and other Web sites.)

g. A *browser* is a software program that is the interface between the user and the Internet and allows users to contact other Web servers.

h. A *Web page* IS a collection of resources located at a single Internet address.

i. *Search engines* are software programs that allow users to search for sites that contain user-specified key words or phrases; a search engine produces a list of Web sites that meet user's search criteria.

j. A *URL* (Uniform Resource Locator) is an Internet *address;* every item on the Internet has a distinct URL. The following list explains the elements of this sample URL: http://www.cdc.gov/travel/vaccinat/html
   1) http: The protocol necessary to access the site
   2) www.cdc.gov: the "domain" or who and what type of organization owns the site
   3) Travel/vaccinate: the "path" within the site to the desired information
   4) html: the language or coding system used in the site

B Methods of finding information on the Internet include:
1. Typing the URL into an address field
2. Searching using a search engine
3. Linking to a site by clicking on hypertext in another site
4. Going directly to a site using a bookmark

C The occupational and environmental health nurse may use the Internet for the following purposes:

1. To obtain current information related to a health issue
2. To stay abreast of current legislation and regulations
3. To share experiences with other occupational health professionals
4. To search and "shop" for products and services to meet the needs of clients
5. To participate in research
6. To obtain continuing education
7. To market services to potential customers

D Although the Internet provides a vast source of information for consumers and practitioners, there are few standards to regulate the quality of information or the credibility of the suppliers of information.

E The following guidelines should be used by Internet users to assess health information available on the Internet:

1. Authors should be clearly identified.
2. Authors should be qualified and their credentials listed.
3. Professional references should be listed.
4. The site should not focus on the sale of services or products.
5. The site owners should indicate that the information offered is not a substitute for services provided directly by a trained professional caregiver.
6. A mechanism to request feedback or more information should be supplied.
7. Confidentiality must be ensured to individuals requesting information.
8. The appearance of the site should be professional.
9. Information provided should be current and the date of last revision noted.
10. Any sources of funding must be identified.
11. If the site is not supported by a government agency, it should bear a mark of recognition by one of several organizations that evaluate health information on the Internet, such as the American Medical Association or the Health on the Net Foundation.

V Intranets

A *Intranets* are private networks developed by companies, universities or other agencies to provide information and services to a prescribed audience using the same technology used on the Internet.

1. Owners of intranet systems prevent unauthorized access to information and services by installing software known as *firewalls*
2. A *firewall* is a software program that is used by owners of a local or wide area network to limit access to designated participants. For example, a company uses a firewall to ensure the security of its intranet and limit access to employees only.

B Companies use intranets to accomplish the following:

1. Centralize services, such as payroll and benefits
2. Allow employees access to company news and business information
3. Distribute information in a timely, efficient manner
4. Post and maintain business directives and policies in a central location
5. Foster the sharing of information among employees, business units, and organizations within the corporation.

C The manager of occupational health services may take advantage of the technology afforded by company intranets to accomplish the following purposes:

1. Distribute health related information to employees via department Web sites or electronic newsletters
2. Share relevant information with departments, such as Benefits, Safety, and Personnel
3. Centralize information such as health-related policies and procedures
4. Automate, expedite, and improve the accuracy of processes such as accident reporting
5. Deliver health related training to employees, and services such as interactive health-risk appraisals
6. Provide employees with links to important Internet sites that contain relevant health and safety information
7. Communicate and share information with external suppliers of services, such as insurance carriers, laboratories, independent medical examiners, or medical supply companies.

VI Office Management Programs

Office management programs represent another category of electronic tools available to the occupational and environmental health nurse.

A Used separately or in combination with health information systems, the Internet, or company intranets, the following office management programs are invaluable when refining information management techniques:

1. *Word processing programs,* such as Microsoft Word and WordPerfect, allow the occupational and environmental health nurse to create text documents, letters, reports, notices, etc.
2. *Spreadsheet programs* create files that allow large amounts of data to be captured, manipulated, and displayed in categorical fashion, such as budgets and other resource management documents.
3. *Relational database systems* allow information to be stored in fields and tables that can be sorted and reported in many combinations. These programs are often used to create forms and questionnaires such as health risk appraisals, training records, exposure questionnaires, and audits.
4. *Presentation programs* allow the occupational and environmental health nurse to create visually effective programs or slide presentations that may contain text, graphics, charts, tables, pictures, and sound. These programs are useful in developing reports, employee training programs, and professional presentations.

B *Communication systems,* including voice and electronic mail, enable the occupational and environmental health nurse to communicate rapidly and efficiently with peers and customers. Tools within this category include the following:

1. *Mail lists,* which allow the user to send the same message to a group of individuals simultaneously
2. *Folders,* which are repositories for saved mail messages on the same topic or from the same sender
3. *Directories,* which are electronic *address books* that enable the user of the mail system to capture and store information about individuals who are contacted often.

VII Implications for Occupational and Environmental Health Nursing

A The ability to manage information efficiently requires occupational and environmental health nurses to integrate information from many sources, including the following:

1. The client
   a. Health status
   b. Illness/injury experience
   c. Work history
   d. Intervention participation
   e. Training and education
2. The company
   a. Benefits information
   b. Salary and hours/shifts worked
   c. Job descriptions, including essential functions
   d. Insurance utilization and experience
   e. Administrative controls
3. Other occupational health and safety departments
   a. Industrial hygiene sampling activity
   b. Safety audits
   c. Personal protective equipment status
   d. Exposure history for individuals, groups, and the organization
   e. OSHA recordable injuries and illnesses
4. Regulatory, legislative, and guideline-setting agencies.
   a. Current regulations related to specific work, tasks, technology, conditions, and environmental agents
   b. Recommendations for addressing potential health and safety issues
   c. Guidelines for establishing effective programs and interventions
   d. Specifications of materials and equipment
   e. Information about specific agents, chemicals, or compounds
5. Outside providers of products and services
   a. Reports and recommendations of providers of clinical services
   b. Support for regulated programs, such as DOT drug testing (Chapters 3 and 14 provide additional information about such programs).
   c. Information from suppliers of health-related equipment and supplies
6. Academic and professional organizations
   a. Current research findings
   b. Literature related to the occupational health setting
   c. Networking with peers within the specialty of occupational health
   d. Advice and consultation about specific health issues
   e. Continuing education for occupational health professionals

B Occupational and environmental health nurses are often required to use a combination of tools to help manage occupational health units; these include the following:

1. Occupational health information systems
2. The Internet
3. Intranets
4. Office management programs

C Occupational and environmental health nurses must be attentive to the legal, ethical, and professional implications of using automated systems to manage occupational health information.

1. To safeguard the security and integrity of health information, the occupational and environmental health nurse must accomplish the following:
    a. Develop policies and procedures regarding the use of all electronic systems and equipment, including computers, fax systems, scanners, and mail systems
    b. Require that all employees with access to health records are trained in the management of health information
    c. Establish and impose penalties for the misuse of the information system and its contents
    d. Establish and maintain audit trails or records to keep track who accesses a record, and when and for what purpose it was accessed
    e. Back up information frequently and store backups in a separate, secure location
    f. Impose "locks" on electronic records that prevent changes to an entry after a predetermined period of time
2. To safeguard the confidentiality of employee health information, the occupational and environmental health nurse must accomplish the following:
    a. Establish and maintain lists of approved users, signatures, titles, and clearance levels, including the following information:
        1) Who may access a record
        2) Who may make an entry to a particular record
        3) Who may read a particular record
        4) Who may retrieve or transmit a record
        5) What fields within a record individuals may view
    b. Require that all employees with access to health records sign a "statement of protection of confidentiality"
    c. Block specific information or restrict access to those with a bona fide "need to know" and those on current user approval lists
    d. Establish and use client identifiers, such as employee numbers, for use during transmission of data
    e. Encode or encrypt sensitive information during transmission
    f. Use multilevel passwords to identify authorized users
    g. Change passwords often on an unscheduled basis

D To manage the transition from manual to automated systems, the occupational and environmental health nurse must accomplish the following:

1. Acknowledge the philosophical as well as the technical changes required
2. Involve as many staff members as practical in all stages of decision making, implementation, and maintenance of information management programs
3. Assess the initial and ongoing training needs of users
4. Recognize that different users learn and adapt at different rates
5. Support users and provide positive feedback for progress made
6. Monitor the benefits and savings of moving from manual to automated methods of managing information
7. Use the technology to highlight the advances being made by the occupational health organization

E Effective information management will increase the ability of the occupational and environmental health nurse to accomplish the following:
1. Manage resources more efficiently
2. Develop more appropriate, higher-quality interventions
3. Communicate more effectively
4. Make better clinical decisions

BIBLIOGRAPHY

Amann, M. (1999). Information management: Computer resources for the occupational and environmental health nurse. *AAOHN Journal, 47(12),* 574-583.

Amann, M. (1997). Occupational health information management systems. In M. Salazar (ed.), *AAOHN core curriculum for occupational health nursing* (pp. 107-112). Philadelphia: Saunders.

American Association of Occupational Health Nurses (1996). Employee health records: Requirements, retention, and access. *AAOHN Advisory.* Atlanta, GA: AAOHN Publications.

Barthel, C., Kalina, C., & Fitko, J. (1998). Business process design: Securing computerized health information files. *AAOHN Journal, 46(12),* 581-586.

Graves, J.R. & Corcoran, S. (1989). The study of nursing informatics. *Image: Journal of Nursing Scholarship, 21(4),* 227-231.

Internet Literacy Consultants Glossary of Internet Terms. (1999). http://www.matisse.net/files/glossary.html

Zielstorff, R., Hudgings, C., & Grobe, S. (1993). *Nest-generation nursing information systems: Essential characteristics for professional practice* (Publication No. NP-83). Washington, D.C.: American Nurses Publishing

Strategies and Approaches to Occupational and Environmental Health Nursing Practice

~

8

Developing, Implementing, and Evaluating a Comprehensive Occupational Health and Safety Program

Karin Myerson and Jane Parker-Conrad

The previous chapters have described the foundations of the occupational health and safety field. This information provides a framework for occupational and environmental health nursing practice. This chapter is intended to identify the strategic processes that are essential to the development, implementation, and evaluation of comprehensive occupational health and safety programs. Chapters 9 through 13 discuss in detail specific components of these programs, and Chapter 14 provides examples of programs that can be used as models in the occupational health setting. Comprehensive health and safety programs include surveillance programs mandated by OSHA standards (e.g., respiratory protection, bloodborne pathogens) and programs that impact the health and productivity of the worker population (e.g., injury/illness prevention programs and case management). Comprehensive health and safety programs are often designed to improve and protect both the work-related and non–work-related health of employees, retirees, and their families. The purpose of these programs is to "assist employees in promoting health, preventing illness, detecting disease at it's earliest stages and rehabilitation" (Wachs & Parker-Conrad, 1990).

I Assessment

Assessment is a process used to gather important health and safety information.

A **Assessment data are used for the following:**
1. Identify areas of need, value, or importance for health programs and topics.
2. Target health and safety behaviors.
3. Describe workers and the work environment.

B **Worker-related assessment may involve the following information:**
1. Description of work and home locations, and demographics of workers, dependents, and retirees
2. Health status of worker population, such as nutritional status, exercise habits, personal behaviors, and lifestyles related to risks (e.g., tobacco use)

3. Health insurance coverage and utilization to determine the major costs and number of health problems affecting workers, their families, and retirees
4. Disability information about type, severity, and cost, to assist in planning specific programs that will focus on early prevention or rehabilitation efforts

C **Environmental assessment at the work site identifies existing and potential health and safety hazards and organizational variables that may affect employees and thus call for special programs.**
1. Examples of work-related information to be collected include the following:
   a. Data concerning exposure to environmental hazards that may affect worker health and safety
   b. Worker injury and illness data
2. Occupational health services activity reports should be reviewed to identify the nature of services provided, who uses the services, and whether nonoccupational problems or concerns are overshadowing time spent on work-related issues or on problems that can be prevented.

D **Other categories of information for workplace assessment include the following (Travers & McDougall, 1995):**
1. Description of the company
   a. Standard Industrial Classification (SIC) Code
   b. Number and type of facilities
   c. Company vision and mission
   d. Organization's culture and values
2. Health service models already in place and available to employees
   a. Available health insurance options
   b. Description of on-site and vendor services
   c. Workers' compensation (self-insured, state funded, or other)
   d. Types of employee programs in place (e.g., employee assistance programs, wellness programs, light duty/alternative work programs)
   e. Safety committee
3. Information included in health records (daily logs, surveillance and monitoring data, disability information, and other)

E **Workplace assessment should include input from multiple sources; for example:**
1. Data from and consultation with other corporate occupational health and safety professionals in the fields of nursing, medicine, safety, and industrial hygiene
2. Data that can be obtained through an insurance company or an area university
3. Information obtained from external occupational medical consultation

F **Assessment tools**
1. The following tools can be used to gather information for the assessment:
   a. Questionnaires
   b. Health risk appraisals
   c. Workplace walk-through reports
   d. Employee health and safety records
   e. Case management reports
   f. Interviews with employees and management
   g. Health insurance claims
   h. Workers' compensation forms

    i. OSHA records/logs

    j. Life insurance records

    k. Medical utilization data

2. The specific tools one uses for the assessment depend on the nature of the initial workplace diagnosis and the factors that led to the original need for the assessment, the financial backing available, the program's goals, and the extent of the study.

3. It is important to determine the specific focus of an assessment; assessments may focus on the following:

    a. Workplace hazard analysis

    b. Health evaluation

    c. Behavior analysis or social concern

    d. Legal/regulatory program compliance issues

    e. Cost savings for the company

    f. Public relations/good will benefits

II Program Planning

Program planning is the recipe for implementing health services goals and objectives and is the blueprint or detailed guideline for directing activities and evaluating all programs and services conducted by or for the occupational health department. (Refer to AAOHN's *SuccessTools, Module Two: Developing Business Expertise,* Chapters 1-3, 1999b.) Program planning includes the following activities:

A **Analyze assessment data and target/prioritize areas where programs need to be developed to benefit the health of company employees.**

1. List strengths and limitations of the worker population and the organization.

2. Review computerized materials and organize data in a manner that will assist in decision making.

3. Select programs that will benefit most individuals and/or the organization's long-term goals (prioritize various data findings).

4. Clarify the process and activities that will provide benefits and assist in reaching short- and long-range goals.

B **Resource identification for program planning activities includes:**

1. *Personnel:* Determine the number and expertise of professionals and other employees needed to develop and implement specific programs. Are additional employees or consultants needed?

2. *Financial resources:* Develop a budget that will include all expenditures for each program.

    a. Divide budget into sections similar to current workplace yearly categories.

    b. Determine direct and indirect costs that will add to existing or expected expenditures.

    c. Identify potential sources of funding for programs and the ideal versus minimum costs required to complete each program.

3. *Equipment:* List the equipment needed for the implementation and final evaluation of the program. Examples include the following:

    a. Audiovisual materials, such as a television, videotape player, camcorder, audio tape recorder/player, and portable overhead projector

      b. Medical equipment and related expenses, such as pulmonary function measurement devices, syringes, needles, and materials for blood analysis and blood pressure measurement

      c. Computers and software needed to produce health risk appraisals, questionnaires, reports, program correspondence, and educational literature

      d. Other miscellaneous materials specific to the data collection, program implementation, or evaluation phase

4. *Supplies and other resources:* Determine what is needed to develop and implement a program.

      a. Obtain paper, computer and fax supplies, and mailing costs as required.

      b. Public relations and marketing may require brochures, posters, television ads, and special incentives (e.g., T-shirts and caps) that help ensure program participation and completion.

5. *Facilities and space* are important.

      a. Determine if in-house facilities are available and adequate or if outside space will be needed.

      b. Estimate the cost of using facilities, which may include heating, air conditioning, and lighting.

C Develop goals and objectives that blend with the organizational philosophy and company culture.

1. Goals and objectives should be developed before presenting a program plan to others for discussion and approval (Box 8-1).

      a. Goals should be presented in broad, general terms that state the expected results of implementing a program.

      b. Objectives are much more specific and should be presented as measurable, limited to a given time period, and relevant to attaining the goal.

2. A program begins with long-term, general goals for the health services department. Short-term objectives are developed to identify what must be accomplished to demonstrate achievement of long term goals.

3. Methods that will be used to accomplish goals and objectives should be identified in the planning phase, for example, educational activities, engineering controls, and administrative practices.

III Program Implementation

Following the planning and approval phases, *program implementation* begins.

A The implementation phase is the transition from program planning to putting the program into operation.

1. The program execution will involve progressive monitoring of activities, personnel, educational processes, and management support.

2. Timetables and schedules should be evaluated periodically to ensure operational success as the programs are developing and to identify who is responsible for their running according to schedule.

3. Progress can be monitored by routinely comparing completed activities with predetermined standards and assignments.

B Program implementation may be done either within the existing health services department or contracted to outside businesses in whole or part.

BOX 8-1

Examples of goals and objectives

Work-Related Program
Goal
To provide health and safety programs for employees to ensure compliance with all mandated Occupational Health and Safety Administration (OSHA) standards.
Objective 1
100% of employees will have recorded evidence that Hepatitis B immunization was provided or offered to all employees who are identified by their job category as having the potential for exposure to blood or blood products.
(Other objectives could target specific OSHA programs such as respiratory protection and hearing conservation)
Objective 2
The company will experience a 10% decrease in reportable injuries in the next 6 months after employees participate in education sessions on health and safety rules in their work area.

Personal Health and Safety Program
Goal
To provide opportunities for employees to participate in health promotion activities to increase their years of healthy life.
Objective 1
30% of employees who do not exercise will report that they participate in moderate daily physical exercise after participation in the exercise education program.
Objective 2
10% of employees who smoke will report that they have stopped smoking for 1 year after participation in the smoking cessation program.
(Other objectives could target specific health issues such as hypertension, weight control, or completion of recommended preventive health examinations after participation in specific health promotion programs offered by the company.)

There are positive and negative aspects of both in-house and vendor-contracted programs.

1. The "pros" of providing in-house programs include the following:
   a. In-house programs are convenient for the working population because they eliminate costly commuting time.
   b. The current staff knows the workplace—the workers, their jobs, and the company culture.
   c. Follow-up is easier for those who need second visits or who fail to show up for appointments.
   d. It is easier to use existing personnel.
2. Problems inherent in in-house programs include the following:
   a. Staff may be so busy with current job duties that they have little energy or motivation to take on additional program activities.
   b. Space for programs is often limited, and finding additional room may prove difficult.

      c. Existing personnel may lack the expertise, experience, or motivation required to conduct educational programs or to provide administration of broader health and safety programs.

    3. The "pros" of vendor-contracted health and safety programs include the following:

      a. Confidentiality (or the perception of it) may be easier to maintain, especially when there is a concern that assessment, utilization, or outcome data may endanger employees' job security.

      b. Interference with existing health services activities and setting priorities is less likely.

      c. Scheduling off-site programs, such as exercise programs, closer to workers' homes could improve program attendance.

    4. The problems inherent to vendor-contracted health and safety programs include the following:

      a. Extra costs may include contractor's travel time, overhead for employees, and nonproductive time spent in setting up programs.

      b. Contract employees do not share the same loyalty to the company as in-house workers and thus are not as vested in program outcomes or long-term program success.

C **Policies and procedures serve as guides to assist in achieving the goals and objectives of the health and safety programs.**

    1. Program policies and procedures provide direction and consistency for the implementation phase and can serve as the basis for program evaluation.

    2. Compliance with company and regulatory guidelines should be maintained with well-developed, well-written, and updated procedures.

      a. Procedures define specific steps or activities that must be followed, provide an excellent avenue for staff orientation, and ensure compliance with protocols and other activities.

      b. Procedures also provide legal backup for both nurse and company should a question arise regarding whether programs/activities are within the scope of practice, consistent with company policy, or compliant with national standards and expectations.

    3. Resources for policies and procedures are available through various agencies and organizations and are useful guidelines; however, these guides should be customized to reflect the goals and priorities of the company and its clients.

D **Barriers (in business environment) to implementation may include the following:**

    1. Political interests that are inconsistent with the program plan
    2. Seasonal variations in production and weather
    3. Union strikes and bargaining or territorial "turfs"
    4. Personnel changes, availability, and expertise
    5. Management changes leading to direction shifts
    6. Equipment delays, availability, or design flaws
    7. Lack of resources needed for implementation

IV The Evaluation Process

The *evaluation process* is used to identify and improve services provided by the occupational and environmental health nurse.

A Evaluation is an integral component of all phases of development and implementation of occupational health and safety programs.

B Methods of evaluation should be appropriate to program goals and objectives as they have been defined.

V Structure, Process, and Outcome

Donabedian (1966) developed the classic three-pronged approach to evaluation that provides an excellent framework for occupational health; the three prongs are *structure, process,* and *outcome* (Table 8-1).

A *Structural elements:* **Examples include management support; physical facilities; supplies and equipment; staff and health resources; worker demographics; and the mission, goals, and objectives to meet the health and safety needs of the work-site community.**

1. Review the management reporting structure and support for the occupational health program, including the following:
   a. Determine who the occupational and environmental health nurse reports to, administratively and professionally.
   b. Participate in the formulation and implementation of administrative procedures.
   c. Participate in the development of policies and procedures applicable to health issues (e.g., return to work, case management, fitness for duty).
   d. Develop the philosophy and written goals and objectives for the occupational health program.
   e. Conduct periodic reviews of the occupational health program to ensure that goals and objectives are being met.
   f. Participate in meetings that address health issues (e.g., safety, management staff, department, and human resource meetings).
   g. Communicate clearly and in writing with management and department heads as needed.
   h. Demonstrate the effectiveness of the health services department in terms of cost, productivity, and return on investment.
   i. Communicate workplace information-distribution lists, upcoming events, and plans to the occupational health staff.

TABLE 8-1

Structure, process, and outcomes: evaluative elements in quality assurance

Structural elements	Process elements	Outcome elements
Physical setting	Management of the operation	Improved health
Philosophy of health by management, employees, health care professionals	Decision-making processes	Compliance with treatment regimens
	Collaboration	Reduced morbidity and mortality
Organizational mission and structure	Nursing interventions/ monitoring	Positive changes in knowledge and attitudes about health
Unit goals and objectives	Services provided	
Human and financial resources	Development of records and reports	Satisfaction with service quality
Operational resources		

Source: Rogers, 1994.

2. Evaluate the suitability of physical facilities provided for the occupational health program; the following features are important:
   a. Central location with easy access for employees
   b. Accessible for ambulance stretchers and other wheeled traffic
   c. Sufficiently spacious to provide examination, treatment and consultation needs
   d. Confidentiality and privacy for clients and for the nurses to complete all aspects of work (telephone consults, examinations, etc.)
   e. Entrance clearly marked "Occupational Health Services" or "Health Unit"
   f. Sink and toilet facilities available and accessible
   g. Convenient and comfortable waiting area
   h. Adequate ventilation, heating, and air conditioning
   i. Access for separate telephone lines for fax, telephone, and computer
   j. Space to maintain supplies and medical records
3. Identify supplies and equipment used by the occupational health program.
   a. Supplies and medications appropriate for the practice are maintained in adequate supply, stored under proper conditions, and not kept beyond expiration dates.
   b. Appropriate medical equipment (e.g., refrigerator, oxygen, otoscope, sphygmomanometers) is available and in good working condition.
   c. Equipment used in performing examinations required by OSHA (e.g., audiometric booths, spirometer) is maintained and calibrated according to federal standards.
   d. Laboratory tests (e.g., cholesterol tests, drug specimen collection) are conducted in accordance with state and federal guidelines.
4. Identify staffing requirements, qualifications, and professional development recommendations.
   a. Copies of professional licenses and required certifications are kept for all staff.
   b. Copies of updated curriculum vitae or resumes are kept on file.
   c. Occupational health staff take advantage of opportunities to grow professionally and to advance the specialty of occupational and environmental health nursing.
   d. Attainment of occupational health nursing certification is supported and encouraged (Certified Occupational Health Nurse [COHN] or Certified Occupational Health Nurse-Specialist [COHN-S]).
   e. Nurses' active membership and involvement in AAOHN, including attendance at the annual American Occupational Health Conference, is encouraged and supported.
   f. Nurses' participation in professional development seminars designed to advance individual practice in occupational and environmental health nursing is supported and encouraged.
   g. Occupational health staff are encouraged to continue formal and informal education.
   h. Professional nursing journals and resources are available.
   i. Nursing responsibilities are defined in a position description. (AAOHN, 1997a)
5. Assess work-site community and ensure that programs, including those required by OSHA, are available to meet the needs of the workers.
   a. Work-force analysis: Number of workers and managers, median age of

population, approximate distribution of population by gender, number of accommodated (ADA-placed) employees on property, and health status of worker population

b. Health and safety hazards, exposures, and OSHA-required programs are identified (e.g., bloodborne pathogens, hearing conservation, respirator usage) (Papp & Miller, 2000).

6. Develop mission, goals, and objectives that meet the health and safety of the workers and the business needs of the company.
   a. Goals and objectives need to be regularly revised and updated.
   b. Mission, goals, and objectives should reflect current issues and practices in occupational health.

B *Process elements* **(e.g., delivery of nursing clinical practice; scope of services and programs; and documentation and recordkeeping abilities)**

1. Nursing clinical practice is appropriate for the occupational health setting, provided the following requirements are met:
   a. Clinical practice is consistent with the following:
      1) State Nurse Practice Act
      2) Pharmacy and Medical Practice Acts
      3) AAOHN Standards of Practice
      4) Published clinical practice guidelines
   b. A policy and procedure manual is written and reflects current occupational health practice.
   c. Occupational and environmental health nursing resources are used to guide clinical practice.

2. The scope of clinical services and programs are designed to meet the needs of the work-site community.
   a. Injury and illness management services include the following:
      1) Care and treatment of occupational injuries and illnesses
      2) Care and treatment of nonoccupational injuries and illnesses
      3) Emergency care for workers and visitors at the facility
      4) Supervision by a registered nurse over the nursing care of all workers
   b. Health promotion and screening programs
      1) Identify the health promotion programs that have been successfully delivered at the work site (e.g., back care, ergonomics, hearing/sight conservation, occupational dermatitis, self-care, hypertension screening).
      2) Evaluate formats used to offer programs (e.g., formal lecture, management meetings, informational pamphlet distribution, posters, and bulletin board or table displays (Chapter 12 provides additional information).
   c. Case management of occupational and nonoccupational injury and illness (including absenteeism) involves the following activities (Chapter 11 provides additional information):
      1) The nurse communicates and collaborates with managers, claims administrators, workers, and medical providers to facilitate appropriate, safe, and timely return to work.
      2) The nurse is familiar with the state's workers' compensation laws.
      3) The nurse reviews health care and response to treatment, including expected normal recovery times (The Medical Disability Advisor, 3rd edition, 1997 is a recommended resource).

4) The nurse recommends an independent medical evaluation when appropriate.
5) The nurse has a working knowledge of medical and health benefit programs offered by the employer.
6) The nurse, together with the manager, identifies temporary modified jobs that support treatment goals.
7) The nurse maintains contact with workers who have sustained an injury or illness.
8) The nurse evaluates workers who are absent from work for more than 5 days with non–work-related illness or injury.

d. Work-site tours for health and safety evaluation are conducted regularly.
1) Health and safety reports are used.
2) Nurse attends meetings of the safety committee to present findings.

e. OSHA surveillance programs, other required programs, and training sessions are completed. Examples: Drug testing for the Department of Transportation (DOT), hearing conservation, respirator approval (OSHA 2000)

f. Employee assistance program (EAP) and/or referrals are available to workers. The nurse is responsible for the following:
1) Identifying how EAP services are provided at the work site.
2) Assessing workers and referring them for appropriate treatment.

g. Immunization programs are offered for prevention, postexposure, and travel (e.g., hepatitis B, influenza, and tetanus

3. Emergency response planning is appropriate for the workplace needs. The program should include a Disaster Plan, Automatic External Defibrillator (AED) Program and First Aid/Responder Team.

a. Disaster Plan
1) Ensure that an emergency response/disaster plan is available.
2) Identify the employees responsible for coordinating and implementing the disaster plan within the facility (there should be a list).
3) Review the disaster plan, then test and revise it as needed.
4) Participate in the planning and implementation of the disaster plan.

b. AED Program
1) Ensure that the AED unit is approved by the U.S. Food and Drug Administration.
2) Ensure that procedures to meet state and local requirements are available.
3) Designate a nurse as the AED program coordinator.

c. First Aid/Responder Team
1) Determine whether the team includes employees at strategic locations and shifts to respond to medical emergencies.
2) Ensure that the first aid team is trained in CPR, first aid, bloodborne pathogens, and AED.
3) Review first aid logs to evaluate the effectiveness/appropriateness of care provided by the First Aid/Responder Team members.

4. Evaluate the documentation and recordkeeping system.
a. Evaluate the quality of documentation and recordkeeping to be sure records are appropriate and clear and that they meet legal reporting requirements.
b. Identify the type of system used for documentation (manual or computer), and ensure that the system has the following characteristics:
1) Documentation is timely and complete

2) Entries on the daily log reflect accurate documentation in the health record.
3) Daily logs are used to summarize clinical activity and trends to report to management.
4) All health records are secured in a locked cabinet.
5) Computerized records are secured by passwords, limiting access to occupational health staff only.
6) Health records are retained according to federal law (exposure records are to be retained for 30 years; health records are retained for the duration of employment plus 30 years).
7) Disclosure of information from a worker's health record is made only with written informed consent of the individual.
8) Work-related injuries and illnesses are shared with the employer only on a need-to-know basis
   c. Review OSHA forms, training logs, and other management reports related to the following:
1) Bloodborne pathogens training
2) Hearing conservation programs
3) Respiratory protection programs

C *Outcome elements:* **Evaluate whether the care provided to a single worker or population of workers achieved expected outcomes or that the processes used are likely to lead to positive outcomes**

1. Health outcomes include the following:
   a. Prevention of preventable illness and injury
   b. Increased compliance with treatment regimens
   c. Increased worker knowledge about self-care
   d. Restoration of function
      1) Physical functions—ambulation, lifting, etc.
      2) Psychological functions—memory, cognition, or mood
      3) Social function—interpersonal relationships, communication
      4) Role function—worker, parent, etc.
   e. Cure or retardation of disease, such as an infection or hypertension
   f. Relief of discomfort
      1) Physical discomfort, such as pain
      2) Psychological discomfort, such as depression
2. Health care outcomes are compared with the cost of health services so that judgments about the value of the health care services can be made for the company. Some examples follow:
   a. Work-site Influenza Immunization Program (immunize healthy adults against influenza to reduce absenteeism)
      1) *Outcome:* The company will have a healthier work force resulting in less absenteeism and improved productivity.
      2) *Cost savings:* A study by Nichol (AAOHN, 1999a) determined a return on investment of $47/employee for their flu immunization program.
   b. Breast Cancer Screening Program (most common malignancy among women in the United States and second leading cause of cancer death) (Caplan & Coughlin, 1998)
      1) *Outcome:* Breast cancer education in the workplace has been shown to have a positive effect on women's knowledge of, and attitudes toward, breast cancers, and on breast self-examination and mammography practices.

2) *Cost savings:* By detecting early malignancies, breast cancer screening reduces mortality in women between the ages of 50 and 69. These programs will result in long-term health savings for the company.
c. Case management (workers' compensation and disability cases)
1) *Outcome:* The most commonly reported outcome of the case management program is the workers' return to work. Quality outcomes such as workers' quality of life and well being after an injury and employee's satisfaction (obtained through interviews) are also important factors to report.
2) *Cost savings:* Lost time and medical costs of case managed cases are often reported as decreased in comparison with non–case-managed cases. It should be noted that Salazar and Graham (1999) reported that there are varied opinions related to the cost effectiveness of case management services, primarily because of the anecdotal nature of case examples. Case management services sometimes may increase cost, but less tangible benefits may justify case management interventions.
3. The measurement of health outcomes begins at the individual level; many individual outcomes may be pooled to assess factors of interest across worker groups.
4. The relationship between good health outcomes and interventions is complex.
a. What nurses do and how well they do it only partially account for a worker's health outcome.
b. It is often impossible to definitively attribute a specific outcome to the performance of the nurse.
c. Other worker-related and community-related factors effect outcomes.
d. The closer in time the measured outcome is to the provided treatment, the more likely it is attributable to the nurse.
1) Outcomes that occur immediately after an intervention are the most likely to be attributable to the treatment (immediate outcome).
2) Outcomes that occur following the nursing intervention, though not immediately, may be related to the treatment (intermediate outcome).
3) An outcome of a nursing intervention that occurs 2 to 5 years following the initial episode of injury or illness is the most difficult to attribute to that treatment (long-term outcome).

VI Methods of Evaluation

A **Techniques for gathering information**
1. Retrospective chart audit
a. Focuses on documented evidence of nursing care provided.
b. Assumes that what is documented is what has been performed.
2. Concurrent document review
a. Critical examination of case management (while care is in progress) and of client outcomes
b. Review of chart, plans for care, immediate feedback
3. Interviewing
a. Verbal interaction: clarifying questions, attitudes, opinions, client satisfaction, and management understanding of health care
b. Important to word questions consistently from worker to worker to decrease bias

4. Questionnaire
   a. Most commonly used tool for program evaluation
   b. Important to write questions clearly and to provide clear directions for completion
5. Observation
   a. Observation of nursing practice related to physical assessment skills, such as occupational history taking, medication administration practices, and treatment plans
   b. Opportunity to provide immediate feedback and validate procedure manual for appropriateness and to determine the relationship of outcomes to actual nursing practices

B **Conducting a quality review**
1. In corporate settings with a number of nurses, a quality-assurance program can be developed by the nurses and used at several different sites.
2. In settings where nurses work alone, develop a quality-review team of interested peers located nearby or form a team of occupational and environmental health nurses representing local AAOHN constituencies.
3. Develop and customize an evaluation tool to identify the specific needs of your company's occupational health program.
4. Use an evaluation tool that reflects current practice in occupational health as a framework to develop your own evaluation tool; consult, for example, AAOHN's *Guidelines for an Occupational Health and Safety Service* (Travers & McDougall, 1995), which provides a comprehensive quality assurance audit tool.

VII Cost-Effective and Cost-Benefit Programs

A **Purposes of cost evaluation**
1. Management's goal for developing or maintaining occupational health services and programs is often to contain costs.
2. Cost-benefit and cost-effectiveness analyses can be used to demonstrate the cost effectiveness of the overall program and the cost benefit of its specific components.
3. Health conditions and safety problems that are having a significant impact on the company's "bottom line" should be targeted for program development, followed by cost-benefit analyses.
4. Cost-effectiveness analysis and cost-benefit analysis are convincing tools for communicating with upper management (refer to AAOHN's *Success Tools, Module One: Measuring and Articulating Value*, 1998).

B **Definition of terms**
1. "*Cost-benefit analysis* looks at return on investment" (AAOHN, 1996).
   A cost-benefit analysis has the following characteristics:
   a. Considers both costs and benefits (or outcomes) of a program in monetary terms
   b. Permits a comparison between unlike elements.
   c. Yields a benefit-to-cost ratio.
2. *Cost-effectiveness analysis* is used to determine which activities or interventions, given alternative approaches, will achieve the program objective and yield the most value or greatest impact on cost" (AAOHN, 1996).

C **Why do a cost analysis?**
1. Cost-benefit and cost-effectiveness analyses, which help determine which

programs or services can produce a benefit that is greater than the cost, are helpful because many administrators are not aware of the true potential of health services or programs for the company or their workers.

2. Demonstrating short-term and long-term costs and benefits
   a. Find cause-and-effect relationships between programs and benefits as noted above, and project how the organization can gain from effective programming in these areas.
   b. Categorize, quantify, and compare benefits and costs.
      1) *Short-term benefits* may include increased morale, productivity, and corporate image.
      2) *Long-term benefits* may include decreased health and life insurance costs, decreased workers' compensation claims, and decreased employee turnover.
      3) *Short-term costs* involve commitment of space, resources, supplies, and equipment, and organizational time and involvement.
      4) *Long-term costs* can include time for participation of management and workers and the ongoing cost of utilities and program maintenance expenses.
   c. Determine the areas of greatest program impact, such as physical impairments, workers' compensation claims, or public relations.
   d. Compare program costs with those of other current company programs and determine how this program compares with their costs and benefits.
   e. Ask whether the proposed health and safety program is a good investment and worthy of everyone's time and effort.
   f. A documentation of workers' compensation costs may help to demonstrate the need for work-related programs in the organization.

D Steps in conducting cost-benefit and cost-effectiveness analyses (AAOHN, 1996).
   1. Determine the program/service for financial analysis.
   2. Formulate the objectives and goals of the program/service.
   3. List alternative ways objectives and goals can be achieved.
   4. Determine costs/benefits for all alternatives.
   5. Determine monetary values for costs/benefits, or determine outcome measures (e.g., absenteeism rates; health services utilization; changes in risk behaviors).
   6. Calculate discounting
      a. Discounting reduces future costs to their present worth.
      b. It answers the question: "What is the cost of providing this service now compared with what it will cost in the future?"

E Resources
   1. See AAOHN *SuccessTools, Module One: Measuring & Articulating Value*, 1998, for specific program examples of determining cost-benefit and cost-effectiveness analysis.
   2. See Guidelines for an Occupational Health and Safety Service (Travers & McDougall, 1995) for a case study on cost effectiveness.

VIII Other Health and Safety Program Considerations

Occupational and environmental health nurses who are actively involved in planning and developing health and safety programs will need to explore many issues to ensure program success and participation.

A Issues that should be addressed in health and safety programs include confidentiality, legal aspects, involvement of advisory committees, and management support.

1. The confidentiality of information collected from or about employees is a major concern, especially as it relates to personal health data, because employees often fear that this information may be used to punish or dismiss them or otherwise endanger their employment.

2. Legal concerns include the company's liability for employees if they become injured when participating in company-sponsored health programs such as Fun Runs and Health Fairs.

3. The involvement of a health and safety advisory committee in program planning, implementation, and evaluation is mandatory.
   a. Labor *and* management representation and input are necessary to ensure the success of programs.
   b. A committee is instrumental in suggesting topics, obtaining peer support, identifying barriers, and identifying resources.

4. Management support must be garnered early in the planning stages to approve the program's financing, workers' involvement, and the program's relevance for the workplace, and to take into account other political and philosophical considerations.

B Occupational and environmental health nurses should consider using a business approach to health and safety program development because the language of business is more easily understood by management; in addition, a *business plan* is helpful in setting up programs and their monitoring success.

1. A business plan can serve the following functions:
   a. Provide an overview of the services included in the comprehensive occupational health and safety program.
   b. Guide the program in its implementation and evaluation.
   c. Provide guidelines for identifying resources required to implement a program.
   d. Communicate ideas and approaches to management and unions.

2. A business plan should be tailored to the individual needs of the organization and the program; the basic components of a business plan are as follows (Helmer, et al., 1995):
   a. *Executive summary:* Summarizes the plan, including the projected return on the investment (ROI).
   b. *Purpose of plan:* Explains what is to be accomplished with the plan.
   c. *Ground rules:* Provides guidelines for the plan by identifying constraints, limitations, and resources; a glossary is needed so there is a common understanding.
   d. *Approach:* Describes how and when the plan will be implemented.
   e. *Requirements:* Describes the specific outcomes that must be accomplished as a result of the plan.
   f. *Scope of work:* Precisely describes the nature of tasks related to the plan, including who is responsible for each task.
   g. *Schedule:* Provides timelines to serve as target dates for each stage of the implementation of the plan.
   h. *Financial:* May be framed as a profit and loss statement; "An accurate projection of costs. . . strengthens the plan and demonstrates to key decision makers that one is serious about the company's 'bottom line'" (Helmer, et al., 1995).

BIBLIOGRAPHY

American Association of Occupational Health Nurses. (1996). *Cost benefit and cost effectiveness analyses (AAOHN Advisory).* Atlanta, GA: AAOHN.

American Association of Occupational Health Nurses. (1997a) *Guidelines for developing job descriptions in occupational & environmental health nursing.* Atlanta, GA: AAOHN Publications.

American Association of Occupational Health Nurses. (1997b). Developing clinical guidelines or protocols for practice. *AAOHN Journal, 45(10)* [Advisory insert].

American Association of Occupational Health Nurses. (1998). *SuccessTools: Strategies for thriving and surviving in business (Module one: Measuring and articulating value).* Atlanta, GA: AAOHN Publications.

American Association of Occupational Health Nurses. (1999a). *SuccessTools: Strategies for thriving and surviving in business (Module two: Developing business expertise).* Atlanta, GA: AAOHN Publications.

American Association of Occupational Health Nurses. (1999b). *Standards of occupational health nursing practice.* Atlanta, GA: AAOHN Publications.

Burton, W.N., Conti, D.J., Chen, C.Y., Schultz, A.B., & Edington, D.W. (1999). The role of health risk factors and disease on worker productivity. *Journal of Occupational and Environmental Medicine, 41(10),* 863-877.

Caplan, L.S. & Coughlin, S.S. (1998) Worksite breast cancer screening programs: A review. *AAOHN Journal, 46(9),* 443-451.

Childre, F. (1997). Nurse managed occupational health services: A primary care model in practice. *AAOHN Journal, 45(10),* 484-490.

Donabedien, A. (1966). Evaluating the quality of medical care. *Milbank Fund Quarterly, 44(3),* 166-206.

Gorksy, R.D., Williamson, D.F., Shaffer, P.A., & Koiplan, J.P. (1996). The 25-year health care costs of women who remain overweight after 40 years of age. *American Journal of Preventive Medicine, 12(3),* 388-394.

Heirich, M. & Dieck, C.J. (2000). Worksite cardiovascular wellness programs as a route to substance abuse prevention. *Journal of Occupational and Environmental Medicine, 42(1),* 47-56.

Helmer, D.C., Dunn, L.M., Eaton, K., Macedonio, C., & Lubritz, L. (1995). Implementing corporate wellness programs: A business approach to program planning. *AAOHN Journal, 43(11),* 558-563.

Hughes, K.J., Glattly, J., & Kelly, D.R. (1998). A stay-at-work plan for injured employees. *Nurse Manager, 29(8),* 42-43.

Konstantinos, K. & Cerspo, J. (1998). Cost-effective hospital based occupational health services: Successful program. *AAOHN Journal, 46(3),* 127-131.

Lukes, E. & Johnson, M. (1999). Hearing conservation: an industry-school partnership. *Journal of School Nursing, 15(2),* 22-25.

Melhorn, M.L., Wilkinson, L., Gardner, P., Horst, W.D., & Silkey, B. (1999). An outcomes study of an occupational medicine intervention program for the reduction of musculoskeletal disorders and cumulative trauma disorders in the workplace. *Journal of Occupational and Environmental Medicine, 421(10),* 833-846.

Meservy, D., Bass, J., & Weldonna, T. (1997). Health surveillance : Effective components of a successful program. *AAOHN Journal, 45(10),* 500-512.

Mignone, J. & Guidotti, T.L. (1999). Support groups for injured workers: Process & outcomes. *Journal of Occupational and Environmental Medicine, 41(12),* 1059-1064.

Occupational Safety and Health Administration (2000). *Screening and Surveillance: A Guide to OSHA Standards.* (OSHA 3162). Washington DC: U. S. Government Printing Office.

O'Donnell, M.P. & Ainsworth, T., (Eds.). (1994). *Health promotion in the workplace.* Albany, NY: Delmar.

Papp, E.M. & Miller, A.S. (2000). Screening and surveillance: OSHA's medical surveillance provisions. *AAOHN Journal, 48(2),* 59-72.

Parker-Conrad, J.E. (1997). Nurse managed occupational health centers: Quality nursing care by occupational health nurses (editorial). *AAOHN Journal, 45(10),* 475-476.

Price, M., Duplessie, K, & Powers, B. (1997). Nurse managed occupational health services without on-site clinical care delivery. A case example. *AAOHN Journal, 45(10),* 496-499.

Quick, J.C. (1998), Introduction to the measurement of stress at work. *Journal of Occupational Health Psychology, 3(5),* 291-293.

Rogers, B. (1994). *Occupational health nursing: Concepts and practice.* Philadelphia: W.B. Saunders.

Rogers, B. (2000). Occupational health surveillance, screening, and prevention. Activities in occupational health nursing practice. *AAOHN Journal, 48(2),* 92-99.

Rogers, B., Randolph, S.A., & Mastroianni, K. (1996*). Occupational health nursing guidelines for primary clinical conditions* (2nd ed.). Boston: OEM Press.

Salazar, M.K. & Graham, K.Y. (1999). Evaluation of a case management program: Summary and integration of findings. *AAOHN Journal, 47(9),* 416-423.

Salazar, M.K., Takaro, T.K., Ertell, K. Gochfeld, M., O'Neill, S.O., Connon, C., & Barnhart, S. (1999). Structure and function of occupational health services within selected department of energy sites. *Journal of Occupational and Environmental Medicine, 41(12),* 1072-1078.

Simonowitz, J.A., (2000). The occupational and environmental health nurse and health surveillance. (Editorial). *AAOHN Journal, 48(2),* 56-58.

Simpson, S.J. (1997). Strategies for comprehensive nurse managed occupational health services: Focusing on work related health problems while maintaining comprehensive care delivery. *AAOHN Journal, 45(10),* 491-495.

Stone, D.S. (2000). Health surveillance for health care workers: A vital role for the occupational and environmental health nurse. *AAOHN Journal, 48(2),* 73-79.

Task force on Community Preventive Services (2000). Introducing the guide to community preventive services. *American Journal of Preventive Medicine. A supplement. 18(1S),* 1-142.

Travers, P.H. & McDougall, C. (1995). *Guidelines for an occupational health and safety service.* Atlanta: AAOHN Publications.

Tsai, J.H., Salazar, M.K., Graham, K.Y., & Grines, J. (1999). Case management for injured workers. A descriptive study using a record review. *AAOHN Journal, 47(9),* 405-415.

U.S. Department of Health and Human Services & Agency for Health Care Policy and Research. (1995). *Using clinical practice guidelines to evaluate quality of care.* AHCPR Pub. No. 95-0046, Vol. 1 and 2. Washington, DC: DHSS.

Wachs, J.E., (1997). Nurse Managed Occupational health centers. *AAOHN Journal, 45(10),* 477-483.

Wachs, J.E. & Parker-Conrad, J.E. (1990). Occupational health nursing in 1990 and the coming decade. *Applied Occupational and Environmental Hygiene, 5(4),* 200-204.

Werner, K.E., Smith, R.J., Smith, D.G., & Fries, B.E. (1996). Health and economic implications of a work-site smoking-cessation program: a simulation analysis. *Journal of Occupational and Environmental Medicine, 38(11),* 981-992.

CHAPTER

9

Prevention of Occupational Injuries and Illnesses

MARILYN HAU

The prevention of occupational illness and injury requires an in-depth knowledge of the work environment and the appropriate skills to recognize and identify actual and potential hazards, evaluate these hazards, and institute appropriate control measures. Prevention and control are on-going processes, requiring continual assessment and evaluation, and the development and refining of programs. This chapter provides a broad overview of techniques and strategies that can be adapted for a variety of health and safety programs. It is the responsibility of occupational and environmental health nurses to determine the particular needs of their organizations and to tailor those programs to their setting.

Recognition and identification

In order to recognize and identify occupational health and safety hazards, occupational and environmental health nurses must know their workplaces and the nature of the work performed; they also need to appreciate the unique attributes, including the risk factors, which may characterize the worker population.

I First Steps in a Prevention Program

The first two steps in a work-site program to prevent illness or injury of the workers are: (1) the recognition or anticipation of hazards, and (2) the clear identification of hazards.

A *Recognition* **is the process of detecting workplace hazards.**

B *Anticipation* **is the foresight to recognize and eliminate hazards in equipment and processes during the planning, process review, and design stages.**

C *Identification* **is the process of defining, describing, and classifying hazards.**

D *Hazard* **is "the potential for harm or damage to people, property, or the environment" (Manuele, 1994).**

   1. Workplace hazards may be classified as physical, chemical, biologic, environmental/mechanical, and psychosocial.

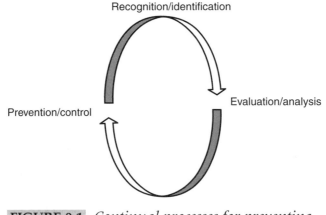

FIGURE 9-1 *Continual processes for preventing injuries and illnesses*

2. Recognizing and identifying hazards requires knowledge of the workers, work site, work practices and processes, and industrial materials used.
3. Sources of information regarding hazards include knowledgeable company representatives; health and safety professionals; professional publications and courses; and direct observation of production processes and workers' activities.

E The overall goal of a prevention program is to recognize and identify hazards, evaluate and analyze these hazards, and select and implement preventive and control measures as a continual process (Fig. 9-1).

II Methods of Identifying Hazards

A A *site survey,* or *walk-through,* is a work-site inspection not related to any particular incident, work area, or piece of equipment.
1. Purpose: to identify unsafe conditions and practices, including items not in compliance with local, state, and federal regulations, including OSHA standards (Box 9-1).
2. Types of walk-through inspections
   a. *Informal inspection:* focuses on routine work, such as inspecting and testing equipment at the beginning of each shift
   b. *Formal inspection:* performed periodically by a team of occupational health and safety professionals; scheduled at convenient times; includes a written report of findings
   c. *General inspection:* may be conducted to ensure compliance with legal requirements or for insurance purposes, corporate or union audits, and fire code compliance
3. A *site survey* follows the flow of work from the beginning to end.
4. A checklist is used to guide the inspection: inspection checklists should be site specific rather than generic.
5. Preinspection activities may include the following:
   a. Determination of inspection time
   b. Meeting with managers and supervisors
   c. Review of previous inspection and accident reports, material safety data sheets, and other relevant records and reports

---

BOX 9-1

A few examples of what to inspect during a site survey

- Atmospheric conditions: dusts, vapors, odors
- Illumination: general and workstations
- First aid and emergency units: eye-wash stations, deluge showers
- Containers: labeling, flammable liquid, waste
- Supplies and materials: caustics, acids, poisons, compressed gases, cryogenics, oxidizers, flammable or spontaneously combustible materials
- Buildings and structures: windows, aisles, floors, stairs, exit signs
- Electrical hazards: extension cords, outlet usage, cord condition, electric gear clearance, shock hazards

- Fire fighting equipment: fire extinguishers, sprinkler systems, standpipes, accessibility, alarms, and testing procedures
- Machinery: guarding of moving parts and pinch points, barrier safety shields, proximity switches, automatic shutoffs
- Material handling: lifting devices, conveyors, lift truck operations, cranes, hoists
- Personal protective equipment: clothing, safety glasses, chemical goggles, gloves, safety shoes, hard hats
- Work practices: eating at the work-station, personal hygiene, adherence to safe operating procedures, housekeeping

---

Source: National Safety Council, 1992

   d. Gathering of essential personal protective equipment needed at site
   e. Gathering of checklists, sampling devices, and other items needed for the inspection
6. Inspection activities may include the following:
   a. Explanation of procedure to supervisors at inspection sites
   b. Observation of employees' work practices
   c. Recording of unsafe conditions and practices, including items out of compliance with OSHA standards
   d. Identification of problems and their causes
   e. Commendation of supervisor and workers when conditions are noted to be safe
   f. Corrective action if an immediate danger, such as a blocked exit, is noted
7. Postinspection activities may include:
   a. Meeting with managers and supervisors
   b. A long-term analysis based on data from both current and previous inspections
   c. Preparation of report
   d. Circulation of report, which should include recommendations for possible solutions and correction priorities
8. Establish an audit system to periodically check for corrected and unresolved problems.

B *Focused inspections* are conducted periodically for the following purposes: to inspect specific processes, equipment, or areas; to investigate an accident;

to evaluate a reported health or safety hazard; or to respond to complaints of such things as a strange odor or loud noise.

1. Individuals or multidisciplinary teams with in-depth knowledge of the process or area should conduct the inspection.
2. Critical parts or operations usually require more-frequent inspections (e.g., light switches, safety valves, cables, belts, fire extinguishers, eyewash stations, or exhaust hoods).
3. Some focused inspections are legally mandated (e.g., elevators, autoclaves, and boilers).
4. A checklist can serve as a useful guide to a focused inspection (Figure 9-2).

C A *records review* or audit may be done alone or as a supplement to other methods of hazard identification.

1. Record audits have the following purposes:
   a. Identify work-site hazards
   b. Better acquaint the occupational and environmental health nurse with the site
   c. Provide historical data for trend analysis and epidemiologic study
   d. Ensure compliance with OSHA standards
2. Although records may indicate the absence or inadequate control of work-site hazards, the recorded information may not reflect the actual circumstance.
3. The following records may be helpful:
   a. Records concerning production and quality-control problems

Electric Forklift Daily Checklist	Truck No.:			Ser. No.:		Check before each shift.			
Date:									
Hour Meter:									
Driver:									
Visual/operation checks	OK	Not OK	OK	Not OK	OK	Not OK	OK	Not OK	OK	Not OK
Obvious damage/leaks									
Tire condition									
Battery plug connect									
Warning lights									
Battery discharge meter									
Horn									
Steering									
Foot brake									
Parking brake									
Hydraulic controls									
Fork operation									
Battery water level									
Seat belts									
Fire extinguisher									
Repairs needed:									
Comments:						Add additional comments on the back			

FIGURE 9-2 *Focused checklist for electric forklift*

Source: Ohio Division of Safety and Hygiene, 1995.

  b. Workers' compensation claims
  c. Employee assistance program utilization reports
  d. Personnel records, including absentee records and job histories
  e. Written hazard-control programs, training records, and records concerning fit-testing and distribution of personal protective equipment
  f. Safety surveys, inspection reports, and exposure monitoring reports
  g. Machine and equipment maintenance logs
  h. Emission and process records
  i. System monitoring and alarm test records
  j. Plans for disaster preparedness and emergency response
  k. Designs and reviews of new or planned facilities, processes, materials, or equipment
  l. Written complaints from workers and minutes of the safety committee meetings
  m. OSHA recordkeeping forms
  n. Other site-specific records that may be identified and examined if deemed appropriate

D *Job hazard analysis*, **also called** *job safety analysis*, **is the process of studying and recording each step of a job to identify existing and potential health and safety hazards and to determine the best way to perform the job to reduce or eliminate these hazards.**

1. Set priorities: begin with the jobs with the highest rates of accident and disabling injuries, jobs where "close calls" have occurred, new jobs, and jobs where changes have been made in processes and procedures.
2. Assess the general conditions under which the job is performed, using a checklist if applicable. Then do the following:
  a. List each step of the job in order of occurrence as you watch the worker performing the job, recording enough information to describe each job action.
  b. Examine each step to determine the existing or potential hazards.
  c. Repeat the job observation as often as necessary until all hazards have been identified.
  d. Review each hazard or potential hazard with the worker performing the job to determine whether the job could be performed in a safer way or whether safety equipment and precautions are needed.
  e. List exactly each new step or method, and identify exactly what the worker needs to know to perform the job safely.
  f. Avoid general warnings such as "be careful."
3. Recommend safe procedures and corrections, including:
  a. Developing a training program
  b. Redesigning equipment, changing tools, adding guards, improving ventilation, or using personal protective equipment
  c. Reducing the necessity or frequency of performing the job
4. Repeat and revise the job hazard/job safety analysis periodically and after an accident or injury. Figure 9-3 presents an example of a job safety analysis form.
5. A job hazard/job safety analysis provides the following benefits (National Safety Council, 1992):
  a. Improves worker hazard awareness.
  b. Increases worker safety training and supervisor/worker communication.
  c. Enhances identification of root causes of accidents.

Job Safety Analysis	Job:		Date:	
Title of worker who performs job:	Foreman/supervisor:		Analysis by:	
Specific work location:	Section:		Reviewed by:	
Required and/or recommended personal protective equipment:				
Sequence of basic job steps	Potential accidents or hazards		Recommended safe job procedures	

FIGURE 9-3 *Job safety analysis form*

Source: Ohio Division of Safety and Hygiene, 1995.

    d. Serves as a valuable tool for ergonomic studies.

    e. Increases the thoroughness of machine inspections.

    f. Helps train new supervisors in unfamiliar jobs.

    g. Determines physical and mental requirements necessary for job performance, a necessity in evaluating job candidates with disabilities.

E *Incident analyses* **are fact-finding procedures to identify the pertinent factors that allow accidents or near misses to occur so similar future incidents can be prevented. A** *near miss* **is an incident that could have resulted in injury or property damage under different circumstances. It should be evaluated to prevent recurrence and a more serious outcome.**

    1. The first step in an incident analysis is to identify immediate causes; this is accomplished via the following steps:

        a. Interviewing workers and collecting physical evidence, including results of any applicable drug screening or alcohol testing, as soon as possible after an accident

        b. Inspecting the scene of the accident or near miss and recording relevant details, using photographs, drawings, and measurements

        c. Interviewing witnesses in private

        d. Being alert to the possibility of attempts to hide injuries or facts because of fear of reprisal, poor evaluations, ruining safety records, discovery of substance abuse, embarrassment, or of implicating others

   e. Using the company's incident investigation form to avoid omitting information
   f. Trying to quote workers' statements in their exact words
   g. Staying objective, avoiding biased statements or questions
2. "Some of the 'root causes' [of incidents] may be:
   a. Lack of management support for safety
   b. Failure to positively reinforce or reward safe behaviors
   c. Lack of preventive maintenance programs
   d. Production output stressed over safety
   e. Low worker morale
   f. Unqualified trainers
   g. Lack of job safety analysis
   h. No assigned responsibility for a function
   i. Unsafe work behaviors without accident experience
   j. Peer values
   k. Poor supervisor/management example" (AAOHN, 1995)
3. Workplace factors that often contribute to incidents include procedures, facilities, communication patterns, and behaviors (Box 9-2).
4. The following benefits are derived from an incident analysis:
   a. Increases health and safety awareness for workers and supervisors
   b. Establishes better rapport between the occupational and environmental health nurse, supervisor, and injured or ill worker
   c. Provides data that can be used for an overall safety program evaluation and prevention of future incidents
   d. Provides essential facts for workers' compensation, OSHA recordkeeping, and insurance claims, such as company fire insurance

F An *incident historical review* is the compilation and analysis of incidents and near misses that have occurred over a selected period of time.
1. Categories of incidents include the following:
   a. Incidents related to specific seasons
   b. Incidents occurring on a particular shift
   c. Incidents occurring to a specific group of workers
   d. Incidents occurring at a specific location or within a specific process
2. The review begins with an analysis of incidents and trends in incidents through review of the following relevant records:
   a. OSHA forms
   b. Safety committee minutes
   c. Accident, incident, or near-miss reports
   d. Logs of daily health service visits
   e. Other periodic reports and records of the health and safety service
   f. Comparison of incident rates with those in similar industries (Box 9-3 presents formulas for calculating incident rates.)
3. The following factors should be considered when evaluating incident trends:
   a. Worker's attitudes **and** behavior: impatience, boredom, recklessness, feeling rushed (as those paid for piecework), insufficiently trained, upset by shift work
   b. Management's attitudes and behavior: emphasis on production over safety, failure to identify hazards and perform corrective actions, failure to enforce safe behavior

BOX 9-2

Examples of immediate causes of incidents

Procedures
nonexistent, not followed, not trained in, not understood, not accurate, impossible to follow

Facilities/Tools/Equipment
personal protective equipment failure, improper design, nonergonomic design, wear/deterioration, lack of proper equipment, poor housekeeping, process equipment failure, missing guards or safety devices

Hazards
manmade, natural source, documented but not repaired, unidentified, identified but accepted, inadequately repaired, presenting a "challenge" to workers

Communication
inadequate planning; breakdown in communication between co-workers, between workers and supervisors, or between contractor and company; confused communications; lack of warning signs; language barriers; illiteracy

Behavior
rushed by supervision, co-worker competition, motivation to finish early, taking shortcuts, no teamwork, heavy client workload, bonus incentives, medication effects, boredom, fatalistic "it can't happen to me" attitude, unauthorized smoking/eating, inattention/distraction, fear of asking for help

Training
none, insufficient, safe work practices not addressed in training, training applied incorrectly, no hands-on training, inadequate follow-up, need for refresher training, training not site-specific

Other Factors
fatigue, lack of sleep, illness, physical stress, repetitive motion, fright, physical incapability, disrupted circadian rhythms because of shift work

Source: AAOHN, in press.

BOX 9-3

Incidence rate calculation

$$\text{Incidence rate} = \frac{\text{Number of new cases/year} \times 200{,}000 \text{ work hours per facility*}}{\text{Number of hours worked at facility/year}}$$

*200,000 work hours is equivalent to 100 employees working 40 hours per week, 50 weeks per year. (Multiplying by 200,000 allows one to compare rates with those of other companies and is a more readily understood number.)

or

$$\text{Incidence rate} = \frac{\text{Number of new cases/year} \times 200{,}000 \text{ work hours}}{\text{Number of people at facility} \times 2000 \text{ hours†}}$$

†2000 hours = 40 hours/week × 50 weeks of work/year

c. Work environment deficiencies: poor lighting, inadequate ventilation, obsolete equipment

G *Chemical inventories* **and** *material safety data sheets* **provide critical information for workers and employers**
   1. They are required by the OSHA 29 CFR 1910.1200 Hazard Communication Standard. (Certain laboratories are required to comply with a similar standard: 29 CFR 1910.1450, which is specific to laboratories.)
   2. They are useful for estimating potential hazards associated with raw materials, products, and other hazardous substances present in the facility.

H *Employee perception surveys/questionnaires* **involve workers directly in hazard recognition and identification; this is important, because the worker most directly involved with the work process often provides insight not otherwise obtained.**
   1. They are most accurate when conducted by an independent, unbiased third party.
   2. They should consist of questions that have been researched and field-tested for reliability.
   3. Results should be shared so all workers may benefit from their co-workers' insight.

I *Process safety reviews* **consist of evaluations performed on activities involving chemicals, including using, storing, manufacturing, handling, or moving chemicals at the site.**
   1. Information is gathered on the hazards of the chemicals, technology, and equipment used in a process, allowing health and safety staff to perform the following activities:
      a. Identify the hazards of new and changed processes
      b. Evaluate processes reviewed within the past 5 years
      c. Review processes related to incidents that had a potential for catastrophic consequences
   2. Process safety reviews serve as a means of determining what could go wrong and what safeguards must be implemented to prevent hazardous chemical releases.
   3. The reviews are mandated by the EPA 40 CFR* Part 68: "Worst Case Scenario" section, and the OSHA 29 CFR 1910.119: Process Safety Management of Highly Hazardous Chemicals for:
      a. Industries using any of more than 130 chemicals in listed quantities
      b. Industries using flammable liquids and gases in quantities of 10,000 pounds or more.

*NOTE: CFR refers to the Code of Federal Regulations, a compilation of final rules and regulations that are originally published in the Federal Register. The CFR is divided into 50 titles representing broad areas subject to federal regulation. Title 29 is labor; Title 40 is protection of the environment.

   4. Methods to determine and evaluate the consequences of the failure of engineering and administrative controls include the following (National Safety Council, 1992; Gressel & Gideon, 1991):
      a. *What if* is a method of thinking in which failure potentials are brainstormed and their causes and effects analyzed.
      b. *Checklists* identify the major hazards and nuisances associated with a particular material.

   c. A *hazard and operability study* (HAZOP) is a formal systematic study of a newly designed facility or operation to assess the potential of individual equipment components to fail, resulting in consequential effects on the overall facility.

   d. *Failure mode and effects analysis* (FMEA) is a "bottom-up" technique in which the failure of a particular process component is assessed for its effects on other components and on the process system as a potential source for accidents.

   e. *Fault tree analysis* is a formalized deductive technique that works backward from a defined accident to identify and graphically display the combination of equipment failures and operational errors that can lead up to the accident.

5. Worker health and safety information, including the health effects of chemicals and the possible need for specific first aid planning, should be evaluated.

J The *ergonomic analysis* **evaluates stresses related to the performance of work so strategies for prevention can be developed.**

1. Preventive strategies include the following:
   a. Redesigning work stations and work equipment (i.e., machine guards)
   b. Improving work environment (e.g., developing a work-rest schedule to prevent heat stress)
   c. Designing warning signs for hazardous equipment and locations
2. The NIOSH Equation for Manual Lifting can be used to identify tasks having a risk of overexertion injuries and low back pain because of lifting and lowering activities.
   a. The guidelines describe an equation that is based on the following variables: horizontal distance; vertical distance; distance of lift; asymmetry of lift; coupling; frequency of lifting (refer to Garg, 1995 for lifting guidelines).
   b. The goal is to design the task so the lifting index is at or below 1.0.
3. Effective ergonomics programs include the following:
   a. Surveillance strategies to assess patterns of exertion injuries
   b. Job hazard analysis/job safety analysis to identify workers at risk
   c. Job design or redesign that considers ergonomic factors
   d. Management and worker training related to the recognition and control of biochemical hazards
   e. Protocol for health management of injured workers

Hazard evaluation and analysis

The next steps to preventing injury and illness are evaluating hazards to determine to what degree a standard has been met, and analyzing identified hazards to determine how hazard controls must be prioritized in terms of human and financial resources.

III Purpose of Hazard Evaluation and Analysis

A The ultimate purpose of hazard evaluation and analysis is to control *all* hazards, existing and potential.

B Hazards that present a high probability of severe injury or illness warrant a greater priority when implementing control measures than do potential hazards that present a remote possibility of less-severe injury or illness.

C Hazard evaluation and analysis serves as an ongoing tool to determine what is working well and what isn't, what deserves commendation and what needs constructive correction.

IV Industry Standards

Industry standards provide a guide for evaluating and analyzing hazards.

A There are two types of industry standards.
1. *Mandatory standards* that establish minimum safety program requirements and maximum levels of permitted exposures; these standards are enforced by government agencies such as OSHA and the Environmental Protection Agency (EPA).
2. *Consensus standards* are voluntary industry standards adopted by agreement among participating members.

B Standards can serve as professional yardsticks against which to measure hazard identification and prevention activities.
1. Occasionally mandatory standards quote consensus standards as their requirements.
2. Standards can carry heavy weight in issues such as insurance company coverage, legal actions, and other issues in which competency and compliance issues are involved.
3. Trade associations, scientific and technical societies, and insurance companies may have certification or compliance requirements that industry can use as a yardstick for hazards and preventive measures.
4. International associations that promulgate consensus standards, often as part of environmental treaties and quality initiatives, are the International Labour Organization and the International Organization for Standardization (ISO 9000 Series, ISO 14000).

C Some standards are inadequate for the following reasons:
1. They may conflict with each other in their requirements, such as the labeling requirements of the Department of Transportation (DOT) versus those of OSHA.
2. Standards in the United States may differ from those of other countries, thus affecting international corporations (Box 9-4).
   a. The processes that are followed, the participants and their extent of involvement, and the legal structures embracing all these standards are different from those of the United States.
   b. It is essential that judgments of other countries not be based on what we have experienced in the United States.
3. Standards may not address an organization's principal risks; thus it is critical that workplaces be assessed for *all* hazards, not just those that are subject to regulation.

D The following must be considered when evaluating the significance of hazards identified.
1. "Low numbers of incidents and injuries do not necessarily mean a hazard-free worksite" (Manuele, 1994).
2. A hazardous event may be rated as catastrophic, critical, marginal, or negligible in its severity; these are subjective categories based on fatalities, injury severity, and financial damage (Manuele, 1994).

BOX 9-4

Examples of processes affecting standards in other countries

European Directives

The Council of the European Union has issued a series of directives intended to ensure harmonization of requirements for the health and safety of individuals. The European directives set out a common framework, for member countries to implement at a national level, of laws, regulations and administrative procedures necessary to comply with their requirements. The European legal instruments can be put into five categories:

- Regulations: binding on all member states and introduced
- Directives: establish principles that are binding on all member states and implemented in accordance with member states arrangements.
- Decisions: binding on those to whom they are addressed.
- Recommendations and Opinions: not binding, but encourage good practice.
- Action Programs: adopted by the Council; indicative of the Council's intention to take measures to achieve its objectives.

Non-European Directives

Other countries also have regulations associated with occupational health and safety issues. These regulations vary widely in nature and complexity. For examples:

- China: China has a significant number of regulations associated with occupational health and safety issues. These regulations vary in different provinces and regions and can be quite complex. In addition, there are many local rules. For example, there are 807 laws, regulations, standards, and rules applicable to Shanghai City.
- Australia: In Australia, standards are determined by the individual states and territories, such as the Queensland Division of Workplace Health and Safety or the Victoria Health and Safety Organisation. A major initiative is self-regulation via a "code of practice," placing a broad duty of care on employers to provide a safe and risk-free workplace.
- Japan: Japanese regulations are determined centrally by the Labor Standards Bureau of the Ministry of Labor. An unusual feature of the Japanese system is that industrial law requires that all employed persons undergo a prescribed occupational medical examination each year (Fleming, Herzstein, & Bunn, 1997).

---

3. The likelihood of a hazardous event is estimated subjectively as frequent, probable, occasional, remote, or improbable.
4. Risk analysis should consider both the probability of an incident occurring and the expected severity of adverse results, thus ranking the risks. Box 9-5 provides a formula for estimating a "risk score," and Fig. 9-4 presents a risk-analysis matrix.
5. Risk analysis should define the people, property, and environment that identified hazards may affect.

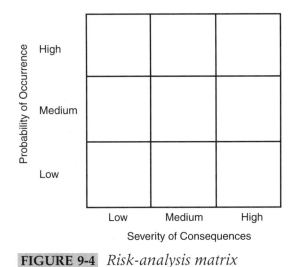

FIGURE 9-4 *Risk-analysis matrix*

BOX 9-5

A formula for estimating risk score

$$R = S \times E \times P$$

where R = Risk Score, S = Severity, E = Exposure, P = Probability

Risk scores can be used to rank the priority of hazards. Assign a value to each variable (for example, by using a scale from 1 to 5); then multiply the potential severity of injury by the frequency of exposure by the probability of exposure to obtain a risk score estimate (Perkinson, 1995).

E **Analysis and evaluation strategies serve as guides for program implementation.**
1. When exposure monitoring indicates that agent action levels have been reached, a worker health surveillance program should be implemented.
2. When worker health data suggest adverse work-site exposures, exposure monitoring may be indicated.
3. Environmental or biological monitoring results that suggest elevated exposure may indicate the need for additional engineering and administrative control measures or for additional training in the proper use of personal protective equipment.

V Exposure Monitoring

Exposure monitoring is the quantitative analysis of work-site exposures to hazards that are recognized, suspected, or anticipated, based on other preliminary hazard identification methods (Weeks, Levy, & Wagner, 1991).

A **Sampling is conducted for all types of exposures.**

1. A sample should represent the workers' exposure or condition that is being evaluated.

2. The following considerations should guide sampling activities:
   a. Whom to sample (those directly or indirectly exposed)
   b. Where to sample (breathing zone, hearing zone, work area, point of operation)
   c. Sampling duration or volume needed
   d. Number and types of samples needed
   e. Sampling period (e.g., day or night, summer or winter)

3. Compare findings with occupational health standards such as OSHA's Permissible exposure limits (PEL), the United Kingdom Health and Safety Executive's Occupational Exposure Limits (OEL), or the American Conference of Governmental Industrial Hygienists' (ACGIH) threshold limit valves (TLVs).

Note: many countries adopt the ACGIH TLVs as their regulatory exposure limits.

4. Interpretation of results must also take the following factors into account (Burgess, 1995):
   a. Exposure levels versus absorbed dose
   b. Sites of entry versus sites of action
   c. Combined effects of two or more substances or sources
   d. Individual susceptibility
   e. Conditions of use in the work environment, including work-site controls in place
   f. Individual worker practices

5. Examples of sampling and analysis problems include the following:
   a. Air pumps and sound-level meters that are not accurately calibrated or that spontaneously change flow rates
   b. Flow rates or exposure circumstances intentionally altered by the subject worker
   c. Color shade changes
   d. Fluctuating environmental conditions
   e. Improper timing, such as sampling when exposure levels are minimal
   f. Problems in quality control, such as failure to submit or download all recorded data or to properly store and analyze samples (Johnson & Bell, 1991; Coffman, 1992)

B **Assessment of noise exposure**

1. Measurements of sound-pressure levels are expressed in terms of decibels (dB).

2. An A-weighted scale combines frequency with intensity to yield dBA measurement (Dobie, 1995).

3. Potential hearing damage can be estimated with a knowledge of the dBA sound level, the duration of exposure during a workday, and the total work-life exposure (Plog, et al., 1996).

4. Personal dosimeters integrate time and noise exposure (Plog, et al., 1996).

5. For engineering controls of noise, sound-pressure levels throughout the frequency spectrum must be measured using an octave band analyzer (Plog, et al., 1996).

6. Internationally, many noise exposure regulations are found in environmental statutes with requirements for community exposure limitations in addition to work-site restrictions.

(Chapter 14 presents an example of a hearing conservation program.)

C Atmospheric monitoring

1. The purpose of atmospheric monitoring is to evaluate, over a given period of time, the presence and concentration of airborne contaminants to which the worker is being exposed.
2. Various methods used to sample gases, vapors, and particulates include the following:
   a. Dosimeter badges
   b. Detector or colorimetric tubes with hand-operated pumps to draw air samples
   c. Electronic direct-reading instruments with sensors
   d. Filters, sorbent tubes, impingers, and other entrapment devices
3. Types of sampling procedures
   a. *Instantaneous* or "grab" sampling collects an air sample over a short period of time ranging from a few seconds to less than two minutes.
   b. The *personal* sample consists of drawing a known volume of air through an appropriate medium located in the worker's breathing zone for a sampling period of from 15 minutes to eight hours.
   c. An *area* sample determines the source of contaminants by creating a "map" of levels present.
   d. Air, chemicals, water, and soil may be monitored by *bulk* sampling.
   e. *Bioaerosol* monitoring for bacteria, viruses, fungi, and other biologicals is performed by methods similar to airborne chemical contaminant monitoring.
   f. *Combustible gas indicators* are direct-reading instruments used to measure explosive levels of gases in confined spaces.
   g. *Oxygen detectors* are direct-reading instruments used to evaluate the percentage of oxygen in the air, especially in confined spaces. (Safe levels established by U.S. standards are from 19.5 % to 23.0% oxygen in air [Ness, 1991].)
4. The sense of smell *or* irritation of the skin, eyes, and upper respiratory system can provide valuable clues to the levels of concentration of the contaminant, but these sensory indicators are unreliable for actual concentration or presence determinations.

D Ionizing radiation monitoring is best carried out by personal dosimetry.

1. Thermal-luminescent dosimeters—the newest being aluminum oxide—or the older film badges are worn by workers, with collection and reading at periodic intervals based on the extent of potential exposure (Breitenstein & Spickard, 1995).
2. Swipe samples, consisting of a wet surface wipe-down and analysis, are taken for evidence of surface contamination by radionuclides (Breitenstein & Spickard, 1995).
3. Area monitoring is accomplished by measuring roentgens per day with the Geiger-Mueller instrument (Geiger counter).
4. Results of radiation measurement are compared with allowable dose standards from the Nuclear Regulatory Commission, EPA, OSHA, and other agencies that regulate radiation protection and measurement.

E Temperature monitoring identifies hazardous extremes in hot or cold environments.

1. Potential for heat stress requires measurement of air temperature by dry-bulb measurement, humidity by natural wet-bulb measurement, and radiant heat by black-globe temperature.

2. Other considerations when measuring for heat stress include fluid and electrolyte balance, training for heat tolerance, drugs, alcohol consumption, age, obesity, and extent of clothing.

3. Proposed occupational health standards for exposure to heat consist of a sliding scale based on the wet-bulb globe temperature, differing for acclimatized and unacclimatized workers.

4. Potential for cold injury requires measurement of air temperature by dry-bulb method plus measurement of wind speed to arrive at a wind-chill factor.

5. Other considerations when measuring for cold injury include exposure to moisture, extent of clothing, and level of exhaustion.

F Surface sampling, or wipe sampling, can be performed to evaluate external surfaces and the worker's skin and clothing for chemical, radiation, and biologic contamination.

G Continuous monitors are alarm units used primarily to detect emergency conditions and trigger evacuation rather than to measure worker exposure (Ness, 1991).

1. Monitors may detect high radiation levels, fire, smoke, flammable atmospheres, oxygen-deficient air, and toxic levels of poisonous gases such as hydrogen sulfide and carbon monoxide.

2. Stationary systems may provide real-time alarm warnings to workers in the area of a hazardous environmental condition.

3. Personal continuous monitors may be worn by workers in areas where potential releases could reach evacuation levels, such as in confined spaces.

4. Portable continuous monitors are similar to personal monitors but may have more display capability and can collect data over a period of time for a specific chemical.

VI Occupational Health Surveillance

Occupational health surveillance consists of the "process of monitoring and collecting data on the health status of worker populations to analyze the effects of workplace exposures and using data to prevent injury and illness" (AAOHN, 1996).

A Surveillance terminology

1. Surveillance applied to populations is called *public health surveillance;* occupational health surveillance is a subset of public health surveillance.

2. Surveillance of individuals, which is sometimes called *medical surveillance,* includes history taking, examination, and monitoring of an individual.

   a. *Medical surveillance* suggests the process of diagnosing and treating; *health surveillance* suggests the process of preventing illness and injury (which is the primary role of occupational and environmental health nurses; thus the term *health surveillance* "is more accurate and reflective of the nature of the activity" (Rogers, 1994).

   b. Biological monitoring and worker surveillance requirements in OSHA standards for specific chemical hazards are listed under "Medical Surveillance."

B The primary goals of occupational health surveillance are as follows (AAOHN, 1996: Levy & Wegman, 1999):

1. Identify the occurrence of injuries and illnesses related to hazard exposure in the work site.

2. Define the magnitude and distribution of occupational disease and injury occurrences.
3. Identify and track trends in disease and injury occurrence as a means of assessing the effectiveness of prevention strategies.
4. Describe specific occupations or industries that would benefit from prevention strategies.
5. Guide the development of engineering and administrative strategies for prevention and control.

C Other benefits to health surveillance include the following:
1. More appropriate therapeutic and rehabilitation activities
2. Appropriate compensation for workers with illnesses resulting from occupational exposures
3. Discovering new relationships between work exposure and disease

D Challenges to the identification and recognition of occupational illness
1. Occupational illnesses often have long latency periods; years and even decades may elapse between time of exposure and occurrence of symptoms.
2. Occupational illness may be indistinguishable from nonoccupational illness (e.g., occupational asthma resembles nonoccupational asthma)
3. Causes of occupational illness are multifactorial; it is difficult to determine the exact cause of illness.
4. Americans are on the move, making it difficult to track exposures.

E The occupational and environmental health nurse is key to providing a quality health surveillance program because he or she (AAOHN, 1996):
1. Is the most frequently available occupational health professional at the work site
2. Is knowledgeable about health surveillance and other occupational health and safety programs
3. Is familiar with the health status of workers
4. Provides cost-effective care

F Occupational and environmental nursing roles related to occupational health surveillance (AAOHN, 1996)
1. Work with company representatives and other occupational health and safety professionals to plan, conduct, supervise, and evaluate the occupational health surveillance program.
2. Conduct and interpret the results of the tests required for occupational health surveillance, and refer employees for additional tests as necessary.
3. Recommend identification, prevention, and control strategies based on test results.
4. Establish and maintain a system of recordkeeping.
5. Evaluate a program's effectiveness; modify the program as needed.
6. Ensure compliance with OSHA regulations.
7. Select, manage, and evaluate vendor-provided health services.

VII Worker Populations Analysis

Worker populations should be viewed not just as a collection of individuals but as a single entity; worker populations include communities and subgroups of workers.

A **Analyzing groups, not just individuals, can detect patterns, trends, changes, and commonalties.**

1. Population data can be used to describe injury and illness trends over time, so patterns with common causes can be identified and prevented.

2. Occupational and environmental health nurses should be alert to group patterns of injury and illness, as follows:
   a. If health visits reveal a cluster of illnesses or injuries, visit the work site to get an understanding of how and why these events may be happening (Weinstock, 1993).
   b. Attempt to identify whether workers with similar complaints perform the same job, work in the same area, or have something else in common (Barnes, 1992).
   c. Monitor trends that may suggest new hazards or the breakdown of prevention and control measures.
   d. Determine whether conditions are improving or worsening (Weinstock, 1993).
   e. Identify the work-site locations involved.
   f. Enlist colleagues from other disciplines e.g., industrial hygiene, engineering), as appropriate.

B *Epidemic events* **are any marked upward fluctuation in disease and injury incidence.**

1. Epidemics are verified when the incidence of a disease or injury exceeds what normally would be expected.

2. An epidemic must have an agent or a cause, in addition to individuals who are susceptible to the illness or injury related to the cause.

3. Management of an epidemic in the work setting should follow these steps:
   a. Identify and arrange for treatment of clients.
   b. Institute control measures to decrease spread of contamination or risk of injury.
   c. Provide workers with appropriate health education.
   d. Establish a program of continued surveillance and monitoring for the infective agent or the source of injury.
   e. Establish a program to prevent recurrence.

C *Epidemic (mass) hysteria* **(also called mass psychogenic illness) is an event in which a group of workers exposed to the same stimulus exhibit common physical symptoms of psychologic origin (Kahn, 1993).**

1. Characteristics of exposure
   a. This illness occurs most often in work settings with physical and emotional stressors, such as boring, repetitive tasks and poor rapport between the work force and company management.
   b. A noxious odor, a substance perceived as toxic, extreme heat, or loud, repetitive noises may serve as triggers (Kahn, 1993).
   c. Transmission of symptoms occurs by sight, sound, or word of mouth rather than by simply being in a common exposure area.

2. Symptom development includes the following characteristics:
   a. An explosive onset of symptoms whose severity is out of proportion to the apparent cause and that can disappear and return rapidly.
   b. A range of symptoms, including headache, nausea, dizziness, chills, difficulty in breathing, and other vague, subjective complaints, divert the worker's attention from hidden stress to external work-site factors (Kahn, 1993).

3. Epidemic stress may be recognized by carrying out the following activities:
   a. Carefully investigate complaints and conduct an exposure analysis of all potential toxicological and biologic causes to rule out a physical basis
   b. Evaluate the work site for psychosocial stressors
   c. Identify workers at high risk for somatoform disorders
4. Other considerations
   a. A careful work-site analysis should be performed; the possibility of physical symptoms must be considered even in the absence of objective findings.
   b. "Hysteria" reactions may be the result of psychosocial stressors in the workplace; this possibility should be investigated.
   c. Treatment consists of first establishing and communicating the lack of connection between the symptoms and the "trigger," then taking measures to reduce occupational stressors.

D Sentinel health event
1. A *sentinel health event* is a disease, disability, or untimely death that is work-related and whose occurrence may accomplish the following:
   a. Provide the impetus for epidemiologic or industrial hygiene studies
   b. Serve as a warning that prevention and control strategies are needed
2. The occurrence of sentinel health events may serve as the stimulus for hazard evaluation and reassessment of control measures.
3. The occupational and environmental health nurse may play an important role in identifying sentinel health events; it is essential that the occupational and environmental health nurse:
   a. Have a thorough knowledge of the work site and its hazards.
   b. Collaborate with professional colleagues within the company when a sentinel health event is suspected.
   c. Participate in continuing education efforts.
   d. Maintain a high index of suspicion for the possibility of a sentinel health event ("gatekeeper" role).
   e. Refer all potentially exposed workers for further evaluation when a work-related problem is suspected (Hau, 1993).

E Multiple chemical sensitivity
1. *Multiple chemical sensitivity* (MCS) has been described as a syndrome that may develop in one or many workers and "affect(s) multiple systems and occur(s) in multiple unrelated environments" (Levy & Wegman, 1999).
   a. Common symptoms of MCS are fatigue, headache, frequent colds, dizziness, nausea, lack of concentration, memory loss, menstrual irregularities, and visual problems (Voelker, 1994).
   b. Often the symptom pattern changes, with some symptoms disappearing and new ones occurring; symptoms can produce total disability.
2. MCS is poorly understood; hence it is a highly controversial phenomenon.
   a. Symptoms are subjective, with no objective evidence of organ system damage or dysfunction.
   b. Health effects described as MCS are related to verifiable environmental exposure.
   c. MCS symptoms are elicited by extremely low exposures to chemicals.
   d. MCS symptoms seem to have a predictable return with environmental stimuli (Sparks, et al., 1994).

3. There is a need for epidemiologic studies and for careful environmental and occupational history-taking to better understand multiple chemical sensitivity.

F **Work-site violence**

1. Because of epidemic growth, workplace violence is creating a new form of job hazard and an increased sense of worker vulnerability.
2. Workplace violence includes harassment, threats, and actual physical assaults in the work site.
3. Recognizing and understanding the potential hazard of work-site violence is a new essential assessment in industry. (Chapter 13 presents additional information on workplace violence.)

Prevention and control

The last steps of work-site programs are to select and implement prevention and control measures. The prevention and control of occupational hazards is central to occupational and environmental health nursing practice.

VIII Identifying Appropriate Prevention and Control Approach

A **Several approaches can be used to prevent and control hazards in the work environment.**

1. Engineering controls include elimination or substitution of materials.
2. Administrative controls include modification of work practices.
3. The use of personal protective equipment

B **Engineering methods are the most preferable means of hazard control; engineering controls do not rely on the human behavior factor to ensure success.**

C **The choice of a control strategy depends on the nature of the workplace, financial and technological feasibility, work tasks, and workers. More than one approach is often required to achieve optimal health and safety.**

IX Prevention and Control Approaches That Focus on Engineering Controls

A *Elimination* **or** *substitution* **of manual tasks and highly hazardous materials is intended to minimize the source of potential exposure by completely removing the hazardous material or replacing it with a less hazardous substitute.**

1. Elimination (or substitution) is the most preferred strategy for control and the method of choice whenever possible.
2. The benefits to health and safety of elimination and substitution often have to be weighed against the technological and economic consequences.
3. When using substitution, care must be taken to ensure that the replacement product does not pose other health or safety risks.
4. Examples of elimination or substitution include the following:
   a. Removing insulation that contains asbestos fibers
   b. Using mechanical or vacuum lifting devices to replace manual lifting
   c. Using a dipping method to coat an object rather than spraying, thus reducing the danger of inhalation

    d. Substituting unbreakable acrylic or thermoplastic product for breakable glass

    e. Using a less toxic and less flammable chemical than one in current use

B *Worksite engineering designs* **are intended to stop hazards at their source or in the path of their transmission and are the preferred strategy when elimination or substitution is not possible.**

  1. Characteristics of workplace designs that promote occupational health and safety include the following:

    a. Appropriate lighting to enable workers to perform their tasks safely

    b. Workstations that are ergonomically designed to reduce the risk factors of repetitive motions, static or awkward postures, forceful exertions, and mechanical pressure on soft tissues

    c. Stairs or platforms with railings, guarded floor and wall openings, and proper floor finishes to reduce slips, trips, and falls

    d. Mats that are specially designed to reduce safety hazards (Box 9-6)

    e. Security designs to reduce the potential for work-site violence (e.g., bullet-proof glass, silent alarms, well-lit parking lots)

    f. Designs that consider the personal comfort of workers (Box 9-7); well-designed workstations can reduce worker stress

  2. Examples of beneficial workplace designs

    a. *Isolation:* provides a barrier between a hazard and those who might be affected by that hazard.

      1) Process isolation: operations handled through remote computer applications in a control room

---

BOX 9-6

Examples of mats designed to reduce safety hazards

- *Fatigue-reducing mats* lessen muscular fatigue and often reduce noise.
- *Slip-resistant mats* protect against slipping on water, oil, ice, or mud.
- *Conductive mats* dissipate static electricity in rooms with high oxygen content, sensitive electronic components, explosives, or volatile liquids.
- *Nonconductive rubber mats* are used in front of switchboards and other high-voltage locations to protect workers from electric shock.

BOX 9-7

Features of stress-reducing workplace designs

- Availability of informal and formal meeting places
- Enclosures accommodating the need for personal space
- Permission to personalize spaces
- Access to daylight/sunlight
- Incorporation of variability through artifacts and cultural symbols, colors, and textures
- Freedom from distractions; visual and auditory privacy

    2) Underground tanks and isolated storage buildings for hazardous materials

    3) Noise barriers

    4) Shields that prevent exposure of nearby persons to welding arcs

  b. *Time-distance–shielding* is the most common approach to protecting workers from ionizing radiation (National Safety Council, 1992)

    1) *Time:* controlling the amount of time exposed to the radiation source, measured in mR/hr

    2) *Distance:* remaining as far away from the radiation source as possible

    3) *Shielding:* placing a barrier impenetrable to radiation between the worker and the source

NOTE: Avoiding ingestion and inhalation of radioactive particulates is also a protection measure, most applicable in the event of radioactive fallout.

C *Automatic systems* **are systems that shut down processes or issue warnings when hazardous conditions develop. They include the following (Cote & Bugbee, 1995):**

1. Fire detectors/alarms, water sprinkler systems, and gas extinguisher systems, such as halon in computer rooms

2. Safety valves, fusible plugs, and rupture discs in boilers and pressure vessels to permit excess pressure relief

3. Automatic fall-protection devices that allow normal descent by a worker in the device, but lock in the event of a rapid descent or fall

4. Circuit breakers, fuses, and other electrical current interruption devices that respond to overcurrents or overloads

5. Explosion detectors that release a suppressant to inhibit further reaction

D *Ventilation* **captures or dilutes airborne contaminants, cleaning the air before or after release (Burton, 1995).**

1. Local exhaust systems: remove contaminated air from the point of origin, away from the worker's breathing zone, through a scrubber or cleaning system to the outside (Burton, 1995)

2. Dilution ventilation: circulates fresh air into the work site to dilute the contaminant air to an acceptable exposure level (Burton, 1995)

3. Filtration: cleans the air before it is released back into the general ventilation or to the outside

4. Other air cleaning methods: electrostatic precipitators, scrubbers, absorbers, and chemical reactors (Burgess, 1995)

E **Storage of hazardous materials**

1. Flammable liquids are stored using bonding and grounding to dissipate static electricity, which could ignite their vapors.

2. Special lead containers are used to store radioactive materials.

3. Refrigerators are used to store heat-sensitive materials or heat-reactive chemicals.

4. Air-reactive chemicals are stored under water. Water-reactive chemicals are stored dry or under oil.

5. Special storage cabinets and safety cans are used to store small amounts of flammable liquids, such as hydrocarbons, gasoline, and kerosene.

6. Puncture-proof sharps containers are used to store contaminated needles and sharps awaiting disposal as hazardous health waste.

7. Certain highly toxic specialty gases, such as silane, must be kept in special gas cabinets.

8. Only the amount of hazardous substance that will actually be used in a reasonable time should be kept.

F **Storage of Equipment**

1. Ladders are secured in storage, often on wall hangers, not propped against a wall.
2. Cylinders of compressed gas, including the oxygen cylinders used by the occupational and environmental health nurse, must be kept upright and secured.
3. Fire extinguishers are mounted in specified locations with recognizable signs and color codes.
4. Products and parts are stored on racks, pallets, and other devices with specified densities, stacking limitations and aisleway clearances.

G *Hazardous energy control* **is used to prevent contact between the worker and hazardous energy sources.**

1. Hazardous energy sources include electricity, chemical reactivity, thermal extremes, mechanical energy, and physical energy.
2. Machine safeguarding to eliminate machine hazards
   a. All moving parts on machines that create pinch points or nip points, such as pulleys, belts, chains, etc., should be guarded during operation. Interlocks preventing machine operation during guard removal should be in place.
   b. Portable power tools, lawnmowers, and grinders should also be guarded (OSHA 3067, 1992).
   c. Methods of safeguarding machines are based on the type of operation, stock size and shape, handling method, and physical layout of the area (OSHA 3067, 1992).
      1) Guards are barriers that prevent access to danger areas (Figs. 9-5 and 9-6).
      2) Devices such as restraints, gates, presence-sensing (optical) devices, and trip controls stop the machine if a hand or other body part is inadvertently placed in the danger area.
3. Electric shock control is accomplished through the following safeguards:
   a. Proper initial installation
   b. The use of grounded outlets, circuit breakers, and disconnects (devices that interrupt current flow when it exceeds the wire's capacity)
   c. The use of ground fault circuit interrupters
   d. Proper insulation
4. Robots are used to perform unsafe, hazardous, highly repetitive, and unpleasant tasks.
5. Lockout/tagout (Fig. 9-7) is used to control hazardous energy sources during the service and maintenance of machinery or equipment that has exhibited unexpected startup or stored energy release (National Safety Council, 1992).
   a. OSHA 29 CFR 1910.147 Control of Hazardous Energy requires the following safety measures regarding a lockout/tagout system:
      1) Employee training
      2) Periodic inspections of the energy control program
      3) Written procedures for identifying all energy sources
      4) A tag warning system
      5) Periodic review and revision of procedures as needed.

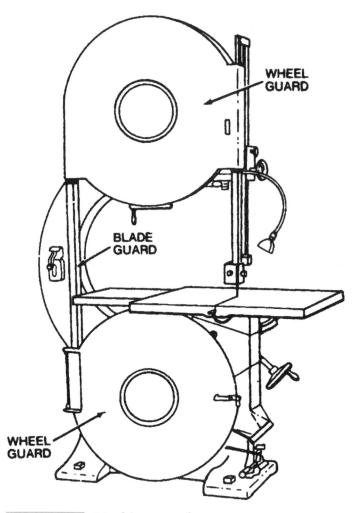

FIGURE 9-5 *Machine guard*

(*Source:* U.S. Department of Labor, 1992)

   b. All energy control devices are placed in the "off" or "safe" position, locked in that position, and tagged with a warning tag.
   c. Chemical process lines are bled out and disconnected or have a line block, called a *blank,* inserted.
   d. Upon work completion, the authorized employee will verify that the equipment has been returned to a safe state of operation before lockout/tagout devices are removed.

H *Mechanical integrity programs* **include preventive maintenance.**
   1. *Preventive maintenance* is the planned, periodic scheduling of equipment and the refurbishing, refitting, inspection, or overhaul of process units to prevent hazardous operating conditions from developing over time and after repeated use (National Safety Council, 1992).
   2. Equipment deficiencies outside the acceptable limits defined by engineering standards must be corrected before further use.

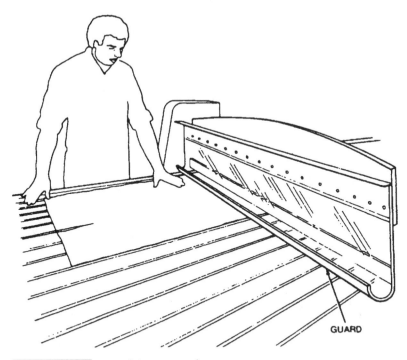

FIGURE 9-6 *Machine guard*

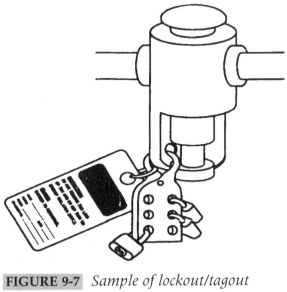

FIGURE 9-7 *Sample of lockout/tagout*
(*Source:* U.S. Department of Labor, 1992)

3. Maintenance materials, spare parts, and equipment suitable for the process application must be maintained in inventory.

X Prevention and Control Approaches That Focus on Administrative Controls

Administrative controls are supervisory and management practices to promote safe work behaviors that eliminate or limit hazard exposures.

A Controlling *work practices* (the manner in which work is performed) is often an important strategy that can limit or reduce a worker's exposure to workplace hazards.

1. Changes in work practices should be accompanied by on-site evaluations to accomplish the following:
   a. Characterize the risks inherent to the tasks.
   b. Ensure that the work practice is appropriate to the task.
   c. Perform a job safety analysis (JSA) on individual work tasks to identify those that may contribute to exposure.
2. It is essential that the workers performing the job participate in the development of safe work practices to maximize the effectiveness of these strategies.
3. Barriers to the implementation of safe work practices
   a. Paying workers by the piece, also called piecework, encourages workers to cut corners for the sake of production output, often sacrificing safe work practices.
   b. Refusing to provide support and funding to safety programs undermines their effectiveness.
   c. Fear of harassment or violence can prevent the adoption of safe work practices.
   d. Incentives that reward productivity may lead to unsafe work practices.
4. Examples of work practice modifications
   a. Vacuuming with equipment that has high-efficiency particulate (HEPA) filters can keep hazardous dusts from being resuspended.
   b. Wet mopping instead of sweeping is another way to minimize contamination from hazardous dusts and particulates.
   c. Using proper body mechanics when bending or lifting can prevent strains and sprains.
   d. The two-person concept (or "buddy system") is a safeguard for workers involved in hazardous operations.
      1) Both persons are exposed to the same hazard simultaneously; each one monitors the other and provides assistance when needed, such as the mutual aid and surveillance employed by power company personnel on live high-voltage systems (National Safety Council, 1992).
      2) One person is exposed to the hazard while the other acts as an attendant to observe and summon help if an emergency develops (Terpin, 1992).

B *Safety committees* with well-defined missions and regular meetings promote illness and injury prevention by engaging in the following activities:

1. Evaluating worker suggestions
2. Promoting accident prevention and safe work practices within each committee member's work area

3. Investigating reported safety deficiencies or assisting in the investigation
4. Reviewing accidents and identifying root causes and prevention methods
5. Performing walk-through surveys and safety inspections
6. Making recommendations on company safety rules
7. Assisting in safety training programs
8. Voting on safety awards recipients
9. Suggesting and promoting safety incentive programs

C *Safety training* **provides specific knowledge, instructions, and skills to enable workers to perform jobs safely while optimizing productivity and motivation.**

1. Training should be site-specific and based on needs identified during hazard identification and evaluation.
2. Training should be provided by effective trainers who are knowledgeable in the subject and available to answer questions and interpret information. Simply showing a videotape to workers is not adequate.
3. Testing and certification are methods for determining competency and ensuring safe performance of various job functions. The following are a few examples of testing and certification programs:
   a. Forklift operator training is often followed by written and performance testing to evaluate for proper, safe forklift operation.
   b. Boiler operators are licensed by the state.
   c. Drivers of certain types and sizes of vehicles must pass a commercial driver's license examination.
   d. Structural welders are usually certified in their skills by the Welder's Institute.
   e. Hazardous materials technicians are certified upon successful completion of the OSHA requirements under 29 CFR 1910.120.

D *Proper scheduling* **can reduce the amount of time any worker is exposed to a hazard or control the timing of the work to avoid the hazard. Examples of proper scheduling include the following:**

1. Schedule work activities that can produce heat stress during cooler parts of the day.
2. Schedule rotations among various job assignments, limiting exposure associated with a single job.
3. Do not schedule workers to perform a new job assignment alone until they have demonstrated adequate job knowledge and performance.

E *Work permits* **are a system to evaluate projects for hazards, specify safe work practices, identify essential personal protective equipment and other safety measures, and provide authorization before any work is done (National Safety Council, 1992).**

1. A Hot Work Permit is used for activities that produce sparks or flames, referred to as *hot work.*
2. A Confined Space Entry Permit is required before working in areas defined as *permit-required confined spaces.*
   a. A *confined space* is an area that is large enough and so configured that an employee can enter and perform assigned work, but has limited or restricted means of access and is not designed for continuous worker occupancy.
   b. A *permit-required confined space* is a confined space with one or more of the following characteristics:
      1) Contains or has a potential to contain a hazardous atmosphere

2) Contains a material that has the potential for engulfing an entrant

3) Has an internal configuration such that an entrant could be trapped or asphyxiated by inwardly converging walls or by a floor that slopes downward and tapers to a smaller cross-section

4) Contains any other recognized serious safety or health hazard

c. Hazards associated with confined spaces that must be evaluated in the permitting process are hazardous atmospheres (oxygen-deficient, flammable, toxic), temperature extremes, engulfment hazards, noise, falling objects, and any other recognized serious hazard.

3. Waste Disposal/Storage Permits may be required for environmental hazardous waste control.

4. Excavation permits may be necessary before digging operations may be performed.

5. Line-breaking Permits may be required before process piping may be opened.

F *Housekeeping* **practices that promote safe working conditions include controlling pests; promptly disposing of waste; keeping floors clear of oil, grease, and water; preventing trip hazards; and properly storing materials, tools. and equipment. Weekly housekeeping inspections are recommended.**

G *Labeling, coding, and posting warning signs* **all help communicate safety issues throughout the work-site.**

1. Some OSHA standards require posting of warning signs in areas where hazards have been identified (e.g., noise or radiation)

2. Safety showers and eyewash stations and alarms are marked with signs and color coding to enhance visibility and rapid access.

3. Exits must be clearly identified with lighted signs; doorways that are not exits must be clearly labeled as such.

4. Color, indicators of direction of flow, and other signs mark controls, piping outlets, and pipelines.

   a. Red—fire protection equipment, danger, and "emergency stops" on equipment

   b. Yellow—trip hazards, flammable-liquid storage cabinets, and materials-handling equipment such as forklifts

   c. Green—location of first-aid and safety equipment

   d. Black on yellow—radiation hazard

   e. Bright blue—inert gases

5. Signs and maps are posted throughout the facility to mark evacuation routes and shelters. General warning signs do not substitute for safe work practices but can serve as cautions and reminders (National Safety Council, 1992).

H *General promotion* **is designed to strengthen and reinforce injury and illness prevention awareness and the attitudes that mold and strengthen it.**

1. Safety newsletters are used to relate safety information directly to each worker.

   a. They impart information and help to boost morale.

   b. To be successful, they should put the spotlight on workers, balancing useful information with recognition of workers' accomplishments.

   c. They can promote safety contests, provide a network for news, offer a management column, and report actual incidents (Willen, 1995).

2. Bulletin boards, which should be visible to everyone, attractive, and eye-catching, can provide a variety of health and safety information.

3. Promotional posters, changed often to avoid over-familiarity, serve as visual reminders of prevention and control programs.
4. Incentive programs are used to motivate workers to work safely and prevent accidents and injuries (Minter, 1995).
   a. Examples of incentive programs include the following:
      1) Contests among departments for the best safety record or best housekeeping performance
      2) Safety awards for companies and plants, offered by organizations such as local safety councils
      3) Safety patches, pins, hard-hat stickers, ball caps, and other apparel bearing positive safety messages
      4) Bonuses to workers, supervisors, and managers when targeted safety goals are reached
   b. Programs should be monitored so workers, supervisors, and managers do not attempt to hide accidents, injuries, and other events to avoid being the cause of a lost record or award.
   c. The primary focus of managers should not be numbers and statistics but rather acknowledging the excellent safety performance of workers.
5. Health promotion programs target lifestyles to lessen workers' vulnerability to work-site exposures and to enhance their ability and capacity to perform job assignments more safely.
   a. Back strengthening through exercise programs can help reduce the incidence of back strain during materials handling.
   b. Smoking cessation programs can reduce risks of synergistic effects of cigarette smoke and asbestos exposure.
   c. Stress management programs can help workers deal with work-related stress.

I *Medical removal* **(removal from exposure for medical reasons) and restricted work programs**
1. Some OSHA regulations have medical removal requirements, which require removal of a worker based on biological monitoring results before clinical health effects appear or end organ systems are injured; these regulations include the lead and cadmium standards.
2. Some employers adopt light-duty programs to return workers gradually to the rigors of full work assignments.
3. Medical removal requirements may have to be employed when a worker becomes sensitized to a work-site hazardous material, such as an isocyanate or an anhydride, and cannot risk any further exposures.

J *Emergency preparedness* **planning and response operations are control measures intended to prevent or minimize harm to persons, property, systems, and the environment in the event of a critical incident.**
1. This strategy may be used for a medical emergency, fire, technologic event (such as a hazardous materials release), or civil event (such as a bomb threat).
2. Phases of an emergency preparedness operation include mitigation, planning, response, and recovery.
   a. In the mitigation phase, the attempt is made to identify and eliminate hazards that have a potential for generating an emergency.
   b. Planning is then conducted to respond effectively in coordination with community response agencies to bring emergency conditions under control and eventually return to normal operations, if possible. (Fig. 9-8.)

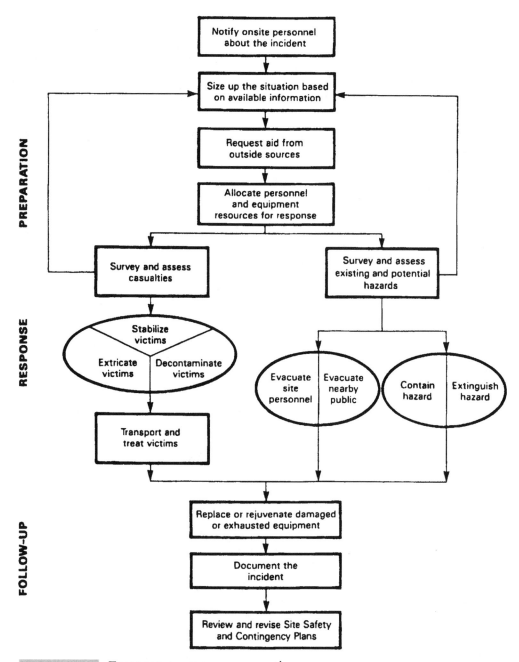

FIGURE 9-8 *Emergency response operations*

c. Critical-incident stress debriefing (CISD) is implemented in the recovery phase to prevent the development of critical-incident stress that typically affects the company's and community's emergency response personnel (McNeely, 1991).
1) Critical-incident stress can develop when providers do not allow themselves to react emotionally to an emergency event.

2) Debriefing enables providers to come to terms with their thoughts and feelings by bringing them out in the open and expressing them.

3) CISD should be conducted within 24 to 72 hours after the event in a nonthreatening environment, confidentially, by trained leaders (Mitchell & Resnick, 1981 cited by Hayes, Goodwin, & Miars, 1990).

4) CISD teams can usually be found through community emergency response agencies, such as the local fire department.

K *Materials and services management* **reduces hazards by establishing effective purchasing systems and preventing substandard equipment, materials, and services from being delivered to the work site.**

1. Training and effective systems ensure that health and safety considerations are applied to the procurement of goods and services; these systems should provide and use lists of all materials, products, machines, equipment, and chemical substances and their required specifications.

2. Goods received are checked against approved lists to ensure proper quality and safety.

3. New equipment and materials are formally reviewed by suitably qualified personnel to identify potential loss exposure and controls to be implemented for them before purchasing.

4. Handling practices and operating and maintenance procedures are developed and communicated before new items are used.

5. Contractor safety records, health and safety programs, training records, and worker certifications are reviewed for hazard potentials and hazard prevention.

L *Special programs* **are available to help employers meet and exceed regulatory requirements.**

1. OSHA's Voluntary Protection Program (Chapter 3)

2. Association-sponsored programs such as the Chemical Manufacturer's Association's "Responsible Care"

3. Proprietary programs such as Dupont's "STOP" program and Det Norske Veritas' "International Safety Rating System"

XI Prevention and Control Approaches That Focus on Personal Protective Equipment

Personal protective equipment (PPE) includes all clothing and accessories worn by the worker and designed to create a barrier against work-site hazards. It is the least desirable control method because of the expense, discomfort, and enforcement problems it creates.

A **Characteristics of personal protective equipment**

1. Workers must be trained in the reasons for wearing PPE; what PPE to wear; how to don, use, and wear PPE; the proper care, maintenance, and useful life of PPE; and any other training requirement involving PPE.

2. The occupational and environmental health nurse should become familiar with the details of the specific PPE used at the facility and with the requirements of the applicable OSHA standard.

a. Typical PPE dispensed by the occupational and environmental health nurse includes eye protection, hearing protection, and skin barrier creams.

b. The occupational and environmental health nurse must take special care to review the research and professional recommendations regarding proper PPE selections and proper fitting.

B **Regulations related to personal protective equipment**
1. The company is required to have a written PPE program and to provide PPE to workers. (Some companies have workers contribute to the cost of prescription safety glasses and safety shoes.)
2. OSHA 29 CFR 1910.132 requires a work-site hazard assessment that has the following characteristics (Roughton, 1995):
    a. Includes a walk-through survey
    b. Requires written certification that the assessment has been performed
    c. Provides a mechanism for ensuring that the need for PPE has been determined and that the PPE selected is appropriate to the hazard

C **Examples of personal protective equipment**
1. 29 CFR 1910.133 requires protective eye and face equipment.
    a. Safety glasses with sideshields are used to protect against flying objects; they must be heat-treated and able to withstand the drop of a 5-pound lead ball without shattering.
    b. Chemical goggles, of vented and air-tight varieties, protect against chemical splashes, vapors, and gases.
    c. Ultraviolet (UV) light protection is most commonly used by welders to protect against the ultraviolet welding arc.
    d. Laser beam protection is necessary to prevent corneal and retinal injuries from exposure to laser beams.
    e. Face shields add further protection against splashes or sparks.
    f. The use of contact lenses, especially while wearing respiratory protection, is under evaluation; there is concern that dirt or other debris can lodge between the lens and the pupil or that soft lenses will absorb chemical contaminants from the air.
2. Hearing protection under 29 CFR 1910.95 requires a written hearing conservation program, including hearing protection and annual audiometric testing for workers exposed to excessive noise. (Chapter 12 presents an example of a hearing conservation program.)
    a. Hearing protection devices include ear plugs, ear muffs, ear molds, and canal caps (Chapter 12).
    b. Hearing aids do not protect against the effects of loud noise, even when the worker cannot hear the noise.
    c. Workers must be shown how to wear hearing protection and how to care for it, and should be observed to ensure that they are using it correctly.
    d. Changes in noise levels may require changes in hearing protection devices.
3. Hand/skin protection is required under 29 CFR 1910.138.
    a. Gloves are selected to protect against heat, cold, abrasion, and chemicals.
    b. Barrier creams are of two varieties, setting up a coating to shield the skin either against water-related exposures or against drying powder-type exposures.
    c. Tapes, similar to adhesive tape, have a gritty or rubbery external surface to protect fingers against abrasion from repeated rubbing or gripping and to aid in gripping.
    d. Sunscreen protects workers from the sun and other UV sources.

   e. Glove boxes, although not strictly PPE, are also used to protect hand exposures, particularly against biological agents.
4. 29 CFR 1910.136 specifies safety shoes for protecting feet from being crushed and fractured.
   a. Boots are used to protect against exposure to water, chemicals, and fire.
   b. Steel-toed shoes protect the toes from hazards such as heavy rolling or falling objects.
   c. Metatarsal plates fit over the shoe and extend protection to the metatarsals from toe-injury hazards.
5. Torso protection is selected according to the specific type of hazard involved.
   a. Chemical-protective clothing may consist of aprons, coveralls, hooded suits, fully encapsulated suits with self-contained breathing apparatus, sleeves, pants, or chaps, and is selected to protect against heat, cold, abrasion, and chemicals.
   b. Radiation protection is provided by lead aprons and protective suits.
   c. Thermal garments include heat-resistant firefighter gear, flash-protection garments, proximity suits for radiant heat, cooling garments and vests using ice packs or circulating cold water, and other garments to protect against extremely hot or cold conditions.
   d. Blast and fragmentation suits are used for protection against small detonations; they do not provide hearing protection.
6. 29 CFR 1910.135 specifies head protection from impact and penetration from falling and flying objects and from limited electric shock and burn hazards.
   a. Hard hats are used in areas where falling and flying objects are a hazard.
   b. Heat-resistant and chemical-resistant hoods are also used.
7. 29 CFR 1910.134 requires respiratory protection when airborne contamination exceeds the TLV or PEL and cannot be eliminated by engineering controls.
   a. Requirements include a written comprehensive respirator program with annual fit testing and worker training.
   b. Respiratory protection is of two types: *supplied air* and *air-purifying.* (Fig. 9-9 presents examples of respiratory equipment, and Fig. 9-10 provides guidelines for selecting respirators.)
      1) Supplied air respirators provide clean air from either a tank (a self-contained breathing apparatus or SCBA) or an air line connected to an air supply.
      2) Air-purifying respirators use a filter or canister to remove hazards from inhaled air; they may be full-mask or half-mask.
   c. Respirator face masks must form a tight seal against the face, requiring fit testing with isoamyl nitrate or irritant smoke as a fit check, prohibiting facial hair growth over 24 hours, and no eyeglass sidebars underneath the mask.
   d. Respirators must be tested for fit by the wearer before each use.
   e. After use, respirators must be properly stored, regularly inspected, and repaired as needed.
   f. A respirator wearer's health status must be reviewed periodically (usually annually) to assess physical and psychological fitness for using the respiratory protection equipment.

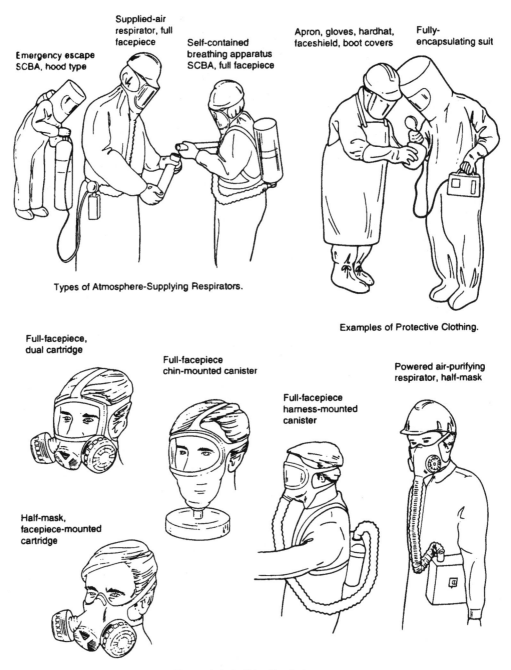

Types of Atmosphere-Supplying Respirators.

Examples of Protective Clothing.

Types of Air-Purifying Respirators.

FIGURE 9-9 *Examples of respiratory equipment*

(*Source:* U.S. Department of Health and Human Services, 1987)

g. The type of respirator to be used depends on the type of air-borne hazard. Respirator and cartridge selection is based on air sampling data performed in an exposure monitoring program.

h. Only NIOSH-approved respirators can be worn.

i. Escape respirator devices allow a person working in a normally safe

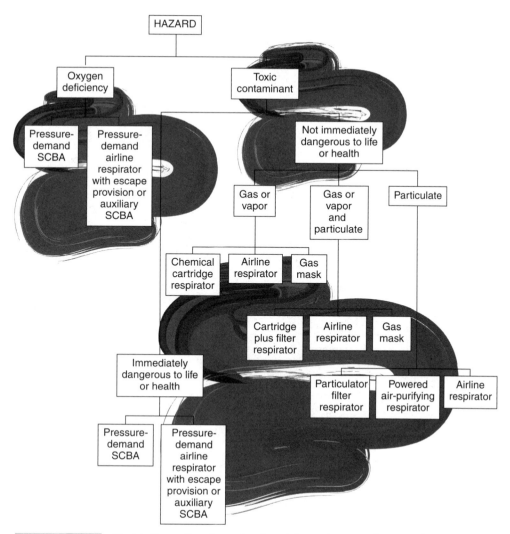

FIGURE 9-10 *Guidelines for the selection of respirators for routine use*

environment sufficient time to escape from suddenly occurring respiratory hazards. They should be used for escape purposes only.

j. Because respirators are uncomfortable or unacceptable to some workers, they may not be worn properly and thus not protect the worker from hazardous exposure.

BIBLIOGRAPHY

American Association of Occupational Health Nurses (AAOHN). (In press). *Incident analysis* [AAOHN Advisory]. Atlanta, GA: AAOHN Publications.

American Association of Occupational Health Nurses (AAOHN). (1996). AAOHN position statement: occupational health surveillance. *AAOHN Journal, 44(8),* 407.

American Association of Occupational Health Nurses (AAOHN). (1995). *Accident Investigation* [AAOHN Advisory]. Atlanta, GA: AAOHN Publications.

American Conference of Governmental Industrial Hygienists. (1994). *1994-1995 Threshold limit values for chemical substances and physical agents and biological exposure indices.* Cincinnati, OH: American Conference of Governmental Industrial Hygienists Technical Affairs Office.

Bang, Ki Moon. (1996). Occupational epidemiology. *Occupational Medicine: State of the Art Reviews, 12(4).* Philadelphia: Hanley & Belfus, Inc.

Barach, P., Small S.D. (2000). Reporting and preventing medical mishaps: lessons from non-medical near miss reporting systems. *British Medical Journal, 320(7237),* 759-763.

Barneo, D.L. (1992). Analysis of group data helps indentify subtle changes in health, hazard status. *Occupational Health and Safety.* 69(12), 30-34.

Breitenstein., B.D., Jr., & Spickard, J.H. (1995). Ionizing radiation. In P.H. Wald and G.M. Stave, (Eds.), *Physical and biological hazards of the workplace.* New York: Van Nostrand Reinhold.

Bradley, W. (1996). Management and prevention of on the job injuries: OHNs make a difference. *AAOHN Journal, 44(8),* 402-405.

Bureau of National Affairs. (1995). Group warned of increasing recognition of multiple chemical sensitivity as illness. *Occupational Safety & Health Reporter, 25(24),* 835-836. Washington, DC: The Bureau of National Affairs, Inc.

Burgess, W.A. (1995). *Recognition of health hazards in industry.* New York: John Wiley & Sons, Inc.

Burton, D.J. (1995). Indoor air quality cases require detective like analyses of facts. *Occupational Health and Safety 64(3),* 23.

Coffman, E. (1992). Sample integrity begins with knowledge of proper collection, storage methods. *Occupational Health and Safety.* Sept. 14, 29.

Cote, A., & Bugbee, P. (1995). *Principles of fire protection.* Quincy, MA: National Fire Protection Association.

De Almeida, I.M., Bindere, M.C., & Fischer, F.M. (2000). Blaming the victim: aspects of the Brazilian case. *International Journal of Health Service, 30(1),* 71-85.

Dessoff, A.L. (1995). Assess risks to control hazards. *Safety + Health, 152(5),* 62-65.

Dobie, R.A. (1995). Noise. In P.H. Wald & G.M. Stave (Eds.), *Physical and biological hazards of the workplace.* New York: Van Nostrand Reinhold.

Eichenberger, J. (1995). How to achieve results through employee committees. *AAOHN Journal, 42(7),* 344-348.

Feyer, A.M., Williamson, A.M. (1991). A classification system for causes of occupational accidents for use in preventive strategies. *Scandinavian Journal of Workplace Environment Health, 17(5).* 302-311.

Fleming, L.E., Herzstein, J.A. & Bunn, W.B. (1997). *Issues in international occupational and environmental medicine.* Boston: OEM Press.

Garg, A. (1995). Revised NIOSH equation for manual lifting: A method for job evaluation. *AAOHN Journal, 43,* 211-216.

Gates, D.M. (1995). Workplace violence. *AAOHN Journal, 43(10),* 536-543.

Geller, E. Scott. (1998). *Incident Analysis.* Neenah, WI: J.J. Keller & Associates, Inc.

Geller, E. Scott. (2000). Maintaining involvement in occupational safety: 14 key points. *Occupational Health & Safety, 69(1),* 72, 74, 76, 85.

Goldberg, A.T. (1996). Finding the root causes of accidents. *Occupational Hazards, 58(11),* 33.

Gressel, M.G., & Gideon, J.A. (1991). An overview of process hazard evaluation techniques. *American Industrial Hygiene Association Journal, 52(4),* 158-163.

Hau, M. (1993). Prevention through sentinel health event recognition. *Preventing occupational injuries, diseases and disability: 1993 national seminar.* Tampa, FL: Seak Legal and Medical Publishers, Inc.

Hau, M.L., and Dierwechter, D.W. (2000). Incident response. In D.B. Cox, (Ed.), *Hazardous materials management.* New York: McGraw-Hill Inc.

Hayes, G., Goodwin, R. & Miars, B. (1990). After disaster. *American Journal of Nursing,* 90(2), 61-64.

Johnson, D.L., & Bell, M.L. (1991). *Sources and control of error in industrial hygiene measurements. AAOHN Journal, 39(8)*, 362-368.

Jones, D.L. (1996). Occupational health services and OSHA compliance. In Law and the workplace. *Occupational Medicine: State of the Art Reviews, 11(1)*. Philadelphia: Hanley & Belfus, Inc.

Kahn, J. (1993). *Mental illness in the workplace*. New York: VanNostrand deinhold.

Keyserling, W.M., Stetson, D.S., Silverstein, B.S., & Brouwer, M.L. A checklist for evaluating ergonomic risk factors associated with upper extremity cumulative trauma disorders. *Ergonomics, 36(7)*, 807-831.

Kurtz, P.H., & Esser, T.E. (1989). A variant of mass (epidemic) psychogenic illness in the agricultural work setting. *Journal of Occupational Medicine, 31(4)*, 331-334.

Levy, B.S., & Wegman, D.M. (1999). Occupational health: Recognizing and preventing work-related disease (4th ed.) Boston: Little, Brown and Company.

Manuele, F.A. (1994). Learn to distinguish between hazards and risks. *Safety + Health. 150(5)*, 70-74.

McNeely, G. (1991). Critical incident stress debriefing. *Texas EMS Messenger*, February/March, 6-9.

Minter, S.G. (1995). A safe approach to incentives. *Occupational Hazards, 57(1)*, 171-172.

Mitchell, J. & Reshick, H.L. (1981). *Emergency Response to Crisis*. Bowie, MD: R.J. BradyCo.

Mullan, R.J., & Murthy, L.I. (1991). Occupational sentinel health events: An updated list for physician recognition and public health surveillance. *American Journal of Industrial Medicine, (19)*, 775-799.

National Safety Council. (1992). *Accident Prevention manual for business & industry: Administration & programs* (10th ed.). Itasca, IL: National Safety Council.

National Safety Council. (1995a). Principles of occupational safety & health for small businesses (POSH). *POSH for small business course*. Itasca, IL: National Safety Council.

National Safety Council. (1995b). *Accident prevention manual for business & industry: Engineering & technology* (10th ed.). Itasca, IL: National Safety Council.

Ness, S.A. (1991). *Air monitoring for toxic exposures*. New York: Van Nostrand Reinhold.

Occupational Safety and Health Administration. (1992). *Concepts and Technigoes of Machine Safeguarding*. (OSHA 3067). Washington DC: U.S. Department of Labor.

Perkins, J.L. (1997). *Modern industrial hygiene* (Vol. I). New York: Van Nostrand Reinhold.

Perkinson, L. (1995). JSA: A new look for an old friend. *Occupational Hazards, 57(8)*, 63-66.

Petersen, D. (1966). *Analyzing safety system effectiveness* (3rd ed.). New York: Van Nostrand Reinhold.

Plog, B.A., Benjamin, G.S., & Kerwin, M.A. (1996). *Fundamentals of industrial hygiene*. Itasca, IL: National Safety Council.

Recipe for an effective safety team. (1995). *Safety Management, 382*, 1-3.

Rempel, D. (1990). Medical surveillance in the workplace: Overview. *Occupational Medicine: State of the Art Reviews, 30*, 435-438. Philadelphia: Hanley & Belfus, Inc.

Rogers, B. (1994). *Occupational health nursing concepts and practice*. Philadelphia: W.B. Saunders Co.

Rogers, B. (1998). Research corner: Research award: PCNPs and occupational illness or injury. *AAOHN Journal, 46(8)*, 412.

Roughton, J.E. (1995). Personal protective equipment: Complying with the standard. *Professional Safety, 40(9)*, 27-30.

Saunders, G.T. (1993). *Laboratory fume hoods*. New York: John Wiley & Sons, Inc.

Senecal, P., & Burke, E. (1994). Root cause analysis: What took us so long? *Occupational Hazards, 556(3)*, 63-65.

Siler, C. (1994). Chemical companies concoct formulas for safety. *Safety + Health, 150(5)*, 50-53.

Smith, S.L. (1994). Near misses: Safety in the shadows. *Occupational Hazards, 56(9)*, 33-36.

Sparks, P.J., Daniell, W., Black, D.W., Kipen, H.M., Altman, L.C., Simon, G.E., & Terr, A.I. (1994). Multiple chemical sensitivity syndrome: A clinical perspective. I. Case definition, theories of pathogenesis, and research needs. *Journal of Occupational Medicine, 36(7)*, 718-730.

Terpin, D. (1992). Taking the risk out of response-confined space entry and rescue. *Industrial Fire World.* 7(1), 16-18, 24.

Travers, P.H., & McDougall, C. (1995). *Guidelines for an occupational health & safety service.* Atlanta, GA: AAOHN Publications.

U.S. Department of Health and Human Services (DHSS). (1994). *Workplace use of back belts—Review and recommendations.* Cincinnati, OH: DHHS (NIOSH) Number 94-122.

Voelker, R. (1994). Does multiple chemical sensitivity exist? *Safety and Health, 150(3)*, 54-58.

Vogel, C. (1991). Cut your losses with JSAs. *Safety & Health, 148(10)*, 38.

Waters, T.R., Putz-Anderson, V., & Garg, A. (1994). *Applications manual for the revised NIOSH lifting equation.* Cincinnati, OH: U.S. Department of Health and Human Services, National Institute for Occupational Safety and Health, Division of Biomedical and Behavioral Science.

Warren, S.B., & Amundson, R.M. (1995). Comprehensive baseline hazard assessments—A team approach. *Professional Safety, 40(7)*, 26-29.

Weeks, J.L., Levy, B.S., & Wagner, G.R. (1991). *Preventing occupational disease and injury.* Washington DC: American Public Health Association.

Weinstock, M.P. (1993). Chasing the missing link. *Occupational Hazard.* 55(9), 116-120.

Willen, J. (1995). How to produce an effective safety newsletter. *Safety and Health, 151(1)*, 46-49.

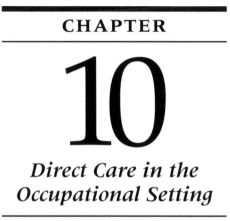

CHAPTER

10

Direct Care in the Occupational Setting

BARBARA BURGEL

Direct care consists of all of the activities involved in the delivery of clinical care to individual clients. These activities include the steps necessary for appropriate clinical decision making, such as taking a health history, conducting a physical examination, and ordering diagnostic or screening studies as well as the actual provision of clinical services. This chapter provides an overview of the processes involved in planning and delivering direct care services in the occupational setting; it concludes with a description of outcomes that can be used to evaluate the effectiveness of services.

I Definition of Terms

A *Direct care* is defined as hands on, clinical care delivery to individual clients.
   1. The range, scope, and depth of these activities vary based on the educational preparation, knowledge, skills, and abilities of the occupational and environmental health nurse.
   2. Licensure laws in each state outline the scope of practice for registered nurses, in addition to advanced practice nursing.

B *Advanced practice nursing* is an umbrella term for a licensed registered nurse prepared at the graduate degree level as either a Clinical Specialist, Nurse Anesthetist, Nurse Midwife or Nurse Practitioner (American Association of Colleges of Nursing [AACN], 1994).

C *Primary care* is defined as an array of integrated and coordinated health services with the following characteristics:
   1. Services are accessible and acceptable to the client.
   2. First-contact, or front-line, services are comprehensive in scope.
   3. Services are coordinated and continuous over time.
   4. Service providers are accountable for the quality and potential effects of the services.
   5. Primary care services are person-centered and holistic, which means they involve all levels of prevention; that is, services are not limited to a single organ or system or to a specific disease process (Nutting, 1991).

D The Institute of Medicine defines *primary care* as the provision of integrated, accessible health care services by clinicians who are accountable for addressing a large majority of personal health care needs, developed in a sustained partnership with clients, and practicing in the context of family and community (Donaldson, et al., 1994).

E *Health care providers* and *clinicians* are additional terms used to describe those who provide clinical care services within their scope of licensure.

II Overview of Direct Care

A Careful planning will determine the range of direct care services needed for a specific industry, and help meet the goals for a healthy work force.
1. The range and scope of direct care services may include the following:
   a. Care for occupational or nonoccupational conditions
   b. First aid, emergency care, minor acute care, chronic illness management, full service primary care, and 24-hour call
   c. Prevention-based services, including health-promotion programs and screening programs such as preplacement programs, immunizations, and health surveillance
   d. Case management of occupational and nonoccupational health problems
   e. Home care and telehealth services
2. Direct care services can be offered to all employees, dependents, and retirees.
3. Health care providers may be employees of the company or independent contractors; contractual arrangements with a health maintenance organization or other organizations for on-site providers may also be developed.
4. Depending on the types of conditions commonly treated, their medical complexity, and the number of anticipated visits, service providers on-site may include the following:
   a. Occupational and environmental health nurses, clinical nurse specialists in occupational health, and adult or family nurse practitioners who specialize in occupational health (Burgel, 1993; AAOHN, 1999)
   b. Family or primary care physicians or doctors of osteopathy who specialize in preventive medicine/occupational medicine
   c. Physical therapist, massage therapist
   d. Mental health professionals
   e. Other providers based on needs assessment
5. The rationale for providing on-site direct care services include the following benefits:
   a. Greater convenience for employees, with less down-time resulting from absence due to sickness and visits to off-site health care providers
   b. Greater opportunity for case management to monitor quality, outcomes, and cost of care
   c. Fast and accurate determination of work-related etiology or aggravation of the symptom or disease
   d. Accommodations, if needed, which are made by on-site providers who are knowledgeable about the work site.
   e. Opportunity to reinforce safe work practices with each employee encounter
   f. Ability to tailor direct care services to the risk profile of the company, and complement/maximize the health benefit plan.

g. Cost savings, which are realized by controlling duplicate health care services and reducing absence resulting from sickness.

h. Opportunity to reinforce a self-care approach to health

6. Determine the need for direct care on-site by evaluating the following factors (Burgel, 1993):

a. Hazard profile of company

b. Geographic proximity of the nearest emergency facility

c. Injury and illness statistics (both occupational and nonoccupational)

d. Demographics of the work force (number of employees, age, gender, length of employment with firm)

e. Health benefit coverage (number of employees with coverage; whether preventive and mental health services are included)

f. Company philosophy about direct care activities for employees

g. Financial and personnel resources

7. There are multiple ethical, legal, and professional considerations for direct care activities in the occupational setting (Burgel, 1996).

a. Ethical considerations

1) Confidentiality of personal health information of workers and their dependents must be ethically and legally safeguarded according to professional codes of conduct and state and federal laws.

2) The direct care provider must balance the "duty to warn" against the right to privacy of the employee or dependent.

3) Limited resources are dedicated to occupational health and safety; if expanded direct care activities are provided at the work site, will occupational health and safety have an even lower priority?

4) Workers have a right to know about the hazards in their work settings and a right to be notified of an exposure or abnormal physical finding.

b. Legal issues

1) Documentation must be done according to professional codes of conduct (Baker, 2000) (Chapter 3, Section VIII).

2) If medications will be dispensed or prescribed, state pharmacy laws must be followed. Advanced practice nurses can prescribe medications in many states.

3) Activities related to the care of clients must comply with OSHA standards, and compliance is needed with state laws for ensuring that direct care providers are free from infectious diseases (rubella, varicella, TB, etc.).

4) Potential liability arises if there is malpractice by the direct care provider. Is workers' compensation the exclusive remedy, or can the injured employee sue the direct care provider for malpractice? Legal advice is needed to clarify the professional malpractice issues for on-site direct care.

c. Professional issues

1) Direct care providers must be competent to perform the direct care activities and must practice within the state's business and professions code and scope of practice.

2) Policies and procedures outlining practice understandings and consultation/referral mechanisms must be clearly delineated.

B **The primary emphasis of direct care activities is health promotion and protection.**
1. Health promotion
   a. Begins with people who are basically healthy
   b. Uses strategies related to personal lifestyle—those personal choices made in a social context—that can have a powerful influence over one's health status (U.S. Preventive Services Task Force, 1996; U.S. Department of Health and Human Services [USDHHS], 2000)
   c. Includes such activities as the promotion of physical exercise and the reduction of the use of alcohol and tobacco
2. Health protection strategies
   a. Strategies that are related to environmental or regulatory measures that confer protection on large population groups
   b. Include food and drug safety and environmental health initiatives (U.S. Preventive Services Task Force, 1996; USDHHS, 2000)
3. The three levels of prevention include primary, secondary, and tertiary measures to protect and promote health and prevent disease (Chapter 12).
4. *Healthy People 2010* (USDHHS, 2000)
   a. Chapter I of *Healthy People 2010* outlines objectives for clinical preventive care, primary care, emergency services, and long term care to meet the goal to improve access to comprehensive, high-quality health care services. The occupational setting is an ideal community-based setting to positively influence many of these objectives.
   b. Chapter 20 of *Healthy People 2010* includes occupational safety and health objectives; all of these objectives include direct care activities with the goal to promote the health and safety of people at work through prevention and early intervention.

C **Health Assessment Competencies**
1. Direct care providers in the occupational setting require the following competencies:
   a. Knowledge of the physical and mental requirements of the job, including an understanding of essential job criteria and reasonable accommodations
   b. Knowledge of the work processes, potential hazards, and any personal protective equipment requirements
   c. Recognition of the link between work-site exposure and adverse health effects, and between worker health status and a safe work environment
   d. Proficiency in history-taking and physical examination techniques
   e. Proficiency in clinical decision making to establish a working diagnosis and outline a clinical management plan to the level of provider scope of practice
   f. Familiarity with clinical practice guidelines and evidence-based practice
   g. An ability to counsel and educate effectively about risk communication, self-care, and lifestyle modification plans
   h. Excellent communication skills to coordinate care, share rationale for treatment, and advocate injured workers and their families through the workers' compensation/disability systems
   i. Ability to manage multiple health and illness conditions
   j. Awareness of the connection between the physical and psychosocial aspects of illness

     k. Knowing when to refer to another discipline (e.g., physical therapist, psychologist, physician)

     l. Documentation strategies that minimize litigation risk (Baker, 2000) and promote communication and continuity of care

2. Operational requirements for direct care activities in an occupational health setting

    a. Facility/equipment requirements

      1) Private space to maintain confidentiality

      2) Patient gowns and sheets

      3) Handwashing facilities

      4) Locked file cabinet for medical records

      5) Small refrigerators (2) for medications (clean) and specimens (dirty). Two refrigerators are desirable but not always possible.

      6) Emergency response equipment, capabilities, and facilities (e.g., oxygen, defibrillator, electrocardiogram capability, starting an intravenous line, allergic response, eyewash, decontamination area)

      7) Equipment to conduct examinations (e.g., clinic table, light source, blood pressure equipment, oto-ophthalmoscope, stethoscope, reflex hammer, tuning forks (256 and 512 Hz), cotton swabs, tongue depressors, peak flow meters, goniometer to measure range of motion, Jamar to measure grip strength, tape measure, gloves)

      8) Screening equipment (e.g., audiometer and sound booth, spirometer)

    b. Supplies

      1) Medications (e.g., vaccinations, prescribed medications, and over-the-counter medications, including herbs and supplements)

      2) Safe needle devices and needle disposal units

      3) Supplies (e.g., splints, ice packs, eye patches, suture kits)

    c. Administrative needs

      1) Systems and supplies for recordkeeping (e.g., intake form, informed consent form, health history questionnaire for initial visit and follow-up, physical examination form for initial visit and follow-up, encounter form, referral form, lab/x-ray forms, prescription pad, physical therapy order forms, reappointment process, medical release form, workers' compensation forms, and OSHA-200 log process [note: in some cases, these forms may be computerized])

      2) Educational materials (e.g., culturally sensitive materials, with simple text and liberal use of diagrams, to manage literacy range; selected consumer-oriented health web sites for self-care education)

      3) List of referrals (e.g., community resources, providers, organizations)

III Health History

A health history provides a database of subjective data that encompasses all aspects of the individual's health, including current and past occupational and environmental exposures.

A **Purposes of a health history**

  1. To establish a health care relationship

  2. To identify active and potential physical and mental health problems

  3. To determine a risk profile for preventable health concerns

B Components of a comprehensive health history

1. Client profile: demographic data, including age, sex, nationality, and job title
2. Chief complaint: reason for visit—illness, injury, or prevention focused
3. History of present illness: includes questions about the seven symptom descriptors and supportive positive and negative data from other sections of the database
   a. Seven symptom descriptors
      1) Location/radiation: Where exactly is the pain/symptom located? Trace where it radiates.
      2) Setting: What were you doing when you noticed the symptom?
      3) Quality: What is the pain like? (sharp/dull/cramping/throbbing)
      4) Quantity/severity: How bad is it? On a 1-10 scale, with 10 being the worst, how would you rate your symptom? What is functional impact of symptom?
      5) Chronology: When did this start? Is it getting better, worse? How long does each episode last?
      6) Aggravating/alleviating factors: What makes it worse? What makes it better?
      7) Associated manifestations: Are there any other symptoms associated with it?
   b. Supportive positive/negative data
      1) Past medical history (e.g., any prior episodes of the same symptom?)
      2) Family history: Does anyone in your family have these symptoms?
      3) Personal/social history: Are there any contributing factors from diet, alcohol, smoking, drug use, exercise? Any new stressors?
      4) Occupational/environmental history: Is there anything in your work or home environment that could be contributing to this symptom?
      5) Review of systems: Are there any related complaints not previously mentioned?
4. Past medical history: prior illnesses, hospitalizations, surgeries, obstetrical history, and current immunization status
5. Medications and allergies: over-the-counter, prescribed and illicit drug use; for allergies, note response to determine if true allergy or a sensitivity
6. Family history: genetic/hereditary risk factors, chronic disease in family, and any significant family problems
7. Personal and social history: status of current relationships; satisfactions, future goals, stressors, and coping style; housing, education, literacy levels, and any financial concerns; violence potential (e.g., is there a gun kept at the home?)
8. Health habits: exercise, alcohol, diet, smoking, illicit drugs, sleep, seat belt use
9. Occupational and environmental health history (section III.D): listing of past and current paid and unpaid positions, including military experience, and any exposures, injuries, impairments
10. Review of systems: a checklist of symptoms, by body system, that may prompt recall of an important symptom within the last six months

C Components of a problem-specific history

1. Client profile
2. Chief complaint
3. History of present illness

4. Key occupational health questions to help determine work-relatedness:
   a. Is the symptom temporally related to work?
   b. Is the symptom temporally related to a change in a work process?
   c. Does the symptom improve/go away when away from work (i.e. on weekends, on vacation, or when the work is modified and the employee is removed from the exposure?)
   d. Do co-workers have similar complaints?
   e. Is the employee exposed to an agent that is known to cause the symptoms?

D Comprehensive occupational/environmental exposure history (ATSDR, 1992; Wegman, Levy, & Halperin, 1995; Twining, 1995) (Fig. 10-1 presents a suggested format.)

1. Purposes
   a. Identifies asymptomatic occupational/environmental illness
   b. Provides epidemiologic correlation between symptoms and activities or exposures
   c. Helps to correctly diagnose occupational or environmental health problems, and stimulates prevention activities at the work site so others are not similarly exposed
   d. Helps prevent aggravation of existing injury/illness
   e. Allows assessment of synergistic risks; for example, whether employee smokes or lives in an urban area with air pollution, and is also exposed to a known pulmonary irritant
   f. Aids in teaching and counseling worker on self-care

2. The employment history/occupational profile includes the following (Twining, 1995):
   a. Name of workplace
   b. Dates worked, and if part-time or full-time work
   c. Type of industry
   d. Description of job duties
   e. Known health hazards in the workplace
   f. Use of personal protective equipment
   g. Time off work for a health problem or injury

3. Selected questions for an occupational exposure inventory includes:
   a. Any skin problems? Any cough, wheezing, or other breathing problems? Any upper extremity or back pain?
   b. Have you changed jobs because of any health problems or injuries?
   c. Have you had any contact with certain chemicals, such as asbestos, acids, ammonia, or benzene? Have you had contact with noise, radiation, heat, or vibration?

4. Selected questions for an environmental history
   a. Have you changed your residence because of a health problem?
   b. Does your spouse have contact with dusts or chemicals at work?
   c. Is pesticide used around your home or in your garden?

5. High yield screening questions (Twining, 1995)
   a. Please describe your job.
   b. Have you ever worked with any health hazard, such as asbestos, chemicals, noise, or repetitive motion?
   c. Do you have any health problems that you believe may be related to your work or home?

Work and Exposure History
Date: _____/_____/_____

Name: _____   SSN: _____–_____–_____

Male _____   Female _____   Birth date:_____/_____/_____
Describe your current job:

What is your job title?

Are you exposed to any of the following health hazards?
Dust _____   Fumes _____   Solvents_____
Chemicals _____   *(if yes, please list):* _____
Noise _____   Vibrations _____   Heat _____   Cold_____
Repetitive motion _____*(if yes, specify type)*
Other types of exposures or concerns: _____

How long have you worked at your current job? _____
Describe a typical workday: _____
_____

Is protective equipment required in your job? Yes _____   No _____   *(If yes, specify type)*
Gloves _____   Goggles/Face shield _____   Hearing protection_____
Safety glasses _____   Mask respirator _____   Air-supplied respirator_____
Coveralls/apron _____   Other types *(list):* _____

Past Employment History

Job	No. of Years	Job Title	Exposures	Protective Equip. *(yes/no; type)*
_____	_____	_____	_____	_____
_____	_____	_____	_____	_____
_____	_____	_____	_____	_____

Additional Activities/Exposures
What are your hobbies? (list): _____
Are chemicals, metals, or other substances involved? *(if yes, please list):* _____
_____

Does anyone in your family work in a job that involves exposure (e.g., lead or asbestos)? Yes _____   No_____
(If yes, please explain): _____
Where do you live? _____
Are there any factories or public dumps near your home? Yes _____   No_____
(If yes, please explain): _____

Smoking History: Do you smoke? Yes _____   No _____   If yes, for how long? _____
Does anyone else in your household smoke? Yes _____   No_____
At home, do you work with:
Household cleaners? Yes _____   No _____*(if yes, please list type):* _____
Pesticides? Yes _____   No _____*(if yes, please list type):* _____
Herbicides Yes _____   No _____*(if yes, please list type):* _____
Are you involved in farming activities? Yes _____   No_____
Do you consider yourself to be in good health? Yes _____   No_____
If no, do you consider your health problems to be related to your work? Please explain.
Does anyone else in your work area have conditions similar to yours? Yes _____   No_____
If yes, please explain.

FIGURE 10-1   *Example of a format for occupational and environmental health history*

Sources: Agency for Toxic Substances and Disease Registry, 1992; Wegman, Levy, & Halperin, 1995; Twining, 1995.

E **Limitations of the health history**
1. Reliability of informant because of language and communication barriers
2. Family and social history may be emotionally charged for the individual
3. Failure of provider to pursue significant data
4. Worker's lack of knowledge about exposures
5. Worker's lack of understanding of the health implications of certain activities
6. Incomplete information—important data not obtained
7. Too much information; hard to interpret

IV The Physical Examination

A **Purposes of the physical examination in the occupational setting**
1. Identify disease
2. Detect disease process in presymptomatic stage
3. Determine biologic markers/target organ measures at baseline; compare measures at time of surveillance
4. Determine any impairment that may impact the ability to do the job or may necessitate an accommodation
5. Document baseline objective findings, if there is prior impairment and potential future apportionment issues

B **Physical examination considerations**
1. The primary purpose of the examination and use of the data will determine the scope of the physical examination. For example, it may be necessary to discuss with the potential employee what is mandatory and what is voluntary in a preplacement evaluation.
2. Examination findings, or absence of findings, should be charted in an objective and nonjudgmental fashion.
3. The ethical principle of nonmaleficence (do no harm) is of primary concern.
4. Findings should be summarized and recorded consistently, so that any abnormalities from baseline can be clearly detected over time.

C **Techniques for physical examination**
1. *Inspection* uses sight to look at the individual and to observe variations from the norm or from previously observed state.
2. *Palpation* uses light and deep touch to feel with hands and fingers to check temperature, moisture, texture, size, pulsation, vibrations, presence of joint swelling, nodules, masses, joint mobility, and organ size and location.
3. *Percussion* is the direct striking of a finger against skin or the indirect striking of a finger against a finger lying against an individual's skin. This technique is used to determine the density, size, and location of underlying organs; sounds range from tympanic to resonant, hyperresonant, dull, or flat.
4. *Auscultation* is the process of listening directly with the bell or the diaphragm of the stethoscope to assess sounds produced by the various organs and tissues.

D **Methods used to conduct the physical examination**
1. The examination should be performed systematically; its scope and depth is dependent on its purpose and the proficiency of the direct care provider.
2. If the person reports a specific symptom—for example, sensory changes in a specific location—more in-depth sensory testing is indicated.

3. Abnormal physical examination findings should be matched with symptoms through a clinical decision making process, with the goal to determine a working diagnosis; or the client can be referred for validation and follow-up to an appropriate health care provider.

4. Laboratory/diagnostic studies: Often, objective laboratory data are obtained at the time of the client encounter (e.g., urinalysis, pulse oximetry reading, or peak flow).

V Clinical Decision Making

A *Clinical decision making* **is the process of analyzing the subjective and objective data, and establishing a working definition of the health problem. This process includes the following steps (Bates, 1995):**

1. Identify the abnormal findings: symptoms, physical signs, laboratory results, and any recent work-site sampling or surveillance results.

2. Cluster these findings into logical groups; for example, numbness into the first and second digits, with atrophy of the thenar muscle in the same hand, with known vibration exposure at work.

3. Localize the findings anatomically; for example, the location of the above symptoms is in the distribution of the median peripheral nerve, but also could be the C6 cervical nerve root

4. Interpret the findings in terms of probable process.
   a. Pathologic—involving an abnormality in a body structure
   b. Pathophysiologic—involving an abnormality in a body function
   c. Psychopathologic—involving a disorder of mood or thinking

5. In occupational health, probable process includes the toxicology of the substance, specifically determining the dose-response and known target organ effect. The material safety data sheet (MSDS) for hazardous chemicals provides additional objective data.

6. Make one or more hypotheses about the nature of the client's problem.
   a. Select the most specific and central findings around which to construct your hypothesis.
   b. Match your findings against all conditions you know can produce them.
   c. Eliminate the hypotheses that fail to explain the findings.
   d. Weigh the probabilities, based on the client's risk profile, extent of exposure, epidemiology of the condition, temporal issues, and toxicology of the exposure.
   e. Consider life threatening "do not miss" conditions and conditions that are treatable.

7. Test the hypothesis. In occupational health, this often includes removal from exposure or modification of work duties, with monitoring for changes in symptoms.

8. Establish a working definition of the problem, the "assessment," and share rationale of how the subjective and objective data and laboratory findings link to support the working diagnosis. It is important to include the client's response to the working diagnosis, and how he or she is coping with this diagnosis.

9. Outline a plan
   a. Diagnostic interventions: What additional laboratory tests or x-ray examinations need to be ordered?

     b. Therapeutic interventions: What will be prescribed today? Include medications, exercise, modified work duties, ice, and splints.

     c. Client education: Describe the education provided at this visit.

     d. Record the date of the follow-up visit, and advise the employee to return sooner to the clinic if condition worsens in any way or if there are questions. Advise the employee regarding urgent care or emergency settings to access, if needed.

  10. The decision making process then repeats itself with follow-up appointments, and the collection of new subjective, objective, and laboratory data. The working diagnoses may be revised and refined over time and the clinical management plan altered, if needed.

  11. In the occupational setting, knowledge of workplace hazards is critical to the decision making process.

B Another approach to clinical decision making includes the above steps, but is augmented by using a cognitive tool to prompt as complete a list of possible diagnoses as possible. This cognitive tool is "VINDICATES."

  1. Vascular

  2. Infectious

  3. Neoplasm

  4. Drug or degenerative

  5. Inflammatory

  6. Congenital

  7. Autoimmune

  8. Trauma

  9. Endocrine

  10. Social/psychosocial

C Examples of prevention opportunities that may result from direct care and clinical decision making in the occupational setting

  1. When an employee presents with a work-related injury, it may signify a breakdown in a control measure. It is therefore critical to do an accident investigation to correct this problem at the root cause so coworkers are not similarly exposed.

  2. When an employee presents with a work-related injury or illness, it may be viewed as a sentinel event. Case-finding screening activities can seek other employees who may have been similarly exposed but are still asymptomatic.

VI Practice Guidelines

Practice guidelines are clinical practice recommendations based on a critical review of research/evidence; their primary aim is to standardize care.

A There are numerous practice guidelines focusing on different aspects of care, including the following:

  1. The diagnosis of a specific health condition

  2. The clinical management of a health condition

  3. Client educational materials for a health condition

B Other purposes of clinical practice guidelines

  1. Reduce variation in practice across geographic regions and across providers

  2. Improve the quality of health care and ensure use of tools and interventions that are based on research/evidenced

3. Promote best practices and cost consciousness
4. Use as a quality assurance/audit tool
5. Assist in the insurance authorization process
6. Facilitate the disability management process
7. Assist in orienting new personnel

C Sources of practice guidelines include:
1. The American College of Occupational and Environmental Medicine guidelines (Harris, 1997)
2. The Agency for Healthcare Research and Quality, in association with the American Association of Health Plans and the American Medical Association, has established a National Clearinghouse for Guidelines (http://www.guideline.gov).
3. The Agency for Healthcare Research and Quality produced three practice guidelines relevant to occupational health: Acute Low Back Pain, Smoking Cessation, and Depression in Primary Care, available through their web site (http://www.ahcpr.gov).
4. The CDC has many guidelines for occupational infectious disease. (http://www.cdc.gov)
5. The occupational and environmental health nurse may also wish to develop or modify selected clinical guidelines; for example, the AAOHN's Advisory called *Developing Clinical Guidelines or Protocols for Practice* (AAOHN, 1997).

D Direct care in occupational health is unique because of regulatory standards that require specific health related examinations or screening tests based on airborne concentrations of a substance and years of exposure (Papp & Miller, 2000). The types of examinations that may be required are as follows:
1. Preplacement examination (e.g., asbestos)
2. Periodic examination (e.g., ethylene oxide)
3. Emergency/exposure examination and tests (e.g., selected carcinogens)
4. Termination examination (e.g., coke oven emissions)
5. Specific screening tests (e.g., spirometry for respiratory protection)

VII Application of Levels of Prevention to Direct Care Activities

A Primary prevention: immunizations
1. Immunizations are widely underutilized as a primary prevention strategy.
2. The CDC has many resources available for the occupational and environmental health nurse, many of which are listed at the web page found at http://www.cdc.gov/nip/publications/ACIP-list.htm
3. The work site is an ideal location for immunizing workers (CDC, 2000). CDC has specific standards for the safe delivery of a vaccination program.

B Primary prevention: the preplacement physical examination
1. Purposes of the preplacement physical following a job offer
   a. Focuses on ability to perform the essential functions of the job
   b. Ensures protection of the worker from known risk factors
   c. Provides information so the worker can be placed in a job that does not compromise the worker's current health status
   d. Assesses the worker's need for accommodation

      e. Identifies any previously undiagnosed health problems

      f. Establishes baseline data such as impairment status, which is important in the event of future apportionment issues

      g. Ensures compliance with federal OSHA standards, the ADA, and other mandated programs such as DOT-required preplacement programs

      h. Introduces the worker to a health care system that is focused on prevention and early detection of disease

  2. Components of the preplacement examination

      a. Job-specific health history (mandatory) and health maintenance questions that may not be relevant to performance of the job (voluntary)

      b. Physical examination of organ systems that are involved in job performance or may be affected by job performance

      c. Appropriate laboratory tests or screenings, based on job requirements (e.g., functional capacity testing, vision testing, spirometry, or selected blood chemistry)

      d. An offer of a vaccine (e.g., hepatitis B vaccination, if exposed to bloodborne pathogens in the course of employment) (Rogers, 1994; Pruitt, 1995)

  3. Tools needed for an effective preplacement examination program

      a. The examiner should have the necessary skills to perform the examination and knowledge of the job requirements.

      b. The examiner must have knowledge of Americans with Disabilities Act (ADA) issues regarding preemployment inquiries about drug and alcohol use, the use of drug testing, and how to interpret direct threat.

      c. The examiner must have knowledge of how the ADA interacts with workers' compensation.

      d. The examiner must have knowledge on the requirements for accommodation, the concept of undue hardship, and the legal issues regarding hiring decisions.

      e. The examiner must be provided a copy of the job analysis that specifies specific requirements, such as climbing ladders, lifting 30 pounds on a continuous basis, reaching 70 inches to push a button to start a machine.

C Secondary prevention: screening

  1. *Screening* is a secondary prevention measure to identify or treat individuals who have a disease or risk factors for a disease but who are not yet experiencing symptoms of the disease (USDHHS, 2000)

  2. Criteria for health screening (U.S. Preventive Services Task Force, 1996)

      a. The disease must be one where early diagnosis and intervention has a positive effect on morbidity and mortality (e.g., a sigmoidoscopy screening to detect colorectal cancer).

      b. The method of administering the test must be acceptable to both the person administering the test and the worker receiving the test.

      c. Efficacy: the test must be able to detect the target condition earlier than it could be detected without screening and with sufficient accuracy to avoid a large number of false negative results (sensitivity) and false positive results (specificity).

      d. The occupational and environmental health nurse should be properly educated to perform the test, recognize abnormal results, and counsel, refer, and provide care for the worker.

  3. Box 10-1 outlines the interventions considered and recommended for the

---

BOX 10-1

Recommendations for periodic health examinations and interventions: ages 25-64

- **Screening**
Blood pressure
Height and weight
Total blood cholesterol (men age 35-64; women age 45-64)
Pap test (women)
Fecal occult blood and/or sigmoidoscopy (>50 yr)
Mammogram +/- clinical breast examination (women 50-69 yr)
Assess for problem drinking
Rubella serology or vaccination history (women of childbearing age)
- **Counseling**
Substance use
Tobacco cessation
Avoid alcohol/drug use while driving, swimming, boating, etc.
Diet and exercise
Limit fat and cholesterol; maintain caloric balance; emphasize grains, fruits, vegetables
Adequate calcium intake;
Regular physical exercise
Injury prevention
Lap/shoulder belts

Motorcycle/bicycle/ATV helmets
Smoke detector
Safe storage/removal of firearms
Sexual behavior
STD prevention: avoid high risk behavior; condoms/female barrier with spermicide
Unintended pregnancy: contraception
Dental health
Regular visits to dental care provider
Floss, brush with fluoride toothpaste daily
Immunizations
Tetanus-diphtheria boosters
Rubella (women of childbearing age)
Chemoprophylaxis
Multivitamin with folic acid (women planning or capable of pregnancy)
Discuss hormone prophylaxis (perimenopausal and postmenopausal women)

Source: U.S. Preventive Services Task Force, 1996

ATV, all terrain vehicle; *STD,* sexually transmitted diseases.

---

periodic health examination for adults, age 25-64 years of age (U.S. Preventive Services Task Force, 1996).

a. Leading causes of death in this age group are malignant neoplasm, heart diseases, motor vehicle and other unintentional injuries, HIV infection, and suicide and homicide.

b. Although the recommended interventions are for the general population, special attention should be paid to the needs of high-risk populations with unique health risks.

D **Secondary prevention: health/medical surveillance**

1. The term *medical surveillance* is used by OSHA to describe the process of determining whether workers are experiencing adverse health effects from exposure to hazards (Papp & Miller, 2000).

2. Medical surveillance refers to the requirements in the OSHA standards for specific clinical activities, including preplacement examinations, periodic

examinations, emergency/exposure examinations, termination examinations, biologic monitoring, and other laboratory or screening tests (Papp & Miller, 2000). (Although the OSHA term is *medical* surveillance, the preferred terminology in occupational and environmental health nursing practice is *health* surveillance to better reflect the purpose and scope of practice.)

3. Occupational health surveillance is the process of monitoring the health status of worker populations to gather data about the effects of workplace exposures and to use the data to prevent illness or injury (AAOHN, 1996a).

4. Purposes of a surveillance examination are as follows:
   a. Protect the worker from exposures that may cause adverse health effects.
   b. Ensure the worker's ability to perform the job activity.
   c. Fulfill governmental surveillance requirements, such as those outlined in the standards for asbestos and lead exposure.
   d. Ensure that environmental controls are working.

5. Five goals of aggregate surveillance activities in occupational health are as follows:
   a. Identify illness, injury, or hazards that represent new opportunities for prevention.
   b. Define the magnitude and distribution of the problem in the work force.
   c. Track trends in the problem's magnitude and assess the effectiveness of prevention efforts.
   d. Target educational and consultation efforts to specific work sites.
   e. Publicly disseminate information to facilitate personal and societal decision and policy making (Wegman, Levy, & Halperin, 1995).

6. Surveillance requires familiarity with the routes of exposure and toxic doses of chemicals. The primary activities involved in surveillance include the following:
   a. Collection of specific exposure data
   b. Selection and application of appropriate medical examinations (Stone, 2000)

7. Occupational and environmental health nurse responsibilities are as follows (Rogers & Livsey, 2000):
   a. Collaboration in the development of surveillance and screening policies (who to test; selection of testing methods based on hazard profile, toxicology, environmental sampling data, and legal requirements; frequency of testing; on-site versus vendor selection for analysis of results; storage of data; reporting of abnormal values; referral plan in response to abnormal values; ethical considerations; policy impact for the work site)
   b. Development of health history questionnaire and physical examination forms
   c. Performance of test examination
   d. Interpretation of test, referral, follow-up, and care plans
   e. Maintenance of confidentiality, record retention, and storage
   f. Health education—recommending changes in personal and work habits
   g. Instruction in self-care techniques for prevention and early detection
   h. Counseling or referral for conditions unrelated to exposure

8. Recognized methods of surveillance include chest x-ray, urinalysis, liver function testing, kidney function studies, complete blood work, audiomet-

ric, spirometry, and other tests needed for specific indicators of organ systems status. The frequency of testing depends on the incidence of disease in a specific target population. A written opinion is required from the person who conducts the examination.

9. OSHA publishes an *Appendix of Screening and Surveillance: A guide to OSHA Standards,* which augments the standards. This can be accessed through the web site found at http://www.osha.gov (Papp & Miller, 2000).

E **Secondary prevention: early diagnosis and treatment of injury and illness (emergency response/first aid, urgent care, chronic care, occupational and nonoccupational)**

1. Anticipate the type of health problems that may present urgently or in event of a disaster.
   a. Disaster preparedness requires a policy and procedure to manage large groups in event of a fire, earthquake, explosion, biologic or bomb threat, or act of violence
   b. Determine extent of direct care provided on site in event of a disaster
   c. Consider establishing Medical Emergency Response Teams
2. First aid:
   a. Eight federal OSHA standards require the provision of first aid. State OSHA programs may have additional requirements.
   b. Consider the scope of first-aid training, the contents of a first-aid kit, and how to respond to shock, bleeding, burns, etc.
3. Urgent care/chronic care
   a. Evaluate each health complaint to determine the following:
      1) Acuity of the condition and need for triage to outside referral
      2) Work causation or aggravation
      3) Ability of the employee to safely do their job with his or her health complaint, and the need for accommodation
      4) Reinforce individual prevention activities
      5) Act on work-site hazard control measures
   b. Go through each step of the clinical decision-making process
      1) Collect and analyze subjective data (health history, including a thorough occupational and environmental history).
      2) Collect and analyze objective data (physical examination, laboratory findings, environmental sampling data).
      3) Formulate assessments (determine whether condition is occupational or nonoccupational, and establish risk profile).
      4) Outline plans (diagnostic, therapeutic, and client-education interventions)
      5) Evaluate and follow up on both the individual and the work site to ensure that preventive measures are implemented and reinforced.
   c. Box 10-2 presents a protocol for the diagnosis and treatment of tendinitis (Burgel, 1998).
4. Many direct care activities require use of over-the-counter or prescribed medications. (Refer to the AAOHN Advisory (AAOHN, 1995) for a summary of over-the counter considerations.)

F **Tertiary prevention: disability and case management**

1. *Case management* is "a process of coordinating an individual client's total health care services to achieve optimal, quality care delivered in a cost-effective manner" (AAOHN, 1996b).

Text continued on p. 267

> **BOX 10-2**
>
> *Protocol for the diagnosis and treatment of tendinitis (Burgel, 1988)*
>
> I. Definition: Tendinitis is an acute or chronic inflammatory pain response after an acute or cumulative trauma to the tendon structures.
>
> II. Database
>
>   A. Subjective information
>
>   1. Age, hand dominance
>   2. Pain diagram, with rating of pain on 1 to 10 scale
>   3. Antecedent events, including nonoccupational risk factors such as trauma, sports, and repetitive activities at home. Describe work activities detailing frequency of fine manipulations, grasps, lifts, reaches, or keystrokes per minute, presence or absence of awkward postures, degree of force used, amount of weight lifted, and whether extremity is resting against sharp edges. Describe tool use, presence of vibration (e.g.:, jackhammer). Describe use of any protective equipment (e.g., antivibration gloves).
>   4. Describe environment: automation versus manual operations, presence or absence of an adjustable work station (e.g., height of work surface, adjustable chair), distance and height of required lift/reach.
>   5. Note symptom course with time off work or vacation.
>   6. Note presence of symptoms in other coworkers with similar job tasks.
>   7. Upper extremity symptoms: Erythema, swelling, locking of digits, numbness, tingling, weakness, nighttime wakening with paresthesias, neck pain
>   8. Past treatments used: nonsteroidal anti-inflammatory drugs, local injections of cortisone, physical therapy modalities, acupuncture, massage, chiropractic treatment, splint use (detail number of hours and for which tasks), assistive devices
>   9. Impact on activities of daily living: family responsibilities assumed by others; modification of repetitive household tasks such as shopping, cooking, vacuuming, and grooming; self-care strategies, including use of lightweight backpacks, "smart-grip" tools, and "quick fixes" to maintain neutral positions
>   10. Past medical history: Arthritis, diabetes, thyroid disorder, pregnancy, medications, allergies to medications, peptic ulcer disease, gastric distress with use of nonsteroidal antiinflammatory agents
>   11. Family history: Arthritis, diabetes, thyroid disorder
>   12. Personal/social history: Exercise (overall conditioning, overtraining, postural awareness), smoking and alcohol (vasoconstriction and impact on healing)
>   13. Past occupational/hobby history: musical instrument, needlework, keyboard/mouse use, hand tool use/vibration.
>
>   B. Objective information
>
>   1. General appearance, noting pain, posture
>   2. Height and weight
>   3. Skin: Erythema, bogginess, swelling, crepitus

BOX 10-2

Protocol for the diagnosis and treatment of tendinitis—cont'd

    4. Musculoskeletal: Bony or soft tissue deformity, muscle atrophy, localized pain to palpation, anatomic distribution of pain/paresthesias, range of motion, special maneuvers (see the table at the end of this box for selected special maneuvers)

    5. Neurologic: Sensory loss mapping, motor strength, deep tendon reflexes, special maneuvers (Phalen's and Tinel's maneuvers for nerve entrapment)

III. Assessment

  A. Determine exact location of tendinitis, its etiology, and whether acute or chronic. If work-related, notify workers' compensation carrier according to State Labor Code.

  B. Rule out nerve entrapment, distal versus spinal cord.

  C. Rule out arthritis presentation.

IV. Plan

  A. Diagnosis

    1. Laboratory, as indicated by the history and physical examination, possibly including the following:

      a. Antinuclear antibody, erythrocyte sedimentation rate, and rheumatoid factor (if you suspect a rheumatologic disorder)

      b. Blood urea nitrogen, creatinine, and liver function tests, if there is a history of prior renal disease, and with prolonged use of nonsteroidal antiinflammatory agents

      c. Thyroid function tests and fasting blood glucose (if you suspect carpal tunnel syndrome)

    2. Other diagnostics: nerve conduction studies with electromyelogram, x-ray, magnetic resonance imaging

  B. Treatment

    1. Nonsteroidal antiinflammatory agents (e.g., Ibuprofen 600 mg TID [three times a day] orally with food)

    2. Cortisone injection if tendonitis is severe, and if one isolated site of pain; the recommendation is not to inject more than three times per year in the same location.

    3. Splint or brace the affected extremity (do not immobilize shoulders for tendinitis). Wean the splint use, as symptoms decrease, to avoid muscle atrophy.

    4. Apply ice after any repetitive activity and at least 2 to 3 times per day for 15 to 20 minutes.

    5. Relative rest based on etiology: omit, decrease by 50%, or modify the offending activity.

    6. After the acute phase, recommend gentle stretching and strengthening exercises to affected area; warm shower before repetitious activity.

  C. Client education (Refer to client education supplement on tendinitis)

  D. Expected client outcomes

    1. Decrease in pain

    2. Increase in function

    3. Increase knowledge about avoidance of repetitious activities and need for overall conditioning

> **BOX 10-2**
>
> *Protocol for the diagnosis and treatment of tendinitis—cont'd*
>
> E. Consultation
>   1. Consult with or refer to an orthopedist or neurologist if there is muscle atrophy or grossly abnormal nerve conduction studies.
>   2. Consult with specialist if symptoms persist beyond 3 to 6 months despite conservative treatment and modification of repetitious activity.
>
> ---
>
> **Client Education Supplement: Treatment for Tendinitis**
> **Description**
> Tendinitis is a painful disorder caused by partial tearing or overstretching of the tendon sheath. Tendons are the fibrous "ropes" that connect muscle to bone. Inflammation is usually caused by a sudden movement that overstretches the tendon, or by small, micro tears to the tendon sheath caused by repetitive movements over time. Numbness and tingling may also occur with tendinitis, and are usually from localized swelling with pressure on a nearby nerve. Known risk factors for tendinitis are awkward postures, frequency of repetitions, amount of weight being lifted, sharp surfaces, and vibration. Treatment is aimed at eliminating these risk factors at home and at work.
>
> **Treatments**
> Rest, ice, compression and elevation (RICE) is the treatment for tendinitis, in addition to using medications such as Ibuprofen, which reduce the inflammation. Consider yourself an athlete as you prepare to do a repetitious activity at home or at work, and do appropriate warm up and cool down exercises every day. Other treatments aimed at prevention of these injuries include:
> Rechoreographing your work and home tasks by doing the following:
> - Slow the speed of your task.
> - Keep your head, neck, wrists, elbows, lumbar spine all in neutral position when doing a task.
> - Divide the task into smaller parts, and scramble the job tasks so your body is not using one set of muscles and tendons for a long period of time.
> - Use long muscles to do the job (e.g., lift your whole arm to shift to a different position on a keyboard, instead of bending at the wrist; turn toward the task, instead of rotating your neck).
> - For every one to two hours of repetitious work, get up and stretch, deep breathe, and change positions.
> - Choose your home exercise to counter your work postures; for example, do the backstroke in swimming if you spend your workday leaning forward over a work surface.
> - Alternate arms and feet, and do not overuse your dominant extremity.
> - Brisk walking with deep breathing is a good exercise for overall conditioning.

BOX 10-2

Protocol for the diagnosis and treatment of tendinitis—cont'd

If your work is causing your tendinitis:
- Notify your supervisor that you have a work-related complaint.
- Discuss your work tasks in detail with your health care provider.
- If you have photos of your work station, show them to your health care provider.
- A work station or work process can be analyzed by an ergonomic specialist, with recommendations to correct any design flaws that could cause a repetitive strain injury.
- Quick fixes can also be tried; for example, raise a computer screen into a better visual field by using old phone books, divide your lifting load in half, or shift more-frequent work tasks closer to your body.

Selected physical assessment maneuvers for work up of tendinitis

Maneuver	Technique	Possible diagnosis
Tinel's at the carpal tunnel	Strike two fingers over carpal tunnel region of wrist; if pain, numbness, or tingling occurs into the 1st, 2nd, 3rd digits, this is a positive Tinel's.	Carpal tunnel syndrome (entrapment of the median nerve)
Phalen's	Flexion of both wrists to 90 degrees for 60 seconds; if pain, numbness, or tingling occurs into the 1st, 2nd, 3rd digits, this is a positive Phalen's,	Carpal tunnel syndrome
Tinel's at the Guyon's canal	Strike two fingers over the hook of hamate above ulnar styloid; if pain, numbness, or tingling occurs into the 4th, 5th digits, this is a positive Tinel's at the Guyon's canal,	Ulnar nerve entrapment or neuritis at the Guyon's canal
Tinel's at the cubital tunnel	Strike two fingers between the medial epicondyle and the olecranon; if pain, numbness, or tingling occurs into the 4th, 5th digits, this is a positive Tinel's at the cubital tunnel.	Ulnar nerve entrapment or neuritis at the cubital tunnel
Finkelstein's test	Client makes fist over flexed thumb and gently ulnar deviates wrist; if pain occurs outside of the first extensor compartment (located just above the radial styloid, on the flexor side of the anatomic snuff box), this is a positive Finkelstein's.	DeQuervain's tendinitis
Resisted wrist extension	Client makes a fist and extends at wrist while resistance is applied downward; if pain occurs in the lateral epicondyle area, this is a positive tennis elbow test	Lateral epicondylitis
Resisted wrist flexion	Client makes a fist and flexes at wrist while resistance is applied upward; if pain occurs in the medial epicondyle area, this is a positive test.	Medial epicondylitis
Palpation of insertion of biceps tendon into shoulder	Client, with elbow flexed at 90 degrees at side, externally rotates shoulder; if pain is palpated at the groove between the greater and lesser tubercles, this is a positive test.	Bicipital shoulder tendinitis

---

BOX 10-3

Waddell's signs for low back pain

These five tests are designed to point toward psychologic causes of low back pain, and if three or more are positive, this is often predictive of medical/surgical treatment failure (Kaiser Permanente Northern California Medical Group, 1996):

1. *Distraction test:* Straight leg raising test may be either diminished or the test negative when the client is distracted. Perform the straight leg test when the client is sitting, and see if the results are different from when the client is supine.
2. *Regional strength test:* When testing muscle strength, there is evidence of cogwheeling or

giving way. Regional sensory testing: diminished sensation fits a stocking glove rather than a dermatomal pattern of sensory loss.

3. *Simulation test:* Axial loading; when the examiner applies pressure on the top of the standing client's head, the client complains of low back pain.
4. *Superficial tenderness:* The skin is tender to alight pinch over a larger than dermatomal area in the lower back.
5. *Overreaction:* Excessive dramatization of the usual expression of pain. Physician reaction: The physician may begin to feel frustrated or angry with the client.

---

2. *Disability management* uses case management strategies to manage the medical care, return to work, and needed accommodations for ill and injured workers with lost time; the goal is to prevent a protracted delay in returning to work (Gliniecki & Burgel, 1995; Harris, 1997).
3. Modified work is an important strategy in disability/case management. Studies examining the impact of modified work found that ill or injured workers who were offered modified work return to work about twice as often as those who are not. (Krause, et al., 1998).
4. Clinical evaluation for substance use and depression/anxiety disorders is important in disability and case management.
5. Several clinical tools can be used to detect malingering or a somatoform disorder. Box 10-3 presents Waddell's signs in clients with low back pain.

VIII Evaluating Outcomes

A Health outcomes are the results or consequences of a process of care. Health outcomes may include the following:
1. Satisfaction with care
2. Use of health care resources
3. Clinical outcomes, such as changes in health status and in the length and quality of life as a result of detecting or treating disease (USDHHS, 2000).

B Examples of health outcome indicators for occupational health are as follows (Rudolph, 1996; Rudolph, 1998):

1. Access to care: Initial treatment for nonemergency work-related conditions will be delivered within 24 hours after the injury is reported.
2. Client satisfaction: x percent of injured workers identified the occupational and environmental health nurse as very to extremely helpful in answering questions about the workers' compensation system on satisfaction survey.
3. Primary prevention: High-risk health care workers will have documentation in their preplacement record of hepatitis B immunity or the offer of vaccination.
4. Secondary prevention: Occupational health history is documented in x percent of medical records of employees with occupational injury; or, chart documentation of ergonomic evaluation within one week of diagnosis of a work-related upper extremity complaint.
5. Tertiary prevention: Sustained return to work, without reinjury, for 90 days after release to return to work; or, litigated cases decreased to x percent after occupational and environmental health nurse case management intervention.

C Use of health outcomes data

1. Focuses resources by (Kosinski, 1998):
   a. Targeting activities
   b. Establishing short and long term goals
   c. Defining responsibilities
   d. Delineating time frames for action items, expected results, and measurements against goals and benchmarks
2. Allows continuous quality improvement
3. Helps justify the occupational and environmental health nurse role, and the value of occupational and environmental health nursing services on-site
4. Documents the scope and depth of direct care activities needed on site: which direct care activities have met the quality outcome standards?

BIBLIOGRAPHY

Agency for Toxic Substances and Disease Registry. (1992). Taking an exposure history. *Case studies in environmental medicine.* Atlanta, GA: U.S. Department of Health and Human Services, National Institute for Occupational Safety and Health.

American Association of Colleges of Nursing. (October 1994). *Position statement: Certification and regulation of advanced practice nurses.* Washington, DC: AACN.

American Association of Occupational Health Nurses. (1995). *Over-the-counter medications.* AAOHN advisory. Atlanta, GA: AAOHN Publications.

American Association of Occupational Health Nurses. (1996a). Occupational health surveillance. AAOHN position statement. Atlanta, GA: AAOHN Publications.

American Association of Occupational Health Nurses. (1996b). The occupational health nurse as case manager. AAOHN position statement. Atlanta, GA: AAOHN Publications.

American Association of Occupational Health Nurses. (1997). Developing clinical guidelines or protocols for practice. AAOHN advisory. Atlanta, GA: AAOHN Publications.

American Association of Occupational Health Nurses. (1999). Nurse Practitioners in occupational and environmental health. AAOHN advisory. Atlanta, GA: AAOHN Publications.

Baker, S.K. (2000). Minimizing litigation risk: Documentation strategies in the occupational health setting. *AAOHN Journal 48(2),* 100-106.

Bates, B. (1995). *A guide to clinical thinking.* Philadelphia: J.B. Lippincott Company.

Burgel, B.J. (1993). *Innovation at the worksite: Delivery of nurse-managed primary health care services.* Washington, DC: American Nurses' Publishing, Inc.

Burgel, B.J. (1996) Primary care at the worksite: Policy issues. *AAOHN Journal 44(5),* 238-243.

Burgel, B.J. (1998). Tendinitis. In G. Collins-Bride & J.M. Saxe, (Eds), *Nurse practitioner/ physician collaborative practice: Clinical guidelines for ambulatory care.* San Francisco: UCSF Nursing Press.

Centers for Disease Control and Prevention. (2000). Adult Immunization Programs in Nontraditional Settings: Quality Standards and Guidance for Program Evaluation, *Morbidity and Mortality Weekly Reports, 49(RR01); March 24, 2000,* 1-13. (http:// www.cdc.gov/epo/mmwr/preview/mmwrhtml/rr4901a1.htm)

Collins-Bride, G. & Saxe, J.M. (Eds) (1998). *Nurse practitioner/physician collaborative practice: clinical guidelines for ambulatory care.* San Francisco: UCSF Nursing Press.

Donaldson, M., Yordy, K., & Vanselow, N. (Eds.). (1994). *Defining primary care: An interim report.* Washington, DC: National Academy Press.

Gliniecki, C.M. & Burgel, B.J. (1995). Temporary work restrictions: Guidelines for the primary care provider. *Nurse Practitioner Forum 6(2),* 79-89.

Goroll, A.H., May, L.A., & Mulley, A.G. (1995*). Primary care medicine: Office evaluation and management of the adult patient* (3rd ed.). Philadelphia: J.B. Lippincott.

Harris, J.S. (Ed). (1997). *Occupational medicine practice guidelines.* American College of Occupational and Environmental Medicine. Beverly, MA: OEM Press.

Kaiser Permanente Northern California Medical Group. (1996). Management of acute low back problems. *Clinical Practice Guidelines.* Oakland, CA: Kaiser Permanente Medical Group.

Kosinski, M. (1998). Effective outcomes management in occupational and environmental health. *AAOHN Journal 46(10),* 500-509.

Krause, N., Dasinger, L.K., & Neuhauser, F. (1998). Modified work and return to work: A review of the literature. *Journal of Occupational Rehabilitation 8(2),* 113-139.

Nutting, P.A. (Ed.) (1991). *A research agenda for primary care: Summary report of a conference* [Pub. AHCPR 91-08]. Washington, DC: DHHS.

Papp, E.M. & Miller, A.S. (2000). Screening and surveillance: OSHA's medical surveillance provisions. *AAOHN Journal 48(2),* 59-72.

Pruitt, R.H. (1995). Preplacement evaluation: Thriving within the A.D.A. guidelines. *AAOHN Journal. 43(3),* 124-130.

Rogers, B. (1994). *Occupational health nursing: Concepts and practice.* Philadelphia: W.B. Saunders Co.

Rogers, B., Randolph, S.A., & Mastroianni, K. (1996). *Occupational health nursing guidelines for primary clinical conditions* (2nd ed.). Beverly, MA: OEM Press.

Rogers, B. & Livsey, K. (2000). Occupational health surveillance, screening and prevention activities in occupational health nursing practice. *AAOHN Journal 48(2),* 92-99.

Rosenstock, L. & Cullen, M. (1994). *Textbook of clinical occupational and environmental medicine.* Philadelphia: W.B. Saunders Co.

Rudolph, L. (1996). A call for quality. *Journal of Occupational and Environmental Medicine 38(4),* 343-344.

Rudolph, L. (1998). Performance measures in occupational medicine: A tool to manage quality. *Occupational Medicine: State of the Art Reviews 13(4),* 747-753.

Stone, D.S. (2000). Health surveillance for health care workers: A vital role for the occupational and environmental nurse. *AAOHN Journal 48(2),* 73-79.

Twining, S. (1995). The Occupational and environmental health history: Guidelines for the primary care nurse practitioner. *Nurse Practitioner Forum 6(2),* 64-71.

U.S. Department of Health and Human Services. (1998). *The clinician's handbook of preventive services* (2nd ed). Washington, DC: International Medical Publishing, Inc.

U.S. Department of Health and Human Services. (2000). *Healthy people 2010: Conference edition*, Vols. I and II.Washington, DC: U.S. Government Printing Office, available at http://www.health.gov/healthypeople

U.S. Preventive Services Task Force. (1996). *Guide to clinical preventive services* (2nd ed.). Baltimore: Williams & Wilkins.

Wegman, D.H., Levy, B.S., & Halperin, W.E. (1995). Recognizing occupational disease, In B.H. Levy & D.H. Wegman (Eds). *Recognizing and preventing work-related disease* (3rd. ed.), Boston: Little, Brown and Company.

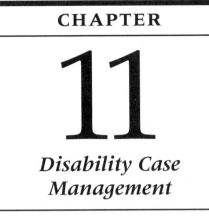

Disability Case Management

MARY LOU WASSEL, JEAN RANDOLPH, KAY BURGERHUFF STEPLER,
AND SANDY WINZELER

Occupational and environmental health nurses routinely coordinate and manage the care of ill and injured workers. Their role as case managers has grown more sophisticated in recent years with the advent of managed care as a primary cost-containment strategy in response to rising health care expenses. This chapter presents an overview of historical and recent trends in disability case management and discusses some of the issues and challenges occupational and environmental health nurses must consider in fulfilling this practice function.

I Case Management

Case Management is a process of coordinating a client's health care services to deliver optimal, quality care in a cost-effective manner. (AAOHN, 1994).

A *Disability case management* **is a broader term referring to the coordination of work-related and non–work-related injury and illness and includes aspects related to group health, workers' compensation, short-term disability, and long-term disability benefits.**

B **Case management is designed to prevent fragmented care and delayed recovery and to facilitate an employee's return to work in appropriate transitional or full duty or to an optimal alternative.**

C **A primary goal of case management is to justify the health care provided with a clear measurement of outcomes; cost savings often result, but the major emphasis should be on optimizing health care outcomes.**

II Important Case Management Terms

A *Benefits*—**Services or monetary compensation owed an individual, as defined by law (i.e., employment benefits or workers' compensation benefits) or based on contractual criteria established in an insurance policy (e.g., long-term disability policy).**

B *Cash Benefits*—**Cash that is paid (as part of workers' compensation benefits) to replace an employee's loss of income or earning capacity due to disability resulting from an occupational injury or illness.**
1. The following four classifications of disability benefits are often used

(additional information about these classifications of disability are in Chapter 3):

a. *Temporary total disability*—tax-free reimbursement for partial wages when a worker is temporarily totally disabled.

b. *Temporary partial disability*—tax-free reimbursement for partial wages when a worker is temporarily partially disabled

c. *Permanent total disability*—tax-free reimbursement for partial wages when a worker is permanently totally disabled

d. *Permanent partial disability*—tax-free reimbursement for partial wages when a worker is permanently partially disabled

2. Benefits are determined and allocated according to state jurisdictional rules.

C *Deductible*—the amount that a member must pay for covered services per specified period (usually the policy year) before the insurer will pay benefits.

D *Earning capacity*—the *potential* wages a worker *could achieve*, given his or her education, skill level, proximity to available work, and other factors.

E *Exclusive remedy*—the legal concept that receipt of workers' compensation benefits is the sole benefit (remedy) for the occupational condition incurred and leaves the employee without an additional course of action against the employer in the form of a tort claim

F *Functional capacity evaluation* (FCE)—a professional assessment to specifically determine a disabled person's residual physical abilities (Shrey & Lacerte, 1997)

G *Gatekeeper*—term commonly used to refer to a primary care provider (PCP) who is responsible for coordinating all of a member's medical care. Also may refer to a type of managed care plan that requires that the member have a formal referral from a PCP in order for other care to be covered by the plan.

H *Indemnity plan*—a traditional insurance program in which the insured person is reimbursed for covered expenses after a deductible is met

I *Independent medical examination*—a second medical opinion related to a worker's health condition that can be legally binding in some jurisdictions

J *Job analysis*—a detailed description of an employee's job duties and physical activities that identifies the essential and nonessential functions of the job

K *Managed care*—a system of health care delivery that influences utilization of services, costs of services, and measures of performance.

L *Maximum medical improvem*ent—the final level to which a person improves/recovers after sustaining a disabling medical condition (may or may not equate to predisability level)

M *Rehabilitation*—treatment provided by multidisciplinary specialists intended to return the employee to optimal function

N *Reserves*—money set aside by a self-insured organization or an insurance carrier to pay the ultimate monetary cost of accidental or business losses.

O *Residual functional capacity* (RFC)—the final determination of a person's physical capabilities or restrictions at the conclusion of recovery from an illness or injury, usually determined from a physical evaluation and review of an FCE test. The RFC determination is compared with the physical demands of the activity to determine the appropriateness of vocational options or limitations in daily living.

P *Risk management*—the process of making and implementing decisions that will minimize the adverse effects of accidental and business losses on an organization (Head, 1997).

Q *Return to work* (RTW)—the desired goal for all workers after an accident or illness.

R *Transitional work*—a temporary job that accommodates the employee's restrictions for a short period during recovery from an accident or illness. Options for transitional work assignments include the following (Fireman's Fund Insurance Company, 1997):

1. *Modified duty,* where an employee's original job is adjusted to accommodate restrictions
2. *Alternative duty,* where the employee performs a different job because restrictions rule out continued performance of original duties

S *Third-party administrator* (TPA)—a company that works with insurance firms, handling all the administrative tasks involved in processing claims. Employers who have become self-insurers, taking on the responsibility of funding their own benefit plans, may use a TPA or oversee payment of claims themselves, via a self-insured, self-administered plan (Mullahy, 1998).

T *Utilization review*—a process that measures use and consumption of available resources (including professional staff, facilities, and services) to determine medical necessity, cost effectiveness, and conformity to criteria for optimal use (Shrey & Lacerte, 1997)

U *Wage loss*—the actual *amount* of monetary losses sustained by a worker due to the inability to work

III Historical Perspective

A *Case management* has been used to describe a variety of strategies for managing health and social services for individuals, families, and work-force populations.

1. Community service coordination, a forerunner of case management, began at the turn of the 20th century in public health programs (American Nurses' Association, 1988).
2. Case management is not a new process, but its scope is expanding and becoming more sophisticated.
3. The current trend in formalized case management began with Medicaid and Medicare demonstration projects in the early 1970s (Case Management Society of America, 1995).
   a. Managed care programs emerged as a strategy to contain health care costs.
   b. As a result, the dual priorities of case management became meeting the client's needs and making good use of community resources.
4. There have been several major shifts in approach for disability case management; from orientation to work adjustment services in the 1970s, to work hardening in the 1980s, and to rehabilitation at the workplace in the 1990s (Shrey & Lacerte, 1997).

B Occupational health nurse case managers have historically been the ideal professionals to coordinate workers' health care services from the onset of illness or injury to the safe return to work or an optimal alternative.

1. Focuses of occupational health case management are as follows:
    a. Providing a safe and healthy workplace
    b. Ensuring that ill or injured workers receive prompt, quality healthcare
    c. Facilitating injured employees' return to work as soon as it is medically safe
2. Occupational and environmental health nurses help injured workers achieve optimal outcomes by using the following (AAOHN 1996):
    a. Expertise in health care delivery
    b. Knowledge of the multitude of service options
    c. Expertise in managing return-to-work programs
    d. Understanding of workers' relationships with their environments

C History has influenced the development and implementation of today's more sophisticated case management services.

1. Today case management requires an understanding of how the health care delivery system is affected by various medical insurance, government, and corporate mechanisms.
2. In the practice setting, case management demands critical thinking skills, clinical knowledge, experience within the health care delivery systems, and knowledge of gaining access to quality, professional resources (Mullahy, 1998).

D Changes in the payment for health care services have historically had the greatest effect on access and delivery.

1. Before World War II, technology was simple and health care dollars were primarily directed toward the treatment of acute illnesses or injuries.
2. After World War II, technology became more complex, and health care expenses for the treatment of chronic, long-term, expensive-to-treat illness and injuries increased dramatically (Rooney, 1990).
    a. The health insurance industry and third-party payment systems emerged.
    b. During postwar economic challenges, it was very common for employers to offer benefits such as pensions, disability benefits, and insurance plans instead of salary increases.
    c. Insurance payments rose as the insurance industry expanded from covering less than 20% of Americans before WWII to greater than 60% by the early 1960s.
    d. It became generally expected that policyholders were entitled to whatever care or treatment licensed health care providers prescribed.
3. Third-party payments rose from covering about 33% of all personal health care costs in 1950 to almost 75% in the 1990s.
4. By the 1990s, most American workers expected their employer-funded insurance benefits to cover the majority of their individual and their family members' health care expenses.
    a. Direct costs for workers' health care expenses and lost wages resulting from occupational illnesses and injuries are generally paid under a variety of employer workers' compensation insurance arrangements.
    b. Costs for non–work-related health care expenses are generally paid under a variety of employer group health insurance arrangements.

E The critical need for effective case management has grown largely as a result of uncontrolled and rising health care costs.

1. By the 1980s, employers were paying for a larger portion of the nation's health care and could no longer tolerate uncontrolled increases in both private and public health care costs that had resulted in double-digit annual increases for their group health and workers' compensation insurance premiums.

2. Corporations found themselves challenged to make a profit in a climate where health care expenses were consuming approximately 15% of the gross national product.

F Managed care as a cost-containment strategy emerged first in the group health insurance arena and later in the workers' compensation area.

1. Managed care incorporates use of preferred provider networks, HMOs, direct contracting, bill audits, utilization review, preadmission authorization, concurrent and retrospective review, second surgical opinions, independent medical exams, and case management.

2. In 1997, nearly 75% of workers who received health benefits from their employers were covered by some type of managed care plan, up from 51% in 1995 (New York Times, 1997 cited in Mullahy, 1998).

3. It has been estimated that more than 110 million Americans are enrolled in formal managed care plans, including a significant number of Medicare and Medicaid recipients as new enrollees.

4. Although managed care programs strive to reach all potential users of health care service, case management is a personalized process that focuses on certain high-risk or high-cost individuals; some of the greatest cost savings are achieved when case management efforts are focused on the 3% to 5% of the client population responsible for 60% to 70% of the expenditures in any health plan (Mullahy, 1998).

5. Decision factors or triggers for using case management are often developed based on the goals of the individual program.

IV Practice Settings for Case Management Services:

A Workplaces/Corporations

B Health care delivery systems (e.g., hospitals, clinics, rehabilitation facilities)

C Provider agencies/facilities (e.g., mental health, home health)

D Managed care organizations, including HMOs

E Public insurance providers (e.g., Medicaid, Medicare)

F Private insurance providers (e.g., workers' compensation, health, long-term care, disability, liability, casualty, auto, and accident)

G Independent case management companies and contractors

V Team Roles and Responsibilities

A The *employee,* who is the central player in the case management process, has the following main responsibilities:

1. Communicating promptly with the employer about the injury or illness and participating in the accident investigation process as appropriate

2. Maintaining contact with the occupational and environmental health nurse

regarding medical care, follow-up appointments, and issues regarding return to work

3. Keeping appointments with all health care providers

B The *occupational and environmental health nurse* is involved in all stages of the case management process. The nurse's responsibilities include the following:

1. Serving as first line contact with the ill or injured employee; this may include assessment, evaluation, and treatment or referral to other health care providers

2. Providing case management, with an emphasis on return to preinjury function (AAOHN, 1994)

3. Acting as a liaison with the employee, other health care professionals, insurers, the employer, and the workers' compensation board, if applicable, on the employee's behalf. (AAOHN, 1996)

4. Working with the employee to establish recovery and rehabilitation goals and objectives

5. Jointly setting a date for return to work; working with the physician to establish a timely and individualized rehabilitation program

6. Communicating with other health care professionals to negotiate care (e.g., home care, hospice) and to assess social support resources

7. Working with the employee to determine if transitional work is available and monitoring employee's progress upon return to work

8. Educating the employee about the limits of the workers' compensation or disability system and referring further questions to the claims manager or human resources, as appropriate

C The *physician* is usually the primary care provider for the seriously injured or ill employee. The physician's responsibilities include the following:

1. Providing timely information regarding diagnosis, treatment, and expected return-to-work date

2. Clarifying any work limitations that may apply upon return to work; approving transitional duty work

3. Being aware of workplace issues, including types of work available and conducting a workplace walk-through assessment as needed to meet this objective

4. Communicating with members of the Return to Work Team, including the occupational and environmental health nurse or claims manager, before making referrals to other specialists for persistent symptoms

D The *employer's* support is critical in an effective case management program, especially in identifying possible transitional duty to expedite return to work. The employer's responsibilities include the following:

1. Investigating the accident or factors impacting illness and injury and reviewing workplace factors, which may need to be changed or modified (e.g., machine modifications, ergonomic improvements)

2. Maintaining contact between supervisor and employee during the disability to promote good will and help maintain the link between the injured employee and the workplace

3. Helping the occupational and environmental health nurse, human resources professionals, and the supervisor identify suitable transitional work

4. Facilitating the worker's return to work as soon as is medically safe

E The *insurer* (whether internal or external), represented by the claims manager, acts as a consultant with all parties during all stages of the claim. Responsibilities of the insurer include the following:

1. Deciding on compensability of the claim
2. Authorizing medical care and payment of bills to providers
3. Ensuring the payment of weekly wages specified in workers' compensation guidelines
4. Responding promptly and accurately to employer's and employee's questions regarding the claim, including referrals, entitlements (e.g., permanent partial disability [PP], temporary total disability [TT], and settlements)
5. Coordinating the flow of information by requesting information from health care providers when necessary
6. Consulting with attorneys, when necessary, regarding specific questions about employees' rights under state workers' compensation law (e.g., controverting or settling a claim)

F *Rehabilitation specialists* (rehabilitation nurses, physical therapists, occupational specialists, and vocational counselors) work with the injured employee during the rehabilitation phases of recovery (AAOHN, 1999). Their major responsibilities include the following:

1. Working with the injured employee so function and strength are regained to meet the goal of return to work
2. Communicating with the team regarding the employee's progress; be aware of "red flags" and issues affecting return to work (Box 11-1 lists several indicators of delayed recovery).
3. Providing specialized programs to facilitate the worker's return to work

---

BOX 11-1
Indicators of delayed recovery

- Time off from the date of injury exceeds 6 months
- Continued subjective complaints without objective findings
- Undiagnosed or untreated depression (either preceding or concurrent with injury)
- Several failures to return to work
- Close to retirement age
- "Doctor shopping"
- Requests for narcotics
- Involvement of an attorney
- A change in the story of injury occurrence
- Unresolved anger at employer about the injury

- Unwillingness to discuss or negotiate an RTW plan
- Other secondary gain issues: disabled partner at home, multiple demands, and entitlement issues
- Income on temporary disability equal to or greater than regular wage scale
- Limited job offerings in the area
- Perceived lack of support from supervisor
- Poor job satisfaction
- History of job performance problems
- Time off without any change in symptoms

Gliniecki & Burgel, 1995.

using such techniques as functional capacity assessments, ergonomic evaluations, work hardening programs, etc.

4. Providing realistic expectations regarding recovery
5. Helping the injured employee manage chronic pain

G The *union* is important in its support of the case management process and the injured or ill employee. Main responsibilities include the following:

1. Working with the employer and the occupational and environmental health nurse to understand and support objectives for the injured employee
2. Helping the injured employee understand his or her responsibilities for return to transitional work
3. Helping the injured employee understand his or her benefits while disabled

VI Steps in Program Development

Establishing an effective case management program requires several important steps: assessment, data analyses and diagnoses, planning, implementation, and evaluation.

A Assessment

1. Gather benefit-utilization data for non–work-related health problems for workers and dependents, specifically for the following:
   a. High-cost cases
   b. Repetitive hospitalizations or extensions of hospital stays
   c. Selected diagnoses (e.g., spinal cord injuries, premature births, cancer, organ transplants, psychiatric diagnoses)
   d. Geographic coverage of workers and dependents
   e. Numerous providers involved in a case
2. Collect the following workers' compensation data by geographic region, department, and job class:
   a. Numbers and costs of first-aid, medical-only, and lost-time cases, and the range of diagnoses
   b. The type of permanent disability awarded and vocational rehabilitation costs
   c. High-reserve cases
   d. Workers' compensation experience rating
   e. Litigation costs (Box 11-2 presents strategies for avoiding litigation.)
   f. Referral data on the number and types of specialty referrals, wait time before seeing specialist, length of physical therapy prescription, etc.
   g. Selected diagnoses (e.g., soft tissue injury, upper-extremity musculoskeletal disorders, low back pain, and stress claims)
3. Review health benefit coverage for workers and dependents for the following:
   a. Preexisting condition exclusions
   b. Mental health benefits (inpatient, outpatient, partial stays)
   c. Home-care coverage
   d. Preauthorization procedures
   e. Second-opinion requirements
   f. Out-of-pocket costs
   g. Prescription coverage
   h. Percentage of workers and dependents not covered by an employer-sponsored health plan
4. Review medical leave-of-absence policies and communication between human resources and the occupational health services.

BOX 11-2

Strategies for avoiding litigation

- Be aware that miscommunication among the parties is one of the largest barriers to efficient case management (AAOHN, 1999).
- Treat injured employees with respect and dignity.
- Respect the employee's right to confidentiality of medical information whenever possible.
- Coach the employer regarding the benefits of instituting a transitional return-to-work program.
- Maintain regular contact among all parties on the health care team to address concerns, treatment, special needs, referrals, etc.

- Maintain contact with the employee to avoid misunderstandings and maintain the bond with the employer.
- Consider a home visit to the employee in cases that have medically complex diagnoses, are deemed catastrophic, or warrant assessment of rehabilitation needs.
- When the employee is hospitalized, consider a visit to the hospital to show support, answer questions, and establish a bond with the employee.

---

5. Assess success of transitional duty program.
    a. Number of successful return-to-work programs
    b. Supervisor cooperation
    c. Number of reinjuries
    d. Overall cost of accommodations

B **Data analyses and diagnoses**
1. Determine regional and programmatic "hot spots" where outcomes and cost have not been well monitored.
2. Conduct a brief, retrospective, cost-effectiveness analysis to determine whether case management could have made a positive impact on a sample of interest.
    a. Select two or three high-cost lost-time cases.
    b. Detail health costs and temporary/permanent disability costs.
    c. Determine the important outcome criteria, based on the natural history of the injury or illness and on published clinical pathways (e.g., a benchmark for an acute low back sprain would be ordering a magnetic resonance imaging [MRI] study *only* when low back pain has caused a limitation for more than four weeks and there is physical examination evidence of nerve root dysfunction [USDHHS, 1994]).
3. Document a range of anticipated cost savings based on the cases identified for case management.
4. If a positive impact of case management can be demonstrated, proceed with formal planning for a pilot project; examples of positive impacts include the following:
    a. Cost savings cover the program's expenses
    b. Less invasive diagnostic procedures are ordered
    c. An improved quality of life results

C Planning

1. Use the following criteria to identify one or two sites to pilot a case management program:
   a. Size of the worker population, number of dependents, and pattern of injury and illness statistics
   b. Opportunity to demonstrate a positive impact within a defined time frame
   c. Management and union support
   d. Strong occupational and environmental health nursing interest and commitment
   e. Strong commitment to primary prevention of work-related hazards
2. Develop a policy statement with program goals, objectives, and timetable.
3. Determine necessary resources (e.g., telephone, computer, fax, modem, car, database management software, and staff) to provide the appropriate level of case management.
4. Network with other disability management professionals in the community.
5. Develop a marketing plan for workers and dependents, including communication with human resources, union, workers' compensation carrier and administrator, community referrals, etc.
6. Consider establishing a task force that will develop strategies to ensure the successful "buy-in" by workers and dependents.
7. Establish evaluation criteria.

D Implementation

1. Initiate a trigger system to notify the occupational health services of cases to be included in the case management pilot.
2. Link the client to the needed services, using appropriate communication skills to share the rationale for treatment choices.
3. Throughout the case management process, use primary, secondary, and tertiary preventive nursing interventions to prevent delayed recovery.
4. Document time spent with client, nature of interactions, anticipated outcome, and cost savings in a computerized database management system.
5. Focus on a realistic return-to-work date.
6. Consider establishing an ongoing committee to assist with return to work and transitional duty.

E Evaluation using a structure, process, and outcomes approach (Fig. 11-1 presents a case management evaluation model)

1. Determine the effects of relevant structural elements on the resolution of cases. Structural elements include the following:
   a. Policies and regulations, including workers' compensation
   b. The characteristics of the delivery system, including the organization of services, personnel involved in service delivery, and financing of services
   c. The characteristics of the injured or ill workers, including their personal attributes, support systems, and attitudes about work
2. Develop methods to ensure that appropriate processes, including the following, are used in the delivery of service:
   a. The interactions among case manager, other service providers, and the injured worker are adequate and appropriate.

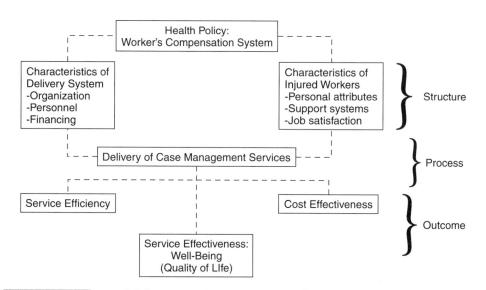

FIGURE 11-1 *Model for case management evaluation*

Source: Aday, L., Begley, C.E., Lairson, D.R. & Slater, C.H., 1993.

   b. Workers are informed and knowledgeable about the structures and processes affecting their cases.

   c. The cause of the injury or illness is analyzed, with the goal to prevent similar occurrences in the future.

3. Assess the outcomes that are affected by case management services; outcomes include service efficiency (timeliness of services), service effectiveness (quality outcomes), and cost effectiveness (dollar outcomes).

   a. Measures of *service efficiency*

     1) A notification system that captures all the cases that meet the case management criteria

     2) Appropriate and accurate entry of data by case managers

     3) Delivery of services within the anticipated time frame, with limited wait time, if referred

     4) Documentation of steady improvement in the worker's condition

     5) An active plan for return to work in a transitional capacity until able to resume full duty of the original job

   b. Measures of *service effectiveness*

     1) The client and family are satisfied with care coordination and communication.

     2) The case manager is satisfied with the implementation of the case management program, including the integration of any suggestions to improve the program.

     3) The important providers and management are satisfied with their collaboration with the case manager to improve care outcomes.

     4) The supervisor is satisfied with the implementation of the transitional duty component of the case management program.

     5) Union leadership is satisfied with a fair and equitable utilization of benefits for workers and their dependents.

   c. *Cost effectiveness* is measured by evaluating direct and indirect costs.

     1) The *direct costs* of accidents include the measurable medical expenses

and payment for lost wages. These costs are fairly easy to quantify, but represent only a fraction of the total cost of accidents when compared with the indirect or hidden costs of accidents. Accurately measuring direct cost savings necessitates the following:

a) Placing a cost value on every intervention
b) Selecting data for a particular work site and comparing several claims that included case management with other claims that were not case managed, trying to control for types of work demands and severity of worker's conditions
c) Evaluating the frequency and costs of office visits, types of diagnostic interventions, numbers and costs of prescriptions, number of inpatient days, and mean length of stay
d) Comparing temporary disability payments
e) Determining the date of injury, date of permanent and stationary status, and amount and percent of any permanent disability award
f) Detailing any vocational rehabilitation costs
g) Listing legal costs (health evaluations, attorney representation)
h) Determining direct cost savings in insurance premiums

2) The *indirect* or hidden costs of accidents are more difficult to measure and represent much greater costs (e.g., time lost by supervisors and other workers, replacement costs for hiring temporary workers or new staff, decreased production levels, lost profits, potential loss of customers, and decreased employee morale). Accurately measuring indirect cost savings necessitates the following:

a) If the worker successfully returned to either transitional or regular work, evaluating of job performance markers (e.g., number of days absent, visits to on-site health services, visits to employee assistance providers, and other appropriate industry-specific productivity data)
b) If the worker did not return to work, evaluating the date of termination and continued costs in the social security/disability system once workers' compensation benefits are depleted
c) Determining the expenses of the case management program, including a percentage of overhead costs and the number of hours of case management time
d) Determining whether savings were realized with the cases analyzed
e) Repeating the cost analysis for a group of claims with similar diagnoses and from a specific department, site, or region
f) Communicating "added value" (quality and outcomes) of case management program to management, union, human resources, and case management staff

NOTE: The Case Study presents examples of scenarios demonstrating these steps.

VII Return to Work (RTW)

A Formalizing the RTW program

1. Companies should have an established RTW Program with a *written* RTW policy statement.
   a. Having a written RTW policy statement will usually require the approval and commitment of upper management.

Case study

	Best-case scenario	Worst-case scenario
Presentation:	A 32-year-old female came into the clinic with a note from her physician after being out of work two days. Her physician has diagnosed left wrist tendinitis and has started her on nonsteroidal antiinflammatories and returned her to work with limited use of the left wrist. The note also stated that the tendinitis was work-related because of the repetitive nature of her work in a manufacturing setting.	A 28-year-old male presented to Employee Health having caught his wrist in a machine at work, sustaining a contusion and a possible ligament injury to his wrist. He was referred to an orthopedist two weeks after the injury.
Clinical findings:	A detailed history and exam revealed the following, which were suspicious for reflex sympathetic dystrophy (RSD): 1. Burning 2. Aching pain, which was out of proportion to the injury and exacerbated by touch and active or passive motion 3. Edema of the hand, soft and pitting 4. Increased warmth and redness of the hand 5. Increased sweating	Symptoms: 1. Severe burning and aching wrist pain 2. Swelling 3. Vasomotor and sudomotor changes 4. Guarding of the affected limb
Treatment/referral:	The employee was unable to return to work. 1. An immediate referral was made to an orthopedist. 2. Notes were faxed to the orthopedist's office, and it was made clear that the diagnosis of RSD needed to be considered. (Phone call to orthopedist was made before sending the fax.) 3. The orthopedist confirmed the diagnosis of RSD with a stellate ganglion block. 4. A physical therapy regimen was initiated while the block was still in effect. 5. Over the next few weeks, more blocks, physical therapy (PT), and different medications were ordered. 6. The employee began to improve and the physician conferred with the employer to determine availability of transitional work.	A diagnosis of RSD was made and the employee received the following referrals and treatment: 1. Referred to a pain clinic 2. Referred to a hand specialist, when a triangulofibrocartilage complex tear was diagnosed by arthrogram/MRI 3. The hand specialist treated the wrist injury. 4. The hand specialist referred the employee to a psychiatrist for depression and adjustment issues, which she felt were secondary to the injury, *without consulting* the pain clinic or the OHNP or insurer. 5. The psychiatrist kept the employee in individual therapy sessions and group therapy and was available for telephone consultations (@ $100 each). 6. Many more medications for anxiety and depression were prescribed.

MRI, magnetic resonance imaging; *OHNP,* occupational health nurse practitioner.

Continued

Case study—cont'd

	Best-case scenario	Worst-case scenario
		7. Three years later, the employee is still being treated by the psychiatrist, who has not released the employee to return to work despite a release from the hand specialist. 8. The employee has, in fact, become extremely dependent on his psychiatric care and has threatened suicide if the therapy is stopped.
Outcome:	1. Two months after the employee's initial presentation to Employee Health, the employee returned to work in a temporary, alternative position. 2. She expanded her workday from 4 to 8 hours over the next 6 weeks. 3. She continued to go to PT and doctors' appointments. 4. 14 weeks after her initial presentation with symptoms, she returned to full duty in her original job. 5. The case was followed for 6 more months to ensure no recurrence of symptoms, after which time it was closed to follow-up. 6. *There was no permanent impairment.*	1. A lack of communication and consultation with the team resulted in uncontrolled referrals and unnecessary expenditures. 2. Continued psychiatric treatment three years after initial injury in spite of orthopedic release to work 3. Total disability, no return to work 4. Attorney involvement and continued legal fees 5. Open case
Direct costs:	Lost wages: $4000 (14 weeks @ $250) Medical: $10,000 Legal Fees $0 Total direct costs: $14,000	Lost wages: Possibly lifetime benefits because of catastrophic claim (37 years to age 65 times 52 weeks @ $250): $481,000 Medical: estimated $300,000 Legal fees: $10,000 (first 3 yrs) Total direct costs: $791,000
Savings	$777,000 potential savings with early recognition of RSD, appropriate referral, and aggressive early treatment	

b. A written RTW policy clarifies management expectations and reinforces a corporate culture in which all employees are valued, will receive prompt, quality health care, and will be returned to either full duty or temporary, transitional duty as soon as is medically safe.

c. Companies will usually have written policies for sick leave, short-term disability, and long-term disability.

d. The corporate RTW policy and procedures should also be included in the employee policy and procedure manual.

e. Having a written RTW policy helps ensure equitable treatment and avoid potentially discriminatory situations where it may be tempting to have one policy for good performers and another policy for challenging performers.

2. The corporate RTW policy and procedures should be communicated to all employees.

3. Labor representatives should be consulted and included when developing or modifying the company's RTW policy and program.

4. Labor representatives can often serve as the occupational and environmental health nurse's advocate in RTW efforts.

B **Preventing lost-time injuries**

1. Even in workplaces with proactive health and safety programs, accidents and injuries do occur.

2. RTW procedures should require prompt notification of supervisors, transportation of the worker to health care treatment, a requirement for accident investigation, and reporting the injury or illness to the insurance carrier.

3. To ensure a safe and healthy workplace, loss prevention and safety programs should address the exposures for the class of business, and focus on loss sources revealed in a thorough analysis of recent, historical loss data obtained from OSHA logs and insurance loss/claims information.

4. Prompt, thorough investigation must be enforced as the primary strategy for learning from accidents and "near misses," directing corrective efforts for faulty processes, and preventing future accidents.

5. Holding supervisors and department managers accountable for safety as a performance measure is one recommended method of ensuring compliance.

C **Addressing injuries and illnesses immediately**

1. Employees are responsible for promptly notifying their supervisor of any injuries or prolonged illnesses.

2. Employers are responsible for immediately notifying their workers' compensation insurance carrier of workplace injuries or illnesses.

3. In work sites where on-site occupational health services are provided, the occupational health professionals should also be notified promptly.

4. Case management ideally begins from the onset of the injury or illness and continues through the safe return to work or an optimal alternative (AAOHN, 1994).

D **Providing timely and quality health care**

1. In situations where the injury or illness occurs "in the course and out of employment" (compensable under workers' compensation laws), employers in most states can direct employees to a panel of preselected health care providers.

2. In an effort to ensure the best health care outcomes, employers or their occupational health professional representatives should preselect a panel of health care professionals who share their commitment to providing prompt, high-quality health care and treatment and returning injured employees to work as soon as is medically safe.

3. Jurisdictional rules dictate how employees access medical care.
   a. Some require channeling within networks
   b. Some require posted panels of providers
   c. Some allow employers to direct all referrals to health care providers
   d. Some allow employers to direct referrals to health care providers under certain provisions or time frames
   e. Some states are designated as employee choice states, and employers are restricted from directing or referring employees to providers.

4. Case managers must maintain current knowledge of changes in workers' compensation laws in their jurisdictional areas.
   a. There are only a few states/jurisdictions that do not assert "exclusive remedy" protection for employers.
   b. Case managers need to know the jurisdictions in which they work to know those situations where exclusive remedy does not apply and an additional claim or suit may be active in conjunction with the workers' compensation claim.

5. Many managed care programs include brokered fee arrangements with a network of health care professional and treatment facilities.
   a. These fee arrangements are among the cost-control strategies for managing benefit costs and insurance premiums.
   b. In addition to providing prompt access to cost-effective care for employees, it is imperative that there also be a process for monitoring and ensuring quality treatment outcomes for employees treated by network or panel health care providers.

6. Developing and fostering trusting relationships with quality health care providers is key to the success of disability case management and an effective RTW program.

E **Promoting a proactive transitional work program**

1. The most important principle of disability case management is *early intervention* (Mullahy, 1998; Shrey & Lacerte, 1997; Donofrio, 1997; Wright & Eggleston, 1997; Hessellund & Cox, 1996); early intervention is likely to result in cost-savings to insurance carriers, employers, and disabled workers; and important psychosocial benefits experienced by clients and their families (Shrey & Lacerte, 1997).

2. Ill or injured employees should be released to return to work as soon as is medically safe.

3. The preferred site for injured employees to rehabilitate in preparation for returning to their original job is their own workplace.

4. This workplace rehabilitation model reduces or eliminates most of the disincentives that result from the worker's lengthy separation from the work site and yields more cost-effective services with better results.

5. The shift in the 1990s toward employers becoming more active participants in rehabilitation efforts is attributed to a reduced labor pool, efforts to minimize costs of injured worker compensation, and the implementation of the ADA, which mandates job modification and accommodation for persons with disabilities (Shrey & Lacerte, 1997).

6. The functional match of an injured or ill worker to the job is the fundamental principle for transitional work programs.
7. Employers can expedite the RTW process by accurately completing a job analysis for each job category.
    a. *Job analysis* is a process that involves a formal analysis of the tasks associated with a specific job or group of jobs; a job analysis specifically identifies what the worker does.
    b. The job analysis should paint an accurate picture of the essential physical and environmental requirements of the job and be made available to treating health care professionals to help determine work return dates and job modification.
    c. Employers and case managers should use the job analysis to determine transitional duty options (modified or alternative work) for employees released to work with medical restrictions.
    d. The terminology *light duty* has developed a negative connotation; the preferred terminology is *transitional work*.
    e. Transitional work is intended to be temporary and progressive, not a permanent job accommodation.
8. After 60 days of temporary transitional work, the RTW team, including the case manager, must evaluate the injured worker's progress, the reality of returning to the original job, and options for a permanent modified position or an alternative position.
9. The permanence of a worker's recovery is determined within six months of entering the case management system, unless there are contributing variables.

F **Occupational illnesses and injuries**
1. Employees who become ill or injured in circumstances that "arise out of and in the course of employment" are eligible for workers' compensation benefits.
2. In addition, preexisting conditions aggravated by employment are compensable in many jurisdictions.
3. The majority of employees who become ill or injured in most workplaces receive medical treatment and return to work before absences result in payment for lost wages.
4. Most lost-time workers' compensation claims result in injured workers returning to full duty in their original position before completing 60 days of transitional work (personal communication, Fireman's Fund Insurance Company, 1998).
5. 1997 data from one large property casualty insurer reflect that approximately 20% or less of workplace injuries result in payments for lost time.

G **Employer disability benefits for nonoccupational illnesses and injuries include the following:**
1. Salary continuance
2. Accumulated sick pay
3. Short-term disability
    a. Conditions and benefit amounts vary per policy.
    b. The benefit is income replacement for a portion of regular earnings as defined by specific policy.
    c. The length of term can vary; it is generally 26 weeks.

    d. This benefit may be statutory in some states.

    e. Employees receiving benefits may be required to provide appropriate documentation from treating medical providers as proof of continued need for benefits, as determined by policy.

    f. Short-term disability can bridge to long-term disability or Social Security Disability Insurance (SSDI).

    g. It may coordinate with Family Medical Leave Act or Americans with Disability Act (DiBenedetto & Haag, 2000).

4. Long-term disability

    a. Income replacement policy; does not cover any medical payments

    b. Policies vary but generally start after 26 weeks.

    c. It is desirable for benefit to coordinate with expiration of short-term disability, but it is not always possible to avoid coverage gaps.

    d. Its emphasis is on vocational rehabilitation; it is also directed at the advocacy of Social Security benefits.

    e. It may coordinate with SSDI, pension, workers' compensation

    f. It is a voluntary benefit, not required by statute.

    g. After the defined period of time (e.g., two years), a policy may require the employee to meet the "any occupation" provision in order to continue to receive LTD benefits.

        1) The "any occupation" provision is a common requirement of some policies, meaning that if the employee is qualified to perform *any* other comparable job or occupation, benefits will cease.

        2) Vocational case managers and experts are often called on to assess the employee's earning capacity to help determine if the employee meets the "any occupation" provision and other criteria and is therefore eligible for long-term disability benefits.

5. Disability nurse case managers play a pivotal role in the following:

    a. Coordinating communications with health care providers, injured workers, and employers

    b. Facilitating the worker's timely return to work

    c. Helping the employee reintegrate into the original job as medical restrictions are lifted

VIII Integrated Disability Management Programs

A Occupational and environmental health nurses recognize that employees' absence from work as a result of either occupational or nonoccupational injuries or illnesses affects the overall work environment and productivity.

B Payments for medical costs and lost wages may be generated from different sources, but all have a common goal of timely, effective return to work.

    1. Employers purchase workers' compensation insurance as mandated by law, and provide health care benefits to be competitive, and to attract and retain employees.

    2. Managed care arrangements have emerged in both the health care and workers' compensation delivery models.

    3. Generally medical costs are lower for nonoccupational injuries than for the same conditions treated under workers' compensation benefits under separate programs (Reese, 1998).

C Integrated disability management programs are being developed with efforts to include the following characteristics:
1. Coordinated workers' compensation, short-term disability, and long-term disability claims administration
2. Single intake and claims-reporting process
3. Coordinated case management of occupational and nonoccupational disability
4. Integrated information management systems
5. Streamlined administrative processes
6. Disability definitions and regulatory compliance issues consistently defined and managed across all programs that meet the organization's needs and objectives (DiBenedetto & Haag, 2000).

D Case managers need to help educate medical providers accustomed to working in a nonoccupational/managed care environment to understand and embrace the more aggressive return-to-work approach of the workers' compensation system. (Reese, 1998)

IX Federal Acts

A There are many regulations that may affect RTW and case management services. These include:
1. Family Medical Leave Act
2. Americans with Disabilities Act
3. Department of Transportation Drug and Alcohol Testing
4. Employee Retirement Income Security Act
5. Consolidated Omnibus Budget Reconciliation Act

B Disability case managers must understand the impact of regulations on their clients' particular situations and craft their case management plans accordingly.

X Delivery Models

A *On-site (in-person) case management*—services provided in-person with the disabled employee at various locations (home, treatment facilities, workplaces, etc.)
1. Advantages of on-site case management
   a. Provides opportunities to establish a firmer, more trusting professional relationship with the employee (Donofrio, 1997).
   b. Allows first-hand observation of the employee's medical condition and his or her response to and compliance with treatment (Alliotta, 1999).
   c. Allows more opportunities to identify personal, familial, environmental, and other factors that may impede the employee's progress in recovery (Donofrio, 1997).
   d. Once a more comprehensive evaluation of all impacting factors is done, more-appropriate interventions can be developed for the case management plan (Donofrio, 1997).
2. Disadvantages of on-site case management
   a. Services are costlier because of the travel and time involved to meet parties involved in the case (Donofrio, 1997).

b. On-site case managers must always justify the benefit of their services in relation to the cost to overcome skepticism of some consumers (Mullahy, 1998).

B *Telephonic case management (TCM)—services provided by telephone by employer representatives or vendor representatives hired to perform the services (Donofrio, 1997)*
1. Advantages of TCM
    a. Allows more-immediate assessment of case management needs.
    b. Establishes at least some level of rapport with the employee and family immediately upon identification of an injury or disabling diagnosis.
    c. Communicates concern for the employee's well being, helping to avoid misunderstandings and feelings of abandonment by the employee.
    d. Allows early opportunity to ease the employee's fears and anxieties by educating them regarding policies, procedures, and jurisdictional requirements, which they need to understand and navigate in the course of their treatment (Aron, 1997; Bechtel, 1998; Donofrio, 1997).
    e. Reduced anxiety in turn reduces the need to seek education from outside sources, such as legal counsel or poorly informed family and friends (Reese, 1998).
    f. Facilitates communication between employee and supervisor to reduce anxiety and resolve concerns the employee may have about job security, relationship with their supervisor, etc. (Aron, 1997).
    g. Allows immediate communication with health care providers to facilitate appropriate treatment, overall case management planning, and interventions (Aron, 1997; Donofrio, 1997; Wright & Eggleston, 1997).
    h. Establishes the telephonic case manager as a coordinator and point of contact for the employee, health care providers, and employer.
    i. Quickly identifies needs requiring on-site evaluation, which otherwise could have been delayed.
    j. Reduces costs compared with on-site case management services, because of the travel and time involved to perform on-site services.
    k. Because of reduced costs, allows employers and insurers to offer services to larger numbers of employees and clientele.
    l. Because it allows earlier intervention, TCM facilitates earlier resolution of cases or identification of severe cases requiring more-comprehensive on-site case management services (Donofrio, 1997).
2. Disadvantages of TCM
    a. Less-personal and less-trusting relationships are established with employees, health care providers, and other parties.
    b. Dependence on verbal information from employees and others may limit the identification of issues that could have been identified with an on-site visit (Donofrio, 1997).
    c. Multiple state licenses may be required for nurses providing case management services over different jurisdictions.
    d. Because of its cost-effectiveness, TCM may be used even when factors indicate more-comprehensive on-site services (e.g., catastrophic cases) (Donofrio, 1997; Wright & Eggleston, 1997).
    e. Telephonic case managers need to be mindful of their liability when providing services in this manner; concerns about liabilities may limit the case manager's ability to provide comprehensive information.
    f. Lack of first-hand understanding by telephonic case managers of the

employer's needs or work environment can limit their effectiveness in some situations.

   g. Although TCM cases are shorter term, the caseload for TCM nurses is often much higher than on-site caseloads, potentially limiting their effectiveness.

   h. A high volume caseload can restrict services to a cursory level, perhaps leading to missed follow-up or confusion of cases.

3. Ethical Considerations

   a. Because on-site case managers have opportunities to develop more-personal relationships with all parties of a case, they need to recognize their own and others' limitations.

   b. Programs limit or dictate the benefits available to the employee.

   c. Case managers need a clear understanding of when they may or may not go outside of a program for other available resources.

   d. If they do obtain resources outside a program, it is important to know under what circumstances and by what source their time will be compensated.

   e. Case managers must be diligent in their ethical conduct and avoid any coercion by referral sources to perform or authorize questionable services.

   f. On-site case management should not be used as a substitute for fraud investigation or surveillance on a case.

BIBLIOGRAPHY

Aday, L., Begley, C.E., Lairson, D.R., & Slater, C.H. (1993). *Evaluating the medical care system: Effectiveness, efficiency, and equity.* Ann Arbor, MI: Health Administration Press.

Alliotta, S. (1999). Patient adherence outcome indicators and measurement in case management and health care. *Care Management.* 5(4), 24-81.

American Association of Occupational Health Nurses. (1994). Advisory: Case Management. *AAOHN Journal, 42(4),* 156A.

American Association of Occupational Health Nurses. (1996). *Position statement: The occupational health nurse as a case manager.* Atlanta, GA: AAOHN.

American Association of Occupational Health Nurses. (1999). *Standards of occupational and environmental health nursing.* Atlanta, GA: AAOHN.

American Nurses Association. (1988). *Nursing case management.* Kansas City, MO: Task Force on Case Management.

Aron, L.J. (1997). What's up with workers' compensation? *Care Management, 3 (3),* 16-20.

Bechtel, G., Newman-Giger, J., & Davidhizar, R. (1998). Case managing patients from other cultures. *Care Management, 4 (5),* 87-91.

Case Management Society of America. (1995). *Standards of practice for case managers.* Little Rock, AR. Case Management Society of America.

Childre, F. (1997). Nurse managed occupational health services: A primary care model in practice. *AAOHN Journal, 45(10),* 484-490.

"Consumers and managed care." *The New York Times,* 9 February 1997, p. 14.

DiBenedetto, D.V. & Haag, A.B. (2000). *Principles of workers' compensation and disability case management,* Vol. 1. Yonkers, NY: DVD & Associates.

Donofrio, J.M. (1997). Telephonic case management: Does it work and who really benefits? *Case Review,* Summer, 34-37.

Fireman's Fund Insurance Company. (1997). *SmartCARE return to work guide.* Novato, CA: Fireman's Fund Insurance Company.

Fireman's Fund Insurance Company. (May 1998). Personal conversation with Judith Arbeit, Regional Claims Manager, and Mary Lou Wassel, Occupational Health Consultant, Southern States Region.

Gliniecki, C.M. & Burgel, B.J. (1995). Temporary work restrictions: Guidelines for the primary care provider. *Nurse Practitioner Forum. 6(2), 79-89.*

Head, G.L. (1997). *Essentials of risk management* (3rd ed.), Vol. 1. Malvern, PA: Insurance Institute of America.

Hessellund, T.A. & Cox, R. (1996). Vocational case managers in early return-to-work agreements. *Care Management. 2(6),* 34-78.

Mullahy, C.M. (1998). *The case manager's handbook* (2nd ed.). Gaithersburg, MD: Aspen Publishers, Inc.

Reese, S. (1998). Integration: The case for blended benefits. *Business and Health, 16(4),* 62-69.

Rooney, E. (1990). Corporate attitudes and responses in rising health care costs. *AAOHN Journal, 38(7),* 304-311.

Salazar, M.K., Graham, K.Y., & Lantz, B. (1999). Evaluating case management services for injured workers: Use of a quality assessment model. *AAOHN Journal, 47(8),* 348-354.

Shrey, D.E. & Lacerte, M. (1997). *Principles and practices of disability management in industry.* Boca Raton, FL: CRC Press LLC.

U.S. Chamber of Commerce. (1999). *Analysis of workers' compensation laws.* Washington, DC: U.S. Chamber of Commerce. (NOTE: This document is prepared and published annually and is an excellent reference for details on workers' compensation laws. To order call toll free, 800-638-6582).

U.S. Department of Health and Human Services. (1994). *Acute low back problems in adults: Assessment and treatment* (AHCPR No. 95-0643). Rockville, MD: Public Health Service, Agency for Health Care, Policy and Research.

Washington State Department of Labor and Industries (1994). *Industrial insurance: glossary.* Olympia, WA: State of Washington Department of Labor and Industries.

Wassel, M.L. (1995). Occupational health nursing and the advent of managed care: Meeting the challenges of the current health care environment. *AAOHN Journal, 43(1),* 23-28.

Wright, L. & Eggleston, M. (1997) Catastrophic case management. *Case Review, 3(3),* 59-61.

Wolfe, G.S. (1998). Cost savings and case management. *Care Management, 4(5),* 5.

CHAPTER

12

Health Promotion and Adult Education

KAY N. CAMPBELL

Health promotion and adult education are essential elements of today's occupational and environmental health practice. The basic principles of adult education provide tools that can be applied to health education and to workplace health promotion. By helping individuals assess their health needs and developing strategies to meet those needs, the occupational and environmental health nurse creates an environment that values and supports healthy workers, thus contributing to the bottom line of the company. Healthy workers are creative, engaged, and productive workers.

I Overview of Health Promotion

Health promotion is a process that supports positive lifestyle changes through corporate policies, individual efforts to lower risk of disease and injury, and the creation of an environment that provides a sense of balance among work, family, personal, health, and social concerns.

A **The evolution of health promotion began with the 19th-century epidemiologic revolution.**
1. 19th century: The focus was on hygiene, sanitation, housing, and working conditions.
2. 20th century: The emphasis was on disease prevention and health.
   a. 1970s: There was recognition that more than half of premature deaths were preventable by lifestyle changes (USDHEW, 1979).
   b. Early 1980s: Comprehensive workplace health promotion programs were instituted to help people change their health behaviors (Lusk, 1997).
3. 1990s to the 21st century: The concept of workplace health promotion has broadened to include not only behavioral and lifestyle change, but also organizational strategies that support healthy work environments.

B **Health promotion activities are conducted by and draw upon the expertise of health professionals from many fields.**
1. Examples of these fields are nursing, health education, medicine, psychology, nutrition, occupational and physical therapy, safety, and ergonomics.
2. Occupational and environmental health nurses are often responsible for developing health promotion programs in work settings.

C Health promotion focuses on the following:
1. Prevention of illness and injury
2. Promotion of personal responsibility for one's health
3. Development of strategies for behavioral change
4. Movement to optimal health by balancing physical, emotional, social, spiritual, and intellectual health
5. Creation of a supportive work environment

D The rationale for health promotion includes the following:
1. Treating preventable illness and injury unnecessarily increases the cost of health care.
2. Health promotion strategies result in improved teamwork, innovation, and creativity within the work force.
3. Health promotion has the potential to improve productivity and quality of life.

E When establishing a workplace health promotion program, a balance of organizational and personal health goals should be achieved through the following:
1. Business goals such as improved employee productivity and morale, reduced health care costs, and recruitment and retention of employees.
2. Health goals such as reduction of major health risks, improved energy and resilience, balanced work and personal life.

F Comprehensive health promotion programs use the following strategies to reduce unnecessary health care utilization (Lusk, 1999):
1. Encouraging appropriate use of health care delivery services
2. Preventing acute illness and injury and delaying development of chronic illness
3. Reducing symptom severity, discomfort, and disability

G Levels of health promotion programming may include the following:
1. Awareness and support programs that increase the level of interest in a health-related topic through newsletters, flyers, posters, seminars, and health fairs
2. Screening programs to help identify high-risk employees
3. Lifestyle behavior change programs designed to help individuals adopt healthy behaviors, such as regular exercise, good nutrition, stress management, and smoking cessation
4. Work-culture enhancement that supports and encourages work/life programs, organizational change efforts, and flexible work alternatives

II National Health Promotion Objectives

A Healthy People 2010: Objectives for Improving Health (USDHHS, 2000): Describes 467 objectives in 28 focus areas by health behavior, disease, or setting.

B Healthy People objectives seek to increase life expectancy and the quality of life and eliminate health disparities.

C The implementation plan to meet these goals include the following:
1. Support gains in knowledge, motivation, and opportunities for better decision making
2. Encourage local and state leaders to accomplish the following:
   a. Develop community and state efforts to promote healthy behaviors

b. Create healthy environments

c. Increase access to high-quality health care

III Health Models

Health models are developed as a means of explaining the concept of health and its relationship to people's health decisions.

A The *Health Belief Model* **was developed by Godfrey Hochbaum, Stephen Kegeles, Howard Leventhal, and Irwin Rosenstock in the 1950s (Rosenstock, 1990).**

1. Major components of the model include the following:

   a. *Perceived susceptibility* is an individual's subjective estimation of his or her own personal risk of developing a specific health problem.

   b. *Perceived severity* refers to an individual's own personal judgment of how serious a health condition may be; perceived susceptibility and perceived severity are often combined into *perceived threat.*

   c. *Perceived benefits* are an individual's estimation of how effective a health recommendation may be in removing the threat.

   d. *Perceived barriers* are an individual's estimation of the obstacles to the performance of a health-related behavior.

2. The likelihood of an action being taken is driven by the positive difference between the perceived barriers and the perceived benefits (O'Donnell & Harris, 1994).

B The *Health Promotion Model* **by Pender (1996) is derived from social learning theory (Section IV.C.) and is organized like the Health Belief Model. It is based on the following premises:**

1. Health promotion is directed at increasing the level of well-being and self-actualization of an individual or group.

2. Health promoting behaviors are continuing activities that must be an integral part of an individual's lifestyle.

3. Health promoting behaviors are viewed as proactive rather than reactive.

C The *Health Promotion Planning Model* **is used to help plan and evaluate health promotion activities (Green & Kreuter, 1999).**

1. Green and Kreuter call the framework for their model PRECEDE; PRECEDE consists of predisposing (attitudes, knowledge), reinforcing (rewards, positive feedback), and enabling factors (resources that facilitate or hinder performance of desired outcome).

2. This model considers the multiple factors that shape health (e.g., behavior, lifestyle, environment).

3. Health promotion education and policy are viewed as important influences on the quality of life.

4. Epidemiologic data provide information about behavior, lifestyle, and the environment.

5. Quality of life is the expected outcome.

D The *Model of Health Promotion Behavior* **assumes that self-efficacy beliefs play a central role regarding health beliefs and behavior (O'Donnell, 1989).**

1. Optimal health represents a balance between physical, emotional, social, spiritual, and intellectual health.

2. Programs are targeted at three levels: awareness, lifestyle and behavioral change, and supportive environments.

IV Behavior Change Theories and Models

As occupational and environmental health nurses work with clients to assist them in changing their lifestyle behaviors, it is critical to have an understanding of behavior change theories. With this knowledge, the nurse will be in a better position to help clients overcome their barriers and move toward successful outcomes.

A **An analysis of psychotherapy theories for behavior change was performed to identify psychotherapeutic principles that relate to helping people change their behavior (Prochaska, 1979).**

1. *Verbal* theories use language and emotions to guide changes in behaviors.
   a. *Consciousness raising* uses the individual's personal experience feedback to stimulate responses.
   b. *Catharsis* allows individuals to express emotions, which produces personal relief and improvement.
   c. *Choosing* gives alternative responses for individuals and self-liberation occurs when they choose an alternative.
2. *Action* or *behavioral* theories use stimuli outside the individual to evoke an action or behavior.
   a. *Conditional stimuli* refers to critical changes made in the stimuli that influence responses; *counter-conditioning* occurs when an individual changes his or her response to a stimulus, and *stimulus control* occurs when the environment is changed.
   b. *Contingency control* refers to managing change by making changes in the environment to cause individuals to change. *Reevaluation* occurs when individuals change in response to consequences without contingency changes in the environment.

B *Transtheoretical Theory*—**Stages of Change Model (Prochaska & DiClemente, 1983), describes interventions tailored to individual responses at specific levels or stages.**

1. The theory was formulated by using numerous psychotherapy theories to develop the stages of change model to produce sustained behavior change.
2. The content of the model varies from client to client depending on the client's history of actions, present environment, and personality.
3. The stages of change include the following: (Table 12-1 presents examples of processes to facilitate change):
   a. Precontemplation: clients are not considering making a change.
   b. Contemplation: clients are beginning to explore or think about making a change.
   c. Planning: clients are determined to stop and begin to develop a plan.
   d. Action: clients modify their behavior, which may also mean they change their environment.
   e. Maintenance continues as the new behavior continues to be practiced.

C *Social Learning Theory* **purports that people's thoughts have a strong effect on their behavior, and their behavior affects their thoughts (O'Donnell & Harris, 1994).**

1. Social Cognitive–Self Efficacy Theory (Bandura, 1986) describes the factors involved in making decisions related to healthy behavior.
   a. These factors include one's personal efficacy (self-efficacy), social and environmental support, and behavioral experiences.

TABLE 12-1

Stages of change model and examples of processes to facilitate change

Stages	Precontem-plation	Contemplation	Planning	Action/maintenance
Psychotherapy theories		Consciousness raising Feedback	Choosing Self-liberation Catharsis	Contingency control Reevaluation Conditional stimuli Stimulus control
Health promotion activities	Posters Invitations to classes Buddy system	Health Fairs Newsletter Brochures Pamphlets Health educa-tion classes Buddy system HRA	Health educa-tion classes Counseling Health Planner	Follow-up contact Environmental supports Health education

Source: Prochaska & DiClemente, 1982.

    b. Self-efficacy is an individual's confidence in his or her ability to perform.
    c. An individual's efficacy expectation determines his or her choice of activity, how much effort he or she will expend, and how persistent he or she will be.
  2. *The Locus of Control Theory:*
    a. An individual's belief (outcome expectation) that his or her own behavior determines reinforcements (outcomes) is called *internal locus of control.*
    b. An individual's belief that reinforcements are controlled by others is called *external locus of control.*
    c. Theoretically, individuals with internal locus of control are more likely to take control of their health and to engage in health promotion activities than are individuals with external locus of control.

D *Transactional Theory* **is characterized by "reciprocal determinism" where individuals change behavior then begin to actively participate with others in the new behavior.**
  1. This experience strengthens the individual's desire to continue the new behavior or find the need to change the environment.
  2. Efficacy and support can modify behavior, and direct experience with the new behavior increases the level of efficacy and support.

E *The Theory of Reasoned Action* **proposes that behavioral intentions are the result of one's attitude and subjective norms (Fishbein & Ajzen, 1975).**
  1. *Attitudes* are determined by beliefs regarding the consequences of a behavior and one's positive or negative evaluation of those consequences.
  2. *Subjective norms* refer to a person's beliefs or perceptions about what others think he or she should do.
  3. *Intentions* are the immediate determinant of behavior.

F *The Theory of Planned Behavior* **builds on the Theory of Reasoned Action; the element added to the Theory of Reasoned Action is the belief that one has the resources to perform the behavior (Ajzen, 1988).**

G *The Theory of Social Behavior* states that the probability of an act occurring in a specific situation is equal to the sum of the person's habit and intention (Triandis, 1999).

H *The Protection Motivation Theory* combines features of the Health Belief Model with self-efficacy theory and other social psychological constructs such as fear, arousal, appraisal, and coping (Prentice-Dunn & Rogers, 1986).

I *The Health Action Process Approach* states that health behavior change takes place over time (Schwarzer, 1992).

V Levels of Prevention

A comprehensive health promotion and health protection program comprises three levels of prevention (Leavell & Clark, 1979):

A *Primary prevention* is aimed at eliminating or reducing the risk of disease through specific actions; examples include immunizations, stress management, smoking avoidance, risk factor appraisal, seat belt use, work-site walk-throughs, and use of personal protective equipment.

B *Secondary prevention* is directed at early case-finding and diagnosis of individuals with disease in order to institute prompt interventions; examples include screening programs, health surveillance, monitoring health and illness trend data, and preplacement and periodic examinations.

C *Tertiary prevention* is directed at rehabilitating and restoring individuals to their maximum health potential; examples include disability case management, early return to work, chronic illness monitoring, and substance abuse rehabilitation.

VI Framework for a Health Promotion Program (Fig. 12-1)

A Health promotion program planning

1. Management should be involved in early stages of planning
   a. Management must understand the value of health promotion and wellness.
      1) Provide management with an estimate of cost savings (including indirect cost savings such as increased productivity, reduced absenteeism, and health care costs) that will be realized as a result of the program.
      2) Use supportive background, including case histories of successful programs, to generate management support.
   b. Management should be kept informed of all program activities and invited to participate in planning as appropriate.
2. Advisory committees representative of the employee population should be formed; representatives include management, line supervisors, union members, the benefits manager, and employee representatives.
   a. The advisory committee provides assistance and advice through all stages of the program, from planning to evaluation.
   b. Workers' involvement in and support of programs at this level are critical to a successful program.
3. To develop appropriate goals and objectives to guide program implementation and evaluation, a well-planned needs assessment must be conducted.
   a. A needs assessment may be used to collect information about the

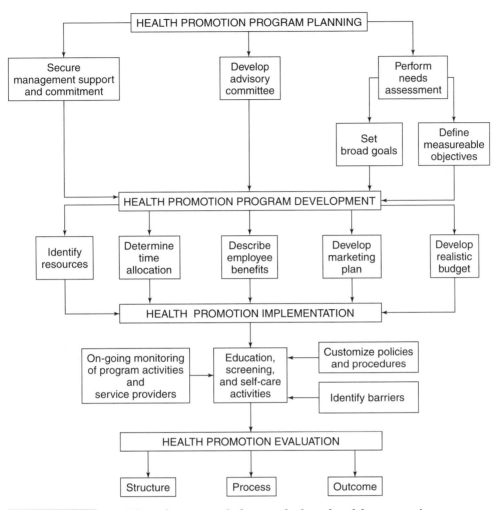

FIGURE 12-1 *Guiding framework for workplace health promotion programs*

Source: Rogers, 1994.

interests and health status of employees through written surveys, interviews, focus groups, or a combination of these methods.

   b. Workers' compensation data, insurance records, absenteeism reports, and other data that reflect health care costs within an organization are an important component of the needs assessment.

   c. A health risk appraisal is an efficient and relatively inexpensive tool that can identify a specific employee's health behavior and risks (Box 12-1).

B Health promotion program development

1. Identify internal and external organizational resources when developing a health promotion program.

   a. Personnel to implement the program.

      1) Programs may be implemented by personnel from health services within the organization, or they may be outsourced.

      2) Programs may require personnel with special skills and knowledge, such as an exercise physiologist to lead an exercise program.

BOX 12-1

Health risk appraisal

- A health risk appraisal (HRA) is a health education tool that is used to compare an individual's health-related behaviors and characteristics with those of the general population by comparing statistics and epidemiologic data. An HRA estimates an individual's life expectancy based on current risk behaviors, and it calculates the amount of risk that could be eliminated by making appropriate behavioral changes.

- A health risk appraisal is easy to administer, confidential, provides information specific to the individual, and is easy to interpret. It includes a section that recommends corrective action, and provides positive feedback for results that demonstrate healthy behaviors.

- A health risk appraisal is used to assess nutrition/weight-management needs, fitness, stress levels, drug and alcohol problems, smoking behaviors, safety behaviors, and cancer signs and risks.

- The benefits of a health risk appraisal include the following:
  - ☐ It provides the health care counselor with a rational teaching aid that can be used as a point of focus during discussions about health and behavior.
  - ☐ It relies on a self-administered questionnaire, simple physiologic measurements, and computer-assisted calculations.
  - ☐ It can be used with large groups because it is efficient and relatively inexpensive.
  - ☐ It is science-based; it uses precise data based on appropriate studies.

---

     3) Personnel from various community agencies, such as the American Cancer Society or the American Red Cross, offer services or programs that can be provided at work sites.

    b. Audiovisual equipment may be essential, as well as other equipment specific to the program (e.g., screening supplies, exercise devices).

    c. Paper, pencils, computer products, and other incidental supplies should be readily available.

    d. The availability of facilities and space appropriate for the purposes of the activity should be determined.

2. Determine the time required to develop the program and for workers to use the program; negotiate with the company for personal versus company time.

3. Investigate the program's existing and potential benefits.

    a. Existing benefits may include insurance incentives for employees who participate in certain activities.

    b. Potential benefits might be negotiated with management; for example, a "wellness" day could be traded for a certain number of sick days.

4. Successful marketing strategies include participation of employees affected by the program.

5. A successful program depends on the inclusion of a realistic and a feasible budget; if costs exceed available resources, the occupational and environmental health nurse will be required to submit a revised budget to management or to adjust the programs to accommodate the available funds.

C **Health promotion program implementation**

1. The primary strategy used in health promotion programs is education; screening and self-care activities are also important elements of a program. (Note: Referral and follow-up procedures must always be included as part of a screening program.)
2. Once a program is implemented, it is continually monitored to assess time frames, costs, and management interest and support; adjustments are made as needed.
3. The advantages and disadvantages of the health service providers (in-house or contracted) should be constantly monitored (Chapter 8 [III: C: 1-4] describes the advantages and disadvantages); if it is determined that disadvantages outweigh the advantages, the providers of services may need to be replaced.
4. Policies and procedures that affect the provision of health promotion services should be customized to meet the needs of the organization.
5. Barriers to program implementation must be identified and considered in future planning.

D **Health promotion program evaluation using structure, process, and outcome**

1. Examples of the structural elements to be considered in the evaluation
   a. Qualifications and adequacy of the staff involved in all phases of the program
   b. Appropriateness of the equipment and supplies used to carry out the program
   c. Demographics of workers who participated in the program
   d. Appropriateness of the facilities
   e. Match of the program with the mission and goals of the organization
   f. Management's commitment to wellness and support of the program
2. Examples of process elements to be considered in an evaluation
   a. The specific activities that characterize the program (e.g., if a diabetic screening program is in place, are the protocols and procedures state-of-the-art and appropriate for this employee population?)
   b. Evidence of collaboration and support among the various personnel involved in the program
   c. A monitoring system adequate to detect the need for changes
   d. Documentation and recordkeeping that meet legal requirements and effectively support communication
3. Examples of outcome elements to be considered in an evaluation
   a. Injury, illness, and absenteeism records
   b. Surveys that evaluate knowledge about self-care (e.g., American Cancer Society screening guidelines) and attitudes about health (i.e., reflected in an expressed desire to participate in healthy behaviors)
   c. Epidemiologic data that reflect behavioral choices related to health (e.g., decreased smoking rates)
   d. Observations of health activities (e.g., increased use of company exercise equipment)

4. Costs and benefits are a critical outcome measure that may determine whether a company will continue to support a program. (Chapter 8 describes steps in conducting cost-effectiveness/cost-benefit analyses.)

VII Lifestyle and Health Promotion

Modifiable lifestyles have been identified as a major cause of premature death in the United States.

A **Addiction behaviors are characterized by compulsion, loss of control, and continued involvement despite adverse consequences.**

1. Tobacco use causes nearly one in five deaths in the United States, making it the most preventable cause of death. The latest trends indicate that 90% of the new smokers are children and teens. Table 12-2 presents a test for measuring nicotine dependence.
2. Alcohol is the most misused drug; one out of every 13 adults in the United States abuses alcohol or is alcoholic. Moderate alcohol use—up to two drinks per day for men and one drink per day for women and older people—is not harmful for most adults. Box 12-2 presents a test for measuring alcohol dependence.
3. Drug misuse includes misuse or abuse of caffeine, alcohol, nicotine, cocaine, heroin, opiates, marijuana, designer drugs (drugs manufactured in an illegal laboratory that mimic a controlled substance), and prescription drugs.

B **Stress is a contributing risk factor to cardiovascular disease; more than half of the visits to health care professionals are for stress-related disorders.**

TABLE 12-2

The Fagerstrom test for nicotine dependence

Questions		Points
1. How soon after you wake in the morning do you smoke your first cigarette?	Within 5 min.	3
	6-30 min.	2
	31-60 min.	1
	After 60 min.	0
2. Do you find it difficult to refrain from smoking in places where it is forbidden, e.g., church, library, cinema?	Yes	1
	No	0
3. Which cigarettes would you most hate to give up?	First one in the A.M.	1
	All others	0
4. How many cigarettes do you smoke per day?	10 or fewer	0
	11-20	1
	21-30	2
	31 or more	3
5. Do you smoke more frequently during the first hours after waking than during the rest of the day?	Yes	1
	No	0
6. Do you smoke even if you are so ill that you are in bed most of the day?	Yes	1
	No	0

Score: 1-6 = Low to moderate dependence
7-11 = High dependence

Heatherton, et al., A revision of the Fagerstrom Tolerance Questionnaire, *British Journal of Addictions*, 1991.

C **Diet is associated with six of the top 10 causes of death: heart disease, stroke, atherosclerosis, non–insulin-dependent diabetes, cancer, and chronic liver disease.**

1. Eating foods low in fat and high in fiber reduces the risk of heart disease and cancer.

2. Low-fat, high-fiber diets also help to control body weight, which is a growing concern, according to the U.S. Public Health Service, because approximately 34% of Americans are overweight (USDHHS, 2000).

D **Regular physical activity helps prevent coronary heart disease, high blood pressure, non–insulin-dependent diabetes mellitus, cancer, osteoporosis, obesity, mental health problems, and low back problems.**

1. Physiologic evidence demonstrates that physical activity improves many biologic measures associated with health and physiologic functioning (USDHHS, 2000).

2. Physical activity can build and maintain healthy bones, muscles, and joints; build endurance and muscular strength, and promote psychologic well-being and self-esteem.

3. Moderate physical activity for at least 30 minutes a day for the majority of the week is recommended for adults.

E **Cancer awareness can lead to early detection and prevention of this disease.**

1. Skin cancer is the most common type of cancer; lung cancer, however, causes the most deaths.

2. Breast cancer is the most common cancer among women in the United States, occurring in one out of nine women; some studies suggest it may be affected by a high-fat diet and excessive alcohol consumption.

3. The risk for uterine cancer increases with age (over 45), obesity, and levels of female hormones.

4. The incidence of prostate cancer increases with age; over 80% of all prostate cancers in men occur after age 65.

F **Alcohol-related traffic accidents are the leading cause of death and spinal cord injuries in young Americans.**

1. Alcohol-related traffic deaths are the second leading cause of teen death.

2. During a typical weekend, an average of one teenager dies each hour in a

---

BOX 12-2

Alcohol and other drug validation question set (CAGE questionnaire)

C Have you ever felt the need to *cut down* on your drinking?

A Have you ever felt *annoyed* by criticism of your drinking?

G Have you ever felt *guilty* about drinking?

E Have you ever used an *eye-opener* or taken a drink the first thing in the morning to steady your nerves or get rid of a hangover?

A positive response to two or more questions creates a high degree of suspicion regarding alcohol dependency.

BOX 12-3

Safe driving tips

- Do not drink alcohol and drive:
  - ☐ Use a designated driver
  - ☐ Use a taxicab
- Use seatbelts consistently
- Use infant/child car seats correctly and consistently

---

car crash and nearly 50% of these crashes involve alcohol. Box 12-3 presents safe-driving tips.

3. Safety also includes preventing falls, fires, and traffic accidents, both on and off the job.

G The World Health Organization (WHO) recognizes infection with the human immunodeficiency virus as a worldwide epidemic, for which prevention is the only control; currently there is no cure, although drug therapies have significantly impacted longevity of those infected with this virus.

H The occupational setting is an ideal location for the development of health promotion programs.

1. Health promotion programs are an essential part of a comprehensive health and safety program in the occupational setting.
2. The timing and type of program will be based on the needs of the worker population (Table 12-3).

VIII Employee Assistance Programs (EAPs)

A An EAP is a work-based mental health program designed to provide support services to employees and, in some cases, employees' families who have personal issues that may affect their well-being and ability to perform their jobs.

1. From the mid 1940s to 1950s, EAPs were designed to deal with alcohol and substance abuse problems.
2. Currently, EAPs address an array of problems, including family, legal, financial, interpersonal, and organizational issues (Travers & McDougall, 1995).
3. The program may include referral, short-term counseling, crisis debriefing, and management coaching.
4. Workplace mental health issues are steadily increasing. EAPs can develop programs to deal with depression, anxiety, and other mental health concerns.

B Standards for programs and professionals providing EAP services are developed by the following:

1. The Employee Assistance Professional Association
2. The Employee Assistance Society of North America

C Objectives of an EAP include the following:

1. To effectively and efficiently provide services for ameliorating mental health problems, as well as alcoholism and other drug-related problems of the work force

TABLE 12-3

Program development in the occupational setting

Health promotion activity	Type of program	When program is appropriate
A. Addictive Behaviors:		
1. Tobacco Use	Smoking cessation Nicotine gum/patches Individual behavioral modification	Smoker wants to quit: Assess dependency for appropriate program and support. (See Table 12-2.)
2. Alcohol and/or Drug Misuse	Awareness Referral Employee assistance Community	Job performance degenerates Absentee pattern appears (see Cage Questionnaire in Table 12-3.)
B. Stress Reduction	Biofeedback Time management Visual imagery Exercise Humor	Company experiences changes (e.g., downsizing) Increased client visits Increased EAP utilization
C. Nutrition	General nutrition Weight management Low fat/low cholesterol Cooking demonstrations Nutrition tables interpretation	Elevated cholesterol level HRA results are out of the norm Reports of high blood pressure Concern about weight
D. Fitness	Recreational Flexibility Strengthening Aerobic	Anytime: everyone benefits from exercise and activity. (Recommended level assessed at preplacement physical)
E. Cancer Awareness		
1. Breast	Cancer awareness Breast self-exam instruction Clinical breast exams Mammography	When worker population includes female workers who are age 20 and older
2. Uterine	Annual pap smears	
3. Prostate	PSA with digital exam	When worker population includes male workers who are age 20 and older
4. Testicular	Testicular self-exam instruction Clinical testicular exams	
5. Skin	Skin cancer awareness	Anytime: All workers can benefit from this knowledge.
6. Colon	Fecal occult blood test Sigmoidoscopy	
F. Safety	Safety awareness education Driving safety Fire awareness safety Carbon monoxide safety	Anytime: Entire worker population can benefit from this information.
G. HIV/AIDS	HIV/AIDS awareness World AIDS Day recognition	Anytime: All workers, particularly those at high risk, can benefit from these activities.

2. To identify employees with job performance problems and to respond to those seeking assistance by directing them toward the best assistance possible and providing continuing support and guidance throughout the problem-solving period

3. To serve as a resource for management and labor in intervening with employees whose personal problems affect their job performance

D **The core methodology of EAPs includes the following steps (Gilbert, 1994):**
1. Identify employees' behavioral problems, based on job performance.
2. Provide expert consultation to employers and managers.
3. Use constructive confrontation appropriately.
4. Create and maintain links between the work organization and community resources.
5. Evaluate the success of employee assistance utilization, primarily on the basis of job performance

E **Criteria for successful programs include the following:**
1. Confidentiality as the cornerstone of the program
2. Accessibility of voluntary self-referral with an on-site or off-site counselor
3. Ability of supervisors to identify and refer employees with problems

F **EAP models include the following:**
1. Internal programs
   a. Staffed by employees of the sponsoring agency
   b. Standard is one staff member for every 2,000 employees
   c. Advantage: familiarity with the culture of the organization
   d. Disadvantage: employee concerns about confidentiality
2. External programs
   a. Contracted by the organization
   b. Services provided by a variety of treatment centers, private companies, and other organizations
   c. Advantage: more accessible to small and medium-sized companies
   d. Disadvantage: may not provide convenient access for employees
3. Combination of internal and external programs

G **The scope of services, which varies among organizations, may include the following (Travers & McDougall, 1995):**
1. Assessment, short-term counseling, and diagnostic and referral services
2. Crisis counseling 7 days a week, 24 hours a day
3. Assistance in the development of a company's mental health policies and benefits program
4. Employee orientation, supervisory training, and union representation
5. Group education programs, such as stress management, conflict resolution, parenting, and organizational change
6. Prepaid alcohol and drug rehabilitation services

H **The role of the occupational and environmental health nurse in providing employee assistance services will depend on the nature of services provided by the organization and on the nurse's knowledge and educational preparation. Occupational and environmental health nurses:**
1. Should be able to detect and recognize signs of potential psychological or emotional distress among employees; stressed employees should be referred as appropriate
2. May provide counseling services related to lifestyle and health behaviors,

personal issues, and work-related problems as part of routine care in the occupational setting; the provision of formal counseling sessions usually requires advanced preparation and credentialing in an appropriate field, such as clinical psychology.

3. Should work with management to ensure that confidential and appropriate employee assistance services are part of a comprehensive occupational health and safety program
4. May provide crisis intervention to an employee (or department) who is then referred to an EAP counselor.
5. May serve as liaison between company management and the EAP
6. May participate in the development of the program from assessment to evaluation

IX Introduction to Adult Education

Adult education principles enable occupational and environmental health nurses to effectively provide adult populations with preventive health information and help them modify lifestyle behaviors.

A Characteristics of adult education
1. Adult education is the purposeful exploration by adults of a field of knowledge, attainment of skills, or a collective reflection upon common experiences.
   a. Explorations take place in group settings.
   b. An individual's personal experiences, skills, and knowledge influence how new ideas are received, new skills acquired, and experiences of others interpreted.
2. Settings for adult education programs include continuing education, training, networks, self-directed learning, distance education, and computer-based and community activity.
3. Participants in adult education are likely to have a variety of learning styles that affect their ability to acquire and retain information.
   a. Using multiple methods of presenting information will maximize the effectiveness of health education programs.
   b. Teaching styles should be adjusted to accommodate the needs of the learner; for example, older workers may require written material with large print and a setting that facilitates their ability to hear the speaker.

B Central principles of effective adult education
1. Participation is voluntary, with adults engaging in learning of their own volition.
2. Facilitation is characterized by a respect among participants for each other's self-worth.
3. Facilitators and learners are engaged in a cooperative group process involving a continuous renegotiation of activities and priorities.
4. Learners and facilitators are involved in a continual process of activity, reflection on activity, collaborative analysis of the activity, new activity, reflection, and so on.
5. Facilitation inspires adults to appreciate that values, beliefs, behaviors, and ideologies are culturally transmitted and to critically reflect on aspects of their professional, personal, and political lives.

C Self-directed learning is the process in which individuals take the initiative in designing learning experiences, diagnosing needs, locating resources, and evaluating learning for themselves (Knowles, 1988).

1. Contracts written by students are the chief mechanism used to enhance self-direction and allow students to diagnose their learning needs, plan activities, and identify and select relevant resources.
2. Techniques for self-directed learning involve the development of problem-solving skills to enhance students' ability to respond to typical problems and challenges.
3. Self-directed learners rely heavily on peer learning groups for support, information exchange, stimulus of new ideas, and locating relevant resources.
4. More time is required for extended exploration of curricular concerns, diagnosis and exploration of perceived needs (of learners) and pre-scribed needs (by educators), and negotiation of an agreed-upon learning plan.

D Teaching involves presenting alternatives, questioning givens, and scrutinizing the self.

1. Characteristics of effective teaching
   a. Set an emotional atmosphere conducive to learning.
   b. Use learners' experiences as educational resources.
   c. Give constructive feedback to students.
   d. Encourage collaboration and participation.
2. The best teaching methods for self-directed learning
   a. Leading discussions that present intellectual challenges in a nonthreatening setting
   b. Forming peer learning groups to experiment with ideas
   c. Encouraging the expression of opinions and alternative interpretations
   d. Providing lectures, demonstrations, independent study, and programmed computer learning

E Adult educational programs are series of learning experiences designed to achieve, in a limited period of time, certain specific instructional objectives. Overall planning includes the following:

1. Identifying the gaps between the learner's current and desired proficiencies
2. Assessing learning needs by the use of questionnaires, conducting individual interviews, observing participants, or consulting with experts
3. Using behavioral objectives to state the intended outcome or proficiency level the learner should obtain as a result of participating in the educational experience (Box 12-4.)
4. Developing a plan that considers the objectives, outcomes, characteristics of the learner, size of the group, available times, equipment, facilities, and budget
5. Evaluating the program in terms of attainment of behaviors
   a. *Summative* evaluations are used to justify the program and focus on the program's worth and impact on the outcomes (e.g., a cost-benefit analysis).
   b. *Formative* evaluations focus on the program's procedures and are used for decision making to make improvements in the program (e.g., standardized tests and inventories).

BOX 12-4

American Association of Occupational Health Nurses, Inc. behavioral objectives

A behavioral objective states what the learner will be able to do on completion of a continuing education activity. A behavioral objective identifies the terminal behavior or outcome of the program.

Objectives are critical to continuing education activity development because they: 1) reflect input from learners relative to educational needs; 2) determine the selection of content and teaching methods; and 3) provide a guide to the evaluation phase.

Be sure that all written objectives:
- Use verbs that describe an ACTION that can be OBSERVED
- Are measurable within the teaching time frame
- Consist of only one action verb per objective
- Describe the learner outcome, not the instructor's process or approach
- Are appropriate for the designated teaching method(s)

Behavioral Terms to Use

apply*	define	distinguish	relate
analyze*	demonstrate*	explain	repeat
choose	describe	identify	revise*
compare	design*	list	select
compile*	develop*	outline	state
conduct*	differentiate	name	summarize
critique*	discuss	recall	synthesize*

*Use these action verbs with teaching methods that involve participants beyond a lecture/discussion approach (e.g., return skills demonstration, written/group exercises, etc).

Avoid using words that describe mental responses that cannot be measured, or terms that are broad, vague, difficult to measure, and permit a variety of interpretation.

Nonbehavioral Terms to Avoid

appreciate	enjoy	perceive
be acquainted with	gain a working knowledge of	recognize
be aware of	grasp the significance of	remember
be familiar with	have knowledge of	sympathize with
comprehend	increased interest in	think
develop an appreciation of	know	understand
develop conceptual thinking	learn	

Source: AAOHN, 1996.

X Philosophies of Adult Education

Adult educators' philosophies and systems of beliefs develop from values, principles, and experience.

A Personal values affect adult educators' approaches to program development.

B Adult educators should develop and use a working philosophy of adult education to accomplish the following:
  1. Provide a point of reference upon which to base activities
  2. Help avoid pitfalls in strategy development

C Recognized philosophies that can guide the adult educator (Table 12-4):
  1. Liberalism: Knowledge is transmitted from expert to novice.
  2. Humanism: Knowledge is acquired voluntarily based on individual needs and is self-directed, experimental, self-evaluated, and facilitative.
  3. Progressivism: Knowledge is accumulated experimentally by use of one's senses and interaction with the world.
  4. Behaviorism: Knowledge is gained by use of scientific method and through programmed learning.
  5. Radicalism: Knowledge is gained through dialogue, dialectical process of reflection and action, problem posing, and critical thinking.
  6. Deconstructionism: Knowledge is achieved through linguistic and literary analysis, by constructing individual reality, using dialectical process of reflection and action, problem posing, and critical thinking.

D Approaches may be eclectic, developed by combining several elements of identified theories, or traditional, developed by adopting one particular theory and building on it.

E Adult education centers on the objectives of the program, needs of participants, curriculum, program content, analysis of the teaching/learning process, and the relationship of the education to the community in which the education takes place.

XI Motivating Adults to Learn

Motivation is the concept that helps explain why people learn as they do. When adults are motivated to learn, they work harder, learn more, have a sense of enjoyment and achievement, and want to continue to learn. Occupational and environmental nurses will be of more assistance to clients if they are able to understand the motivational needs of health promotion program participants.

A Characteristics of instructors who are able to motivate (Wlodkowski, 1998):
  1. They are experts who present instructional material in a logical and orderly manner, thus providing clarity to difficult and new information, and are prepared to convey their knowledge through instruction.
  2. They use motivation to arouse behavior, give direction or purpose to behavior, cause behavior to persist, and influence the learner to choose a particular behavior.
  3. They have a realistic understanding of the needs and expectations of adults that influence their motivation to learn.
  4. They teach in a manner that expresses care for the learner and knowledge of the subject, together with the intent to encourage similar feelings in the learner.

TABLE 12-4

Adult education philosophies: comparative analysis and summary evaluation (CASE) of philosophies

Analytical components		Philosophies					
	Liberalism	Humanism	Progressivism	Behaviorism	Radicalism	Deconstructionism
Origins	Circa, 4th Century B.C., Ancient Greeks, rise of republic-democratic state, classic ideals, Judeo-Christian, and western origins	16th Century Western origins (Greco-Roman) and Eastern influences (Buddhism and Confucianism), 18th century enlightenment and existentialism of 20th century	16th century European rationalist, empirical, and scientific thought; 19th Century pragmatism/romanticism, and the industrial revolution	18th Century Darwinism, scientific realism, positivism, rise of empiricism, and 20th Century school of American psychology	Anarchists of 1800s, the Freudian left, Marxists, socialists, Christianity, liberation theology, radical feminism, labor movement, and existentialism	Radical-analytic concepts initiated in France—gained increased notice in U.S. (intellectual circles) in 1970s, 1980s and 1990s
Purposes	To enlighten the citizenry, pursue absolute truth, attain wisdom, foster development of individual as good virtuous being, and support a democratic society	To enhance personal growth, self-fulfillment, and development of the whole person, and to achieve individual autonomy	To develop individual abilities and social consciousness, foster a practical understanding of the world, and maintain the democratic state while promoting social reform	To control overt behavior of the organism and scientifically condition individuals to operate within their environment	To develop the process by which revolutionary personal, political, social, and economic changes are brought about	To construct reality in terms of the individual acting within a specific socio-political climate, and to construct and critically approach reality
Instructional Strategies	Knowledge is transmitted from expert to novice: Socratic method (discussion and dialogue-problem posing and response) lecture and classical readings	Knowledge is acquired voluntarily based on individual needs; and is self-directed, experimental, self-evaluated and facilitative	Knowledge is accumulated experimentally by use of one's senses and interaction with world, experience, by scientific methods, and by problem solving techniques	Knowledge is provided by use of scientific method, and through programmed learning: using strict sequence of stimulus and response to reinforce desired behaviors and to extinguish the undesirable	Knowledge is gained through dialogue, dialectical process of reflection and action, problem posing, and critical thinking	Knowledge is achieved through linguistic literary analysis, by constructing individual reality, using dialectical process of reflection and action, problem posing and critical thinking

Continued

Synopsis developed from Dr. Nancy E. Hagan, "Philosophy and Adult Education" by Robert M. Ward.

TABLE 12-4

Adult education philosophies: comparative analysis and summary evaluation (CASE) of philosophies—cont'd

Analytical components	Philosophies					
	Liberalism	Humanism	Progressivism	Behaviorism	Radicalism	Deconstructionism
Teacher/Learner Relationship	Vertical: Pedagogical (pedantic)	More horizontal than vertical: A collaborative facilitative process	More horizontal than vertical: a reciprocal process	Vertical: Teacher-controlled and directed	Horizontal: Teacher-learner equality	Vertical: Learner focused
Relationship Between Individual, Society, and State	Education is to produce an informed citizenry supportive of the democratic state	Education is to develop self-actualized citizenry who will indirectly support democratic state	Education is to focus on individual-social development which will generally support the democratic state and will directly influence social changes	Education is to be used to control the environment so as to direct the behavior of individuals within society, thereby supporting the current controlling systems in authority	Education is to produce socially and politically aware individuals who are capable of bringing about social and political change in existing governing systems	Education is concerned with the development of the individual's critical thinking and with the exposure of oppression, and in turn, political action to bring about changes in existing governing/ruling systems.
Relationship to Political and Economic Systems	Highly subject to political climate and economic conditions, i.e. in last century and a half, government has supported need of productive workhorse rather then enlightened populace	Political/economic climate does not substantially affect humanistic programs inasmuch as most are individual and small group matters vs. large social-political movements	Political/economic climate may have substantial effect on support of social reforms which may have an effect and be affected by politics	Politics and economics play a significant role in the design of the state, which, in turn, directly affects overt behavior	Highly affected and may significantly affect politics and economy, which are critical elements in social change	Political and economic forms are tool of critical analysis which may, in turn, affect political and economic forms

Representative Proponents and Movements	Socrates, Plato, Augustine, Thomas Aquinas, Thomas Jefferson, Everett Dean Martin, and Jacques Maritain; Franklin's Junto, founding of early American Universities, lyceums, Chautauqua, university extension programs, Great Books Program, and Elderhostel	Maslow, Rogers, May, Tough, McKenzie, and Brookfield; Human potential seminars, encounter-type groups, training groups (T-groups), Knowles' andragogy, counseling, self-directed learning projects	John Dewey, Eduard Lindeman, Benne, Bergevin and Jane Addams; Settlement houses in urban areas for immigrants; land grant universities, Cooperative Extension Service, citizenship education and community development, community colleges, adult basic education, and vocational education	J.B. Watson, E.L. Thorndike, and B.F. Skinner; Binary computer programs and skills, programmed learning, competency-based education, and behavior modification	Ivan Illich, John Ohlinger, Paulo Freire, Gramsci, Habermas, and Mezlrow; Horton's Highlander Folk School, Freire's literacy training used in Third-World countries, and popular education	Jacques Derrida, Paul de Man, J. Harris Miller, Barbara Johnson, Stanley Fish, Annabel Patterson, and Jane Tompkins; Cultural diversity and pluralism
Criticisms	Anti-vocational stance, often considered elitist, oppressive, and ethno-centric	Normlessness, lack of standards for learning process, no accountability, and exaggerated emphasis on learner's needs	Experiential learning alone may be inadequate; antiintellectualism and indefinite role of teacher	Big-brother image; individual has no control over external forces, individual is a pawn; discounts higher cognitive processes; reduction-istic and dehumanizing; discounts faith, emotion, and beliefs	Belief that revolutionary approach is only method to change society; challenges all aspects of culture and its structures, polarizes relationships between oppressors and the oppressed	All western values are intrinsically oppressive; only political action can free people from dominant ideology or hegemony; oppressive, unyielding—totally negates absolutes: all is relative, and anti-liberal stance
Contributions	Significant influence in mainstream adult education; instrumental in development of early American universities, numerous adult education programs and other institutions	Strong emphasis on individual learner and self-development; instrumental in providing adult education with a more humane face; and strong force in adult education	Significant role in social movement and reforms fostered integration of immigrants into society; focused attention on experiential learning and scientific methodology	Developments in programmed learning, contract learning, behavior modification programs, accountability; competency-based education; extensive use in continuing professional education and in training and development	Significant role in raising critical consciousness and producing social change	Emphasis on critical examination of language, recognition of various cultural groups, and acknowledgment of diversity

B Definitions of motivating factors (Wlodkowski, 1998)

1. An *attitude* is a combination of concepts, information, and emotions that result in a predisposition to respond favorably or unfavorably to particular people, groups, ideas, events, and objectives.
   a. Attitudes may be acquired through experience, direct instruction, or identification of role behavior.
   b. Attitudes can be modified by a new experience.
2. A *need* is a condition experienced by the individual as an internal (intrinsic) or external (extrinsic) force.
   a. A need leads the person to move in the direction of a goal.
   b. Identifying and addressing the learner's needs enhances motivation.
3. *Stimulation* is any change in perception or experience with the environment that makes people active.
   a. Stimulation sustains adult learning behavior.
   b. Attention, interest, and involvement are goals for learner participation.
4. An *affect* is the emotional experience of feeling, concerns, and passions that influence behaviors; when appropriate, the instructor should relate content and instructional procedures to learners' concerns.
5. *Competence* and *self-confidence* are motivating forces in learning; consistent feedback to learners regarding their mastery, progress, and responsibility will enhance their learning.
6. *Reinforcement* is a positive or negative response to an individual's behavior that affects the probability of the behavior's recurrence.

XII Teaching Methods and Techniques

(Table 12-5)

A *Learning contract:* a formal agreement written by the learner detailing conditions of learning, including timelines and written evaluation

B *Lecture:* a planned oral discourse on a particular subject by a qualified person

C *Discussion:* an exchange of ideas between teacher and learner about subjects and issues

D *Mentorship:* an informal role in which the teaching function is primarily a means to advancement and secondarily a contribution to the learner

E *Case study:* an in-depth study of a representative problem or situation

F *Demonstration:* a presentation showing how something works and the procedures followed when using it

G *Simulation:* a method of obtaining skills, competence, or knowledge by participating in activities similar to a real-life activity of interest

H *Forum:* an open discussion with one or more resource persons and an entire group

I *Panel:* a small group of three to six persons who have a purposeful discussion of a topic about which they have specialized knowledge; discussion is in presence of an audience

J *Symposium:* a series of presentations by two to five persons of notable authority on different aspects of the same or closely related themes

K *Computer-enhanced education:* use of computers as an enhancement to teacher-learner interaction

TABLE 12-5

Teaching methods and techniques

	Definition	Purpose	Specifics	Advantages	Limitations
Learning Contracts	Formal agreement written by learner detailing what will be learned, how learning will be accomplished, timeline, and written evaluation	Individualizes the learning process	Components include objectives, resources and strategies, target dates for completion, evidence of accomplishment, and evaluation strategies	Flexible; learners control the process; preferred methods	Uncomfortable for learners and teacher if not used before; learners question quality of learning; teacher placed at risk for excess time pressures
Lecture	A planned oral discourse on a particular subject by a highly qualified individual	Cognitive transfer of information from teacher; framework for learning activities; identifies, explains, and clarifies different concepts, problems or ideas; challenges beliefs, attitudes, and behaviors; and stimulates the audience to further inquiry	Preparation includes preplanning, organization, compliance with time constraints, handouts and practice	Precise and orderly format; popular; useful when no handouts; use for large groups; forum for one-on-one and enhances listening	Audience is exposed to one view; biased information may be given; discourages learners from the teaching/learning interaction; not able to determine impact on audience; speaker may not know audience level of knowledge or experience; evaluated on entertainment value rather than content
Discussion	Allows learners and teacher to talk about subjects and issues	Allows cognitive and affective exploration of issues	Prepare by setting discussion themes; providing resource materials; evoking consensual rules; personalizing discussion topics; and attending to group composition	Most favored, inclusive, and participatory	May uncover emotional issues which may need to be dealt with before further learning can take place
Mentorship	Designates an informal role in which the teaching function is recognized primarily as a means to personal and institutional advancement and only secondarily as contribution to the overall well-being of the protégé	Promotes the development of the learner	Role of the mentor involves being supportive, challenging, and visionary	Promotes critical thinking; develops personal power and independence; provides a role model	Provides an environment where power may be misused, emotional dependence fostered and favoritism practiced. Hero worship, values conflicts, and feelings of abandonment may be experienced

Continued

TABLE 12-5

Teaching methods and techniques—cont'd

	Definition	Purpose	Specifics	Advantages	Limitations
Case Study	An in-depth study of a problem or situation	Presents real life examples for study	Types include: case reports, analysis, and discussion Design the study by focusing on the problem; developing supporting materials; reviewing; and field testing the case	Causes critical thinking; develops decision-making and problem-solving skills; and is participatory	Long preparation time; requires a facilitator to think on the spot
Demonstration	Presents how something works and the procedures followed in using it	Arouses interest and motivation; directs attention; supports verbal explanation; enables economical use of time and resources; and provides step-by-step guidelines in performing tasks or improving skills	Types include: instructional, participant volunteers, and full participation Roles Teachers must be technically expert; able to analyze process and break into small steps; and have all materials ready for use Learner must practice each step, communicate problems, and practice deficiencies	Illustrates point to enable learners to comprehend complex and difficult materials in a short time; reduces gaps between the learner and practice; and provides variety to facilitate different learning styles	Discourages some learners; difficult to isolate tasks, skills, and procedures into step-by-step manuals; time consuming; uses only small groups; limited individualized feedback

| Simulation | A technique that enables learners to obtain skills, competence, or knowledge by becoming involved in activities that are similar to those in real life | An attempt to address real problems under real-life conditions and discuss them; develops complex cognitive skills such as decision making, evaluating, and synthesizing; impacts the learners' values, beliefs, and attitudes; induces empathy; sharpens interpersonal communication skills; and help learners unlearn negative attitudes or behaviors | Types include: role play, case study, and critical incident Steps are experience, sharing, processing, generalizing, and application Roles Facilitator should explain the purpose; give short, clear, and understandable instructions; provide relevant, real-life situations; involve problem solving appropriate to the level of the learner; have adequate interaction with learners; and give appropriate feedback. Learners should participate in all activities; develop an attitude of sharing and support; have open feedback with facilitators, and apply knowledge, skills, or attitudes to personal life situations | An opportunity to apply learning to a new situation; participatory; no consequences of wrong decisions; immediate feedback; generates new ideas and changed attitudes; and is cost effective | Negative learning may occur if situation too complex; teacher must be proficient; expensive to design and conduct; time consuming |

L Distance education: communication between teacher and learner occurs through print, writing, telephone, or electronic media

M Nominal group technique: a type of group process that emphasizes the way people learn as contrasted to what they learn

N Brainstorming: a sharing of free-flowing ideas that is intended to stimulate creative thinking and the development of new ideas

XIII Effective Presentations

Presentations involve the preparation and delivery of critical subject matter in a logical and condensed form, leading to effective communication (Morrisey & Sechrest, 1997).

A Elements of a presentation

1. The goal of any presentation is effective communication, which means getting the message across in a manner that accomplishes the stated objectives.
2. Audience needs must be identified in order to reach the goals; audience needs are the determining factor in the selection of appropriate resource materials.
3. Meaningful content is supported by presentation aids, presentation techniques, and logistical details.

B Types of presentations

1. *Persuasive* or selling presentations pique the interest of potential participants, convince management to approve programs, or sell existing customers on the benefits of making changes.
2. *Explanatory* presentations make new information available or refresh an audience's understanding of a given topic by providing a general overview or description of a new development.
3. *Instructional* presentations teach how to use something, such as a new procedure or piece of equipment.
4. An *oral report* brings the audience up to date on a subject they already know something about, by providing details suited to the needs and interest of the audience.

C Preparing the presentation

1. Establish written behavioral objectives, stating specific expected results and measurable accomplishments (Box 12-4).
2. Audience analysis
   a. Identify the objectives for the audience.
   b. Develop an overall approach to achieve objectives.
   c. Describe the social and demographic characteristics of the audience.
   d. Select appropriate information and techniques.
3. Prepare a preliminary plan consisting of no more than five main ideas or concepts, and discuss it with the officials who are planning the event.
   a. The plan is a guide for the presenter, keeping ideas channeled, focusing on points to be emphasized, and preventing the omission of information.
   b. Know the audience: If possible, determine the number of participants, where they work, what type of work they do, and their attitudes toward the subject.
   c. Make modifications as necessary before the presentation.

4. When selecting resource information, determine the purpose of the presentation material to be covered and the level of detail needed to meet the audience's needs.
   a. Questions to be answered
      1) What is the purpose of this presentation?
      2) What do the participants expect and need from this presentation?
      3) What should be covered? What should be eliminated?
      4) What amount of detail is necessary?
      5) Will members of the audience have limitations (e.g., physical disabilities, language limitations, illiteracy, or other barriers to learning) that require adjustments?
      6) What can be withheld from the presentation but offered as a resource?
5. Organize the materials into the introduction, body, and conclusion of the presentation.
   a. The introduction should include the following:
      1) A direct statement concerning the subject of the presentation and its importance
      2) Some audience interest linked to the subject
      3) Examples leading directly to the subject
      4) Strong quotations related to the subject
      5) Important statistics that emphasize a point
      6) Strong or anecdotal information illustrating the subject
   b. The body of the presentation should consider the following:
      1) Visual illustrations as important aids to support the content
      2) Reiteration, statistics, comparisons, analogies, and expert testimony to present the main ideas
   c. The conclusion should consist of the following:
      1) A summary of the main ideas
      2) A review of the purpose of the presentation
      3) An appeal for audience action
6. Practice the presentation aloud to yourself, videotape or audiotape the practice session, or give a pilot presentation.
7. Evaluation
   a. Evaluation is a critical component in assessing the effectiveness and efficiency of a program intervention in achieving a predetermined objective.
   b. Evaluations cannot be accomplished without taking into account people and their environments.
   c. By using the planning process data, measurable objectives, and program participants, a meaningful evaluation can be undertaken.

D **Development and use of audiovisuals**
1. People retain about 30% of what they hear; about 20% of what they see; and about 50% of what they both hear and see; visual aids are used in a presentation to facilitate learning.
2. Characteristics of effective visual aids
   a. Each aid represents one key concept.
   b. They are appropriate to the audience.
   c. Text is restricted to a maximum of six words per line and 10 lines per visual, consisting of short phrases and key words rather than complete sentences.

     d. They use color or contrast to highlight important points.

     e. They represent facts accurately.

     f. They should be checked for spelling and accuracy; they can be unconvincing if inaccurate or misspelled.

3. To maintain quality, the presentation should contain no more than one visual for every 2 minutes of presentation time; the presentation, not the visuals, should be the center of attention.

4. Guidelines for using media include visibility and audibility, ease of operation, and accessibility.

     a. Consider room size, number of people, any distracting noises, seating arrangement, visual obstacles, and lighting.

     b. Organize the equipment before the presentation; arrange presentation components in sequence, and designate someone to help with lighting, if needed.

     c. Select aids based on availability, cost, and convenience.

5. Specific tools used in teaching include an overhead projector, slides, video, flip charts, handouts, audio recorder, chalkboards, computer visuals (e.g., Internet, PowerPoint), and models. (Table 12-6 lists advantages and disadvantages of each.)

6. Aids to further understanding (Note: When using any of the aids listed in this section, it is important to consider that all nonoriginal material may be subject to copyright.)

     a. The purpose of a chart is to direct thinking, clarify points, summarize information, and show trends, relationships, and comparisons. There are numerous types of charts (Box 12-5).

     b. Illustrations, diagrams, and maps clarify points, emphasize trends, get attention, or show relationships or differences.

     c. Exhibits show finished products, demonstrate the results of good and bad practices, attract attention, arouse and hold interest, and adequately illustrate an idea.

     d. Manuals, pamphlets, outlines, and bulletins provide standard information and guidelines as well as reference and background material.

     e. Cartoons, posters, and signs attract attention, arouse interest and often promote critical thinking.

     f. Photographs and illustrations from textbooks or magazines tie the discussion to actual situations and people, illustrate the immediate relevance of a topic, or show local activities.

     g. Examples and stories relieve tension, fix an idea, get attention, illustrate a point, clarify a situation, or break away from a delicate subject.

     h. Field trips present a subject in its natural setting, stimulate interest, blend theory with practical application, and provide additional material for study (Morrisey & Sechrest, 1997).

E **Logistics: preparing for a presentation**

1. Invite the audience to the presentation by letter, memo, phone call, formal announcement, electronic mail, or word of mouth.

2. Room set-up options depend on the size and shape of the meeting room, size and nature of the audience, type of presentation, delivery method, and kind of participation wanted from the audience.

     a. *Auditorium* style is used for large groups when there is no need for the audience to write or consult reference materials and when audience

TABLE 12-6

Specific media tools

	Definition	Advantages	Disadvantages
Overhead Projector	An electric device designed to project transparent materials as large as 10 by 10 inches and as small as 2 by 2 inches	The projected image is visible in a lighted room and transparencies are made inexpensively	Teachers must be able to talk and use transparencies simultaneously; machines require electric outlet and bulb
Slides	A small piece of film on which a single pictorial graphic image has been placed for still projection	Convenient to use, easy to obtain in high quality, relatively inexpensive, easy to use with no more than 5 to 6 lines per slide, and can be made from anything that is drawn, painted, written, typewritten, printed, or photographed	Slides must be viewed in a darkened room; each presentation requires filing, storing, and organizing slides
Video	Motion on tape shown on a television monitor with sound	Provides a common stimulus for students, with specific examples which achieve identification and involvement of the viewer with characters and situations presented	Expensive; not all information being presented may be consistent with what is being presented; must be shown in a darkened room and equipment often fails
Flip Charts	A series of bound sheets of paper or poster-board that can be flipped over, one at a time, to show a series of thoughts, pictures, outline points, questions, cartoons, or symbols	Portable, economical, and versatile; can be prepared ahead of time and used repeatedly	Not useful with large audiences; do not store easily; good handwriting skills are needed to develop
Handouts	Printed or duplicated material given to learners, such as outlines, job descriptions, bulletins, cartoons, charts, and problems	Allows learners to receive the same information and to be able to review or reference after presentation	A supplement, not a substitute for presentation; may distract from the main point or confuse the learner
Audio Recorder	Recorded sound on a magnetic tape	Flexible timing and interruption of instruction; inexpensive, reusable, and easy to use; and tape is useful in large and small groups	Poorly prepared or used materials may distract or discourage learners
Chalkboard	A board whose writing surface is specially treated for use with chalk	Minimal cost; allows for spontaneity, audience involvement, and on-the-spot revisions	Not a permanent record; it has limited use in a large group
Models	Scaled representation, which may be equal in size, smaller, or larger than original	A model shows clearly and quickly "how" and "why" something works and permits close up observation, investigation, and analysis	Commercial models are costly to purchase; require large storage space, special atmospheric conditions, or extreme care in handling

Source: Adapted from Morrisey & Sechrest, 1987.

BOX 12-5

Types of charts

- *Highlight charts* present a direct copy or emphasize a point.
- *Time sequence charts* show relationships over time.
- *Organizational charts* indicate the relationships among individuals, departments, and jobs.
- *Cause-and-effect charts* illustrate causal relationships.
- *Flow charts* show the relation of parts to the finished whole or to the direction of movement of a process (e.g., PERT [Program Evaluation and Review Technique] charts).
- *Inventory charts* show a picture of an object with its parts labeled off to the side.
- *Dissection charts* present enlarged, transparent, or cut-away views of an object.

- *Diagrammatic* or *schematic charts* provide a simple portrayal of a complex subject by means of symbols.
- *Multibar graphs* represent comparable data using horizontal or vertical bars.
- *Divided-bar graphs* show the relation of parts to the whole by using a single bar divided into parts by lines.
- *Line graphs* display information using a horizontal scale and a vertical scale.
- *Pie graphs* show relations of parts to the whole, like a divided-bar graph.
- *Pictographs* represent comparable quantities in a given time by use of symbols such as a stack of coins representing comparable costs.

Source: Morrisey & Sechrest, 1987.

    participation is limited to a question-and-answer period; generally, no tables or writing areas are available for participants.

  b. *Classroom* style is useful for relatively formal situations where participants need to write or actively use reference materials; tables or desks are provided.

  c. *Horseshoe,* or U-shaped, style is useful when eye contact with the audience and relatively informal discussions are desirable and participants may write or use materials easily; this is most desirable for small groups.

  d. *Buzz* style is useful when small-group discussions are conducted as part of the presentation; these discussions can be held easily at small tables distributed around in the room.

  e. *Chevron* or herringbone style is useful for group discussions, creating a more formal climate than buzz style and a less formal climate than classroom style; rectangular tables are preferred.

3. Equipment that may be needed includes a table for projection equipment, lap top computers (for PowerPoint presentations), slide and overhead projectors, extension cords, spare bulbs, flip chart, and markers. Consider backup slides or transparencies when using the computer.

4. Always check equipment, room temperature, and lighting; put slides, transparencies, and handouts in order; hide displays that should be out of

sight before presentation; number transparencies or slides in order in case they become mixed up.

5. Coordinate arrangements at the presentation site by giving clear instructions regarding the specific needs; arrange for shipping materials in advance; arrive early to prepare the room; and always know how to operate equipment personally.

6. Announce "housekeeping" details before the presentation begins: rules regarding smoking, eating, or drinking; rest room locations; time and location of breaks; and registration requirements.

F **Deliver the presentation**

1. Effective communication is a two-way process, involving both the speaker and the listener, that leads to some form of action or response.

2. In the communication process, the listener is the more important of the two members.

3. Platform techniques, such as eye contact with the audience, appropriate dress, confidence, and relaxed hand movements are important behaviors to exhibit.
   a. Gestures can be effective if they are properly synchronized with certain words or phrases and are not overused.
   b. Body movements are effective in releasing some of the speakers' tension, drawing attention back to the speaker from the visual aid, and changing the pace of the presentation.
   c. Facial expressions should be lively, varied, and appropriate to the mood of the audience.
   d. Concentrate on reducing distracting mannerisms such as lip licking, nose patting, ear tugging, stretching, or playing with pens, rubber bands, or paper clips.

4. Develop good voice quality: a natural, conversational pitch and injection; a level of volume that can be heard by all; a rate and tempo that varies enough to maintain the audience's interest; and deliberate pauses, used as needed.
   a. "Uh" results when the thought process interrupts the speech process and is eliminated with increased familiarity with the subject.
   b. Trailing sentences or loss of voice at the end of sentences lose the audience.
   c. Faulty pronunciation and poor enunciation can be corrected by checking the dictionary for correct pronunciations and by adopting a manner of speaking that is clear, precise, and easy to listen to.

5. Tools facilitate the delivery of a speaker's message.
   a. A lectern provides a surface on which notes may be placed; provides an out-of-sight storage space for aids and handouts; gives a resting place for hands; establishes a type of relationship with the audience.
      1) Remaining behind the lectern establishes a formal relation with the audience.
      2) Moving to the side or front of the lectern removes the barriers and is less formal.
   b. The pointer draws attention to specific items on a visual aid and should be put down when not in use.
   c. The podium or lavaliere microphones should be used in practice until the presenter is speaking comfortably in a natural voice and with equipment at the proper height or on the lapel close to the mouth.

6. Learning to deal with audiences' questions is a vital skill for presenters.
   a. Conducting question-and-answer sessions involves accepting the question as a compliment from the participant, being prepared for possible questions, paraphrasing the question to ensure that everyone understands it, making the question relevant to the discussion, and trying to give a correct answer.
   b. Dealing with some difficult situations requires experience.
      1) Arguments should be postponed until after the session because they limit the participation of the rest of the audience.
      2) "Curves" or "loaded" questions may be intended to put the speaker on the spot, so end the discussion quickly and move on.
      3) Long-winded questioners should be handled by picking out a word or an idea that is being expressed and show its relationship to the presentation; or, as a last resort only, cut the questioner off in the interest of time.
      4) The audience grows tired very quickly of a questioner who takes over to make a speech; the presenter should take control of the situation by asking the questioner to ask the question and then move on.
      5) A question may come up for which the speaker has no answer; in that case, the speaker should admit it and ask the group if they have an answer.

G Always finish the presentation or program by evaluating the process and content.
1. Allow participants to rate the instructor.
2. Participants should evaluate whether the program addressed the stated goals and objectives and their own personal objectives.
3. Participants should be evaluated to determine the knowledge they gained during the presentation; this could be done using a pretest/posttest format.

BIBLIOGRAPHY

Ajzen, I. (1988). *Attitudes, personality, and behavior.* Chicago, IL: Dorsey Press.

Bandura, A. (1986). *Social foundations of thought and action: A social cognitive theory.* Englewood Cliffs, NJ: Prentice-Hall.

Fishbein, M. & Ajzen, I. (1975). *Belief, attitude, intention and behavior: An introduction to theory and research.* Reading, MA: Addison-Wesley.

Galbraith, M.W. (Ed.). (1998). *Adult learning methods.* Malabar, FL: Krieger Publishing Company.

Gilbert, B. (1994). Employee assistance programs: History and program description. *AAOHN Journal, 42(10),* 488–493.

Glynn, T.J. & Manley, M.W. (1995). *How to help your patients stop smoking* (NIH publication No. 95-3064). Bethesda, MO: National Cancer Institute, National Institutes of Health.

Green, L. & Kreuter, M. (1999). *Health promotion planning: An educational and environmental approach.* Mountain View, CA: Mayfield Publishing Company.

Heatherton, T.F., Kozlowski, L.T., Frecker, R.C., & Fagerstrom, K.O. (1991). The Fagerstrom Test for Nicotine Dependence: A revision of the Fagerstrom Tolerance Questionnaire. *British Journal of Addictions,* 86:1119-1127.

Knowles, M.S. (1988). *Self-directed learning: A guide for learners and teachers.* New York: Cambridge Books.

Leavell, H. & Clark, E. (1979). *Preventive medicine for the doctor in the community.* New York: McGraw Hill.

Lusk, S.L. (1997). Health promotion and disease prevention in the worksite. *Annual Review of Nursing Research, 15,* 187-213.

Lusk, S.L. (1999). Demand management programs. *AAOHN Journal, 47(6),* 277-279.

Morrisey, G.L. & Sechrest, T.L. (1997). *Effective business and technical presentations* (3rd ed.). Reading, MA: Addison-Wesley Publishing Co., Inc.

O'Donnell, M.D. (1989). Definition of health promotion: Part III: Expanding the definition. *American Journal of Health Promotion, 3(3),* 5.

O'Donnell, M.D. & Harris, J. (1994). *Health promotion in the workplace* (2nd ed.). New York: Delmar Publishers, Inc.

Pender, N. (1996). *Health promotion in nursing practice* (3rd ed.). Stamford, CT: Appleton & Lange.

Prentice-Dunn, S. & Rogers, R.W. (1986). Protection motivation theory and preventive health: Beyond the health belief model. *Health education research: Theory and practice 1, (3),* 153–161.

Prochaska, J.O. (1979). *Systems of psychotherapy: A transtheoretical analysis.* Homewood, Illinois: Dorsey Press.

Prochaska, J.O. & DiClemente, C.C. (1983). Stages and processes of self-change of smoking: Towards an integrative model of change. *Journal of Consulting and Clinical Psychology 51(3),* 390–395.

Prochaska, J.O. & DiClemente, C.C. (1982). Transtheoretical theory: Toward a more integrative model of change. *Psychotherapy: Theory, Research and Practice 19(3),* 276-288.

Rosenstock, I.M. (1990). The health belief model: Explaining health behavior through expectancies. In K. Glanz, F.M. Lewis, & B.K. Rimer (Eds.), *Health behavior and health education: Theory, research, and practice.* San Francisco: Jossey-Bass, pp. 39-62.

Schwarzer, R. (1992). Adaptation and maintenance of health behaviors: A critical review of theoretical approaches. In Schwarzer, R. (Ed.), *Self-efficacy: Thought control of action.* New York: Hemisphere.

Travers, P.H. & McDougall, C. (1995). *Guidelines for an occupational health & safety service.* Atlanta: AAOHN Publications.

Triandis, H.C. (1999). Values, attitudes, and interpersonal behavior. In M.N. Page (Ed.), *Nebraska Symposium on Motivation, 1979.* Lincoln, NE: University of Nebraska Press, pp. 195-259.

U.S. Department of Health, Education, and Welfare. (1979). *Healthy people: Surgeon General's report on health promotion and disease.* Washington, DC: USDHEW.

United States Department of Health and Human Services. (2000). *Healthy people 2010: Volume I and Volume II* (DHHS Publication No. 2000-0152). Washington, DC: U.S. Government Printing Office.

Wlodkowski, R.J. (1998). *Enhancing adult motivation to learn.* San Francisco: Jossey-Bass, Inc.

13

Managing Psychosocial Factors in the Occupational Setting

MARY K. SALAZAR AND RANDAL D. BEATON

The quality of one's work life is a reflection of a multitude of psychosocial factors in the workplace. Knowledge and recognition of these factors is essential to the development of effective and efficient occupational health and safety services. This chapter provides an overview of the various dimensions of psychosocial factors. It also describes methods to assess and respond to them, and concludes with a discussion of techniques that can be used to evaluate stress reduction programs.

I Overview of Psychosocial Factors

Psychosocial factors are directly related to the structure of work, organizational characteristics, interpersonal relationships at work, the meaning of work, and the characteristics of the workers themselves.

A Structure of work
1. The structure of work refers to how work is organized; it includes workload, pace of work, hours and scheduling, and the level of monotony or challenge inherent in work processes.
2. The organization of work will determine whether the workers' talents, knowledge, and other personal resources are properly used.

B Organizational characteristics
1. Organizational culture and climate set the tone for worker communication patterns, prioritization of tasks, worker behavior, and the nature of worker interactions. (Chapter 6 provides more information about climate and culture.)
2. The various work environments (physical, biologic, chemical, mechanic, and psychosocial) affects workers' perceptions of health, safety, and security within their organizations.
3. Other organizational structures include organizational mission and philosophy, the size of the organization, its physical arrangement, and its service or product.

C Interpersonal relationships and work
1. Relationships with managers and supervisors are determined by the management styles that prevail in an organization (Chapter 6); management styles determine the level of communication, decision-making power, and level of control experienced by the worker.
2. Co-worker relationships can be supportive, nonsupportive, or conflictual (Beaton et al., 1997).
3. New styles of labor, such as computerized recordkeeping, electronic communication, and computer and video monitoring have threatened workers' ability to have interpersonal relationships with co-workers and supervisors.

D The meaning of work (Salazar & Graham, 1999)
1. Work has been described as being important to the individual's sense of self-worth and identity.
2. Work may be viewed as an important responsibility, and a means to 'not be a burden' on others.
3. Work is a way to support one's family.
4. Work is a symbol of personal achievement and values.
5. Work is a central part of most people's lives.

E Characteristics of workers (Salazar & Graham, 1999)
1. *Personal attributes* include the demographic attributes of workers, their personality traits, feelings about work, spirituality, and levels of motivation.
2. *Social networks,* especially family support, may affect workers' attitudes about work, their response to occupational illness and injury, and their ability to return to work when an injury or illness occurs.
3. A worker's level of *job satisfaction* is related to the structure of work, the organizational culture and climate, and interpersonal relationships at work.

II Psychosocial Hazards

Although psychosocial hazards tend to be more nebulous and less tangible than other categories of hazards, they nevertheless exert a pervasive influence on health and safety.

A Workplace violence has been identified as an important health and safety issue in the modern day workplace.
1. Homicide is the second leading cause of job-related death among all workers in the United States; and is the leading cause of workplace fatalities among women (OSHA, 1999).
   a. An average of 20 workers are murdered each week, accounting for 12% of all fatal work injuries and 31% of occupational deaths among women (NIOSH, 1996; OSHA, 1999; U.S. Department of Labor, 1998).
   b. Robbery is the primary motive for job-related homicide, accounting for 85% of deaths.
   c. Disputes among co-workers and with customers account for about 10% of the total number of deaths.
   d. Sales workers experience the highest number of homicides, followed by taxi drivers, chauffeurs, and law enforcement officers; although they do not have the highest number of deaths, taxi drivers have the highest risk at 41.4 per 100,000 persons.

2. There are approximately 2 million assaults and threats of violence against American workers each year (OSHA, 1999).
   a. Unlike homicides, nonfatal workplace assaults are distributed almost equally between men (44%) and women (56%).
   b. Retail sales workers are the most common victims, with an average of 330,000 attacks each year; this is followed by police officers, who experience an average of 234,000 attacks each year.
   c. Although fatal events are most often associated with robberies, nonfatal violence is more likely to result from anger or frustration of customers, clients, or co-workers.
   d. Most nonfatal workplace assaults occur in service settings such as hospitals, nursing homes, and social service agencies. Forty-eight percent of nonfatal assaults in the workplace are committed by health care patients (NIOSH, 1996).
3. According to NIOSH (1996), risk factors for workplace violence include the following:
   a. Contact with the public
   b. Exchange of money
   c. Delivery of passengers, goods, or services
   d. Having a mobile workplace, such as a taxicab or a police cruiser
   e. Working with unstable or volatile persons in health care, social services, or criminal justice settings
   f. Working alone or in small numbers
   g. Working late at night or during early morning hours
   h. Working in high crime areas
   i. Guarding valuable property or possessions
   j. Working in community-based settings
4. The Occupational Safety and Health Administration has developed recommendations for engineering and administrative controls that can be used to prevent workplace violence (Box 13-1).

B **Mistreatment and harassment**
1. Workplace mistreatment or harassment is any act against an employee that creates a hostile work environment and negatively affects the employee, either physically or psychologically.
   a. These acts of workplace mistreatment include all types of physical or verbal threats, coercion, intimidation, and all forms of harassment; mistreatment also includes excessive use of memoranda or inappropriate use of electronic mail (Spratlen, 1994).
   b. Every workday, an estimated 43,800 U.S. workers are mistreated or harassed.
   c. Coworkers account for most of the harassment, followed by customers.
2. Sexual harassment consists of any "unwanted verbal or physical sexual advance"; this can range from "sexual comments and suggestions, to pressure for sexual favors, accompanied by threats concerning one's job, to physical assault, including rape" (Levy & Wegman, 1999).
   a. "Studies indicate that 40 to 60 percent of women have experienced some form of sexual harassment at work" (Levy & Wegman, 1999).
   b. Victims of sexual harassment may become anxious, depressed, or physically ill. Some quit their jobs or request transfers; others may take undue amounts of sick or leave time (MacLennan, 1992).

BOX 13-1

Examples of violence prevention and control measures

Engineering controls and workplace adaptations

- Security systems for use by staff: panic buttons, handheld noise devices, cellular phones
- Metal detectors at high-risk doorways
- Closed circuit video recording in high-risk areas
- Curved mirrors in hallway intersections and secluded areas
- Bullet-resistant, shatterproof glass in reception, triage, and admitting areas
- Furniture arrangement to avoid entrapment of staff
- Limitation or elimination of items that can be used as weapons
- Two exits provided whenever possible
- Bright lighting indoors, outdoors, and in parking areas
- Lockable, secure rest rooms for staff, separate from visitor facilities
- Locks on rarely used doors, in accordance with local fire codes
- Vehicles used in the field maintained in good working condition

Administrative and work practice controls

- Conduct periodic workplace safety and security analyses
- Establish a zero-tolerance violence policy
- Establish a trained response team to respond to emergencies
- Ensure adequate and qualified staffing at all times
- Provide management and administrative support during emergencies
- Control access to areas other than waiting rooms or lobbies
- Prohibit employees from working alone in high-risk areas
- Use adequate numbers of properly trained security personnel
- Provide security escort to parking lots
- Develop specific policies and procedures for off-site workers' safety
- Train workers in de-escalation and personal protection techniques

Source: USDL, OSHA, 1996

---

   c. The rank of workplace harassers in one study were managers (13.9%), supervisors (30.6%), colleagues (48.6%) and someone from outside of the workplace (6.9%) (MacLennan, 1992).

C **Unemployment and underemployment**

  1. "Unemployment is more destructive to physical and mental health than all but the most dangerous jobs" (Levenstein et al., 1999).

    a. Studies have found a link between unemployment and heart disease, liver disease, suicide, and other stress-related diseases.

    b. Unemployment affects not only the worker, but also the worker's family. For example, domestic violence is two to three times higher in families with unemployed men than in households of fully employed men.

2. The underemployed include contingent, temporary, or part-time workers; an increasing percentage of employers are employing temporary and part-time workers.
   a. In 1990, there were 5 million involuntary part-time workers; that is, workers who would prefer to be working full time.
   b. Temporary or contingent workers are less likely than permanent workers to have life insurance or employer-provided pensions.
   c. These workers experience stress because of lower wages and lack of job security; they are also more likely to have inadequate occupational health and safety services such as safety training.
3. Downsizing is an intentional reduction of a work force as a means of improving efficiency and effectiveness within an organization (Moore, 1999).
   a. Studies suggest that "survivors" of downsizing (those individuals who were not laid off when the reduction occurred) experience increased workloads, lowered trust in management, diminishing job security, and decreased morale.
   b. One study found that 5 years after downsizing, workers were depressed, insecure, and angry at management (Noer, 1993).
   c. Other effects of downsizing include increased turnover and absenteeism and decreased work performance.
   d. Multiple health effects related to threats to employment security have been reported, including sleep disorders, increased blood pressure, and increases in cholesterol levels (Ferrie et al., 1998).

D Shift work (NIOSH, 1997)
1. Approximately 15.5 million Americans are shift workers, working evenings, nights, or rotating shifts.
2. Research suggests that a forward rotation of shifts (from day to evening to nights) is better than a backward rotation in terms of helping workers adjust to changes in sleep patterns (Box 13-2).
3. Short-term effects of shift work include sleep deprivation and disturbances of circadian rhythms, which results in decreased work performance and increase risk of accidents.
4. Long-term effects of shift work include gastrointestinal disturbances and heart disease.
5. "Poor working conditions add to the strain of shiftwork. Adequate lighting, clean air, proper heat and air conditioning, and reduced noise will avoid adding to the shiftworker's burden" (NIOSH, 1997).
6. Shift workers may be more sensitive to toxic substances because of changes in circadian rhythms.

E Characteristics of work
1. *Workload* refers to the total information load that a worker is required to perceive and interpret while performing tasks (Baker & Karasek, 1999).
   a. *Overload* occurs when the information processing load is greater than the worker's information processing capability
   b. *Underload* occurs when the information processing is not challenging enough for the worker; underload results in monotonous, boring work.
2. *Role stress* results from an interpretation of one's role within an organizations (Kahn & Boulding, 1964; Baker & Karasek, 1999).
   a. *Role conflict* occurs when a worker experiences conflicting demands, or

---

BOX 13-2

Suggestions for improving shift work schedules

- Avoid permanent (fixed and nonrotating) night shifts; most workers never really get used to nights.
- Keep consecutive night shifts to a minimum (2 to 4 days in a row before a couple of days off).
- Avoid quick shift changes (less than 10 hours between shifts).
- Allow some free weekends, at least two each month.
- Avoid several days of work followed by minivacations; this can be very fatiguing.

- Keep long work shifts and overtime to a minimum; if working 12-hour shifts, two or three in a row should be the maximum.
- Consider different lengths for shifts, possibly shorter shifts when there are lighter workloads.
- Examine start-end times; flextime may help workers cover their child care needs.
- Keep the schedule regular and predictable; this assists in planning.
- Examine rest breaks; shift workers may need more than the standard coffee and lunch breaks.

Source: NIOSH, 1997

---

when a worker is required to perform a task that is outside of the perceived requirements; as many as 48% of workers are affected by role conflict at some time in their work life.

b. *Role ambiguity* results from lack of clarity about the scope and responsibilities of the job; about 35% to 60% of U.S. workers are affected by role ambiguity.

F Stresses in the modern workplace

1. Electronic performance monitoring, which has become increasingly common in the modern workplace, has been related to increased anxiety, depression, anger, and fatigue among monitored workers (Stiles, 1994).
2. New technologies have increased the speed of production, putting pressure on workers to perform rapid and repetitive motions.
3. Automated machinery and robots have eliminated or threatened some jobs; some workers' jobs have become de-skilled as a result of new high-tech equipment and machinery.
4. Increased globalization of workplaces has lead to the development of multinational companies, increased competition, and decreased profitability.
   a. As a result of globalization, occupational health and safety problems have become ubiquitous, affecting workers nationally and internationally.
   b. Because of decreased profitability, management is no longer willing to honor its "social contract" with workers. ("'Social contract' is management's commitment to maintain decent wages and working conditions in return for some job security and a rising standard of living." [Levenstein et al., 1999]).
   c. For a sizable portion of U.S. workers, international competition has

resulted in lower wages, compulsory overtime, and an increased pace of work accompanied by decreased attention to occupational health and safety (Levenstein et al., 1999).

5. Home-based telework has become an increasingly attractive option to employers and workers (Standen, Daniels, & Lamond, 1999).
    a. It is estimated that 21 million workers telecommute for some part of their work week (NIOSH, 1999).
    b. The effects of telework and telecommuting on the psychologic well-being of workers are complex and significant.
    c. It has been hypothesized that employer's expectations of greater performance and accountability of teleworkers has the potential to increase job pressures.
    d. There is a need for continued research to identify and manage the potential psychologic effects of working at home.

III Occupational Stress

A Definitions

1. *Occupational stress* is "the harmful physical and emotional responses that occur when the requirements of the job do not match the capabilities, resources, or needs of the worker." (NIOSH, 1999).
    a. Stress can be either a positive (eustress) or a negative (distress) influence on one's sense of well-being (Selye, 1974).
    b. *Stressors* refer to the physical or psychologic demands or stimuli to which an individual or worker group must adjust.
2. A *stress reaction* occurs when there is a mismatch between the work conditions and the individual worker (Levy & Wegman, 1999).
    a. *Acute stress reaction* refers to the initial and relatively brief fight-or-flight reaction to a stressor.
    b. *Chronic stress reactions* are long-term stress reactions or strains that involve the mobilization of the neuroendocrine and neurotransmitter systems affecting every organ system; they may be manifested as physiologic, psychologic, or behavioral chronic stress responses.

B Facts about occupational stress

1. A NIOSH (1988) report identified work-related psychologic disorders as one of the top 10 occupational health risks for U.S. workers.
2. A Northwest National Life survey in 1991 found that 40% of U.S. employees surveyed viewed their jobs as "very or extremely stressful."
3. St. Paul Fire and Marine Insurance Company (1992, cited in NIOSH, 1999) concluded that ". . . problems at work are more strongly associated with health complaints than any other life stressor."
4. Nearly 50% of states in the United States allow workers' compensation claims for emotional disorders and stress-related disability.

C Job conditions that may lead to stress (NIOSH, 1999)

1. Excessive workload, lack of rest breaks, long work hours, shift work, and monotonous and boring tasks
2. Management style that precludes worker's participation in decision-making and results in poor communication between workers and supervisors or workers and co-workers
3. Interpersonal relationships that result in "poor social environment and lack of support from co-workers and supervisors"

4. Work roles with "conflicting and uncertain job expectations, too much responsibility, and too 'many hats to wear'"
5. Career concerns, which results in "job insecurity and lack of opportunity for growth, advancement, or promotion"
6. Environmental conditions, such as "unpleasant and dangerous physical conditions"

IV Effects of Stress on Workers

Stress is manifested by an array of physiologic, psychologic, and behavioral disorders.

A Psychologic disorders among workers

1. Depression is one of the most prevalent psychologic conditions observed in the occupational setting (Sears et al., 2000).
   a. One study found that depressed workers had between 1.5 and 3.2 more short-term work-disability days in a 30-day period than other workers (Kessler et al., 1999).
   b. Depression is more prevalent in certain occupations, particularly care-giving occupations such as hospice nurses, physicians, and social workers.
2. Sleep disorders are most commonly reported among shift workers and workers who work long hours; sleep disorders have been correlated with physiologic symptoms such as gastrointestinal disturbances and heart disease.
3. "Burnout is a psychological syndrome of emotional exhaustion, depersonalization, and reduced personal accomplishment" (Maslach, 1993).
   a. *Emotional exhaustion* refers to feelings of being emotionally overextended and depleted of one's emotional resources.
   b. *Depersonalization* refers to a negative, callous, or excessively detached response to other people.
   c. *Reduced personal accomplishment* refers to a decline in one's feelings of competence and successful achievement in one's work.
4. Substance abuse has been directly correlated with the amount of stress experienced by workers; for example, one study demonstrated a direct relationship between job complexity and increased use of substances (Oldham & Gordon, 1999).

B Physiologic responses to stress

Epidemiologic research has documented a relationship between job conditions and certain types of physiologic responses, including the following:

1. Cardiovascular disease such as hypertension and myocardial infarctions
2. Musculoskeletal disorders resulting in headaches, myofascial back pain, and upper extremity cumulative trauma disorders
   a. Studies have found a relationship between dissatisfaction with work status and the risk of low back pain.
   b. Psychosocial factors have been identified as the "best predictor of chronicity" of musculoskeletal pain; pain-related disability has its genesis in the first few days or weeks after a problem (injury) occurs (Kendall, 1999).
3. Gastrointestinal conditions such as peptic ulcers, gastritis, and other digestive disorders

4. Impaired immune functioning; for example, one study found that even a few months of high levels of job stress increased an individual's susceptibility to common cold viral infections

C Behavioral responses

1. Inordinate workplace stress may lead to work performance decrements, decreased attention/concentration, increased distractibility, increased muscle tension, and poor judgment.

2. Other behavioral responses include irritation, self-neglect (e.g., poor nutrition, lack of exercise), and interpersonal conflict.

3. In more extreme cases, homicide or suicide may be a behavioral response.

V Effects of Stress on Organizations

Organizations experience both tangible and intangible effects from stress.

A Studies have demonstrated that stressful working conditions are associated with increased absenteeism, tardiness, and intentions by workers to quit their jobs (NIOSH, 1997).

B Work performance is measured by productivity and the quality of work.

1. Research suggests that policies benefiting worker health also benefit the bottom line because of better productivity and fewer performance errors.

2. Healthy organizations are those organizations with low rates of illness, injuries, and disabilities that are competitive in the marketplace.

3. Examples of characteristics that are associated with low-stress work and high levels of productivity (NIOSH, 1999)
   a. Recognition of employees for good work performance
   b. Opportunities for career development
   c. An organizational culture that values the individual worker
   d. Management actions that are consistent with organizational values

C Estimates of losses to the U.S. economy because of stress-related illnesses, injuries, worker's compensation claims, and decreased productivity were calculated to equal $160 billion annually (Jeffress, 1998).

VI Occupational Stress Models

Multiple conceptualizations of occupational stress have resulted in the development of many occupational stress models over the years.

A Social psychological models examined the influence of role conflict and role ambiguity on job satisfaction and occupational strain indices (Kahn & Boulding, 1964).

B The person-environment fit (P-E) postulates that stress occurs because of a poor fit between the subjective person and the subjective environment (French et al., 1982).

1. According to the P-E model, a mismatch is present in one of two forms:
   a. Between the demands of the job and a persons' ability to meet those demands
   b. Between the motives of the person (e.g., income, self-actualization) and the environmental supplies to satisfy those motives

2. A deficiency of this model is that it has limited ability to predict what objective conditions result in stress.

C The demand-control (D-C) model categorizes occupations on the basis of psychologic demands and job control (also called *decision latitude*) (Karasek & Theorell, 1990).

1. The D-C model purports that strain occurs when there is an imbalance between the demands of the job and the worker's decision latitude.
2. The amount of control that a worker has is now recognized as a decisive factor in the development of occupational stress.

D Systems models view occupational stress from an organizational systems perspective.

1. The NIOSH Systems model uses comprehensive schemata to examine the interaction of work and nonwork stressors (Hurrell & McLaney, 1988).
   a. A combination of job stressors, nonwork factors, individual factors, and buffer factors predict acute reactions.
   b. Acute reactions are categorized as physiologic, psychologic, and behavioral effects.
   c. Outcomes include work-related disabilities and other diagnosed problems.
2. The ecological model (Salazar & Beaton, 2000) offers a method of examining stress in the context in which the stress occurs (Section VII).
3. These system approaches are consistent with the position that dealing with occupational stress requires looking beyond the individual worker or worker groups to the conditions of work.

VII An Ecologic Approach to Occupational Stress

A Ecologic theory is a type of systems theory that describes multiple layers of influence.

1. Ecologic theory evolved from biologic and social sciences.
   a. Its biologic origins date back to 1859 when Darwin described the complex interrelationships between organisms and their environments.
   b. The term *human ecology* was coined in the 1920s in a sociologic context in an attempt to systematically apply the basic theoretic scheme of plant and animal ecology to the study of human communities (Hawley, 1950).
2. In the 1970s, Bronfenbrenner generated a new wave of interest in using an ecological approach to examine human problems.
   a. Bronfenbrenner (1977) felt that the study of humans requires the "examination of multiperson systems not limited to a single setting and must take into account aspects of the environment beyond the immediate situation containing the subject."
   b. Bronfenbrenner believed that human relationships and interactions could be best understood when they were viewed in context, and that the context could be viewed at various levels of organizational complexity.
3. The basic premises of ecologic theory are as follows:
   a. Systems are complex and interrelated.
   b. Everything is connected to everything else.
   c. Change is constant.
   d. Systems are dynamic.

B The ecologic model offers a method of examining stress that goes beyond the individual worker to the context in which the stress occurs.

1. This approach is consistent with the position that dealing with occupational stress requires a workplace approach.

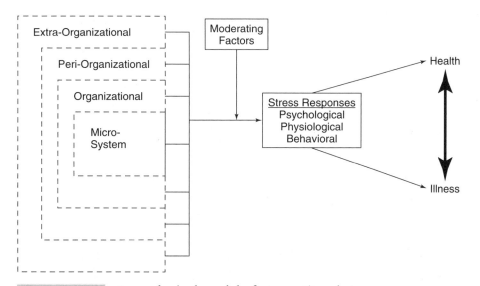

FIGURE 13-1 *An ecological model of occupational stress*
Salazar, 2000.

2. The model goes one step further, proposing that the broader context in which the organization is embedded may also influence the occurrence of stress in the workplace.

C **The ecologic model of occupational stress (Fig. 13-1) includes four nested levels of occupational stressors: the microsystems, the organizational system, the peri-organizational system, and the extra-organizational system (Salazar & Beaton, 2000).**

1. The *microsystem* consists of the environment immediately surrounding the worker or group of workers. It includes the physical features of the environment, the interactions that a worker experiences, and the activities that occur there.

2. The *organizational system* is made up of the multiple structures and functions that constitute a work organization. Examples of organizational structures are labor unions, the size of the organization, its physical arrangement, and of course, its service or product.

3. The *peri-organizational system* refers to the forces within the societal system in which the individual and organization are imbedded that have an immediate affect on the work organization. These include regional economic conditions, the political climate, prevailing social conditions, and the general health of the community that relate directly to the organization.

4. The *extra-organizational system* includes the cultures, societal norms, traditions, and government and economic policies that directly or indirectly affect workers. Direct effects are related to government policies, regulations, and standards.

D **Moderating factors serve as a means to ameliorate or intercept the effects of the identified stressors. They include the personal attributes, coping strategies, and social support systems of the worker.**

E **A multitude of physiologic, psychologic, and behavioral stress responses can result from the interaction of multiple stressors (Section IV).**

F **The health-illness continuum describes the outcomes that result from the interaction of the ecosystems, moderating factors, and stress responses.**

1. These outcomes can be positive (health) or negative (illness), or anywhere between.
   a. The "health" end of the continuum might be related to the sense of esteem and personal satisfaction that one derives from work.
   b. The "illness" end of the continuum includes ulcers, hypertension, angina, chronic headaches, cardiovascular diseases (e.g., myocardial infarction), and a multitude of mental health disorders.
2. Occupational and environmental health nurses are in a prime position to determine where workers are on the health-illness continuum; the ecologic model can then serve as a useful tool to identify and assess stress-related problems.

VIII Managing Psychosocial Factors in the Workplace

Managing occupational stress is a cyclic process; it includes multiple steps between identifying the sources of stress and evaluating the intervention.

A **Principles underlying programs**

1. There are two prevailing approaches to workplace stress: the worker approach and workplace approach.
   a. *Worker approach* includes stress management, EAPs, and counseling strategies that are designed to improve workers' ability to cope with their occupational stressors.
   b. In contrast to the worker approach, the organizational *workplace approach* is based on the principle of improving working conditions (and decreasing occupational stressor exposures) for all workers (Box 13-3).
      1) This approach addresses the root causes of identified stress in the workplace by designing strategies that reduce or eliminate identified stressors.
      2) As a result of years of research and experience, NIOSH favors this approach.
2. Comprehensive stress-prevention programs involve a combination of organizational change (workplace approaches) and individual stress management (worker approaches) to prevent or ameliorate job stress to create a healthier workplace.

B **Assessing psychosocial factors**

1. A first step in managing psychosocial factors in the workplace is to identify the job conditions that can lead to stress (Section III.C. provides a list of job conditions).
   a. The sources of occupational stress in a given workplace can be assessed using a variety of approaches, including interviews of the major stakeholders of a workplace organization, an employee survey, and observations at the workplace.
   b. Group discussions with management, labor representatives, and employees can provide valuable and rich information about the problem.
2. The second step in the management of psychosocial factors is to measure the stress reactions; both subjective and objective indices of occupational strain should be assessed.
   a. Subjective indices include self-reports of stress-related symptoms, job

---

BOX 13-3

Approaches to organizational change to prevent job stress

Workload
- Ensure that the workload is in line with the worker's capabilities and resources.
- Avoid underload as well as overload.
- Increase control over the pace of work.

Work Schedule
- Establish work schedules that are compatible with workers' demands and responsibilities outside the job.
- Use flextime, job sharing, or a compressed work week to allow flexibility.

Work Roles
- Clearly define workers' roles and responsibilities.
- Avoid conflicts related to expectations of workers.

Content
- Design jobs to provide meaning, stimulation, and opportunities for workers to use their skills.

- Rotate jobs to increase stimulation and challenge.

Participation/Control
- Give workers opportunities to participate in decisions and actions affecting their jobs.
- Develop strategies to encourage positive interpersonal relations with co-workers and supervisors.

Job Future
- Improve communications; reduce uncertainty about career development and future employment prospects.
- Keep workers informed about decisions that will affect their positions, including the potential for promotions and mechanisms for professional growth.

Social Environment
- Provide opportunities for social interaction among workers.

Source: Sauter, Murphy, & Hurrell, 1990.

---

satisfaction, and perceptions of workplace morale, including the following (Baker & Karasek, 1999):
1) Symptoms and motivations related to work conditions
2) Anxiety, depression, and other emotional reactions
3) Cognitive functioning and work performance
4) Behavioral changes such as sleep disturbances and substance abuse
5) Physiologic measures such as blood pressure monitoring, measuring the metabolites of catecholamines, and galvanic skin responses
6) Other symptoms or diseases that are related to stress
   b. Objective indices include turnover rates, health care costs, absenteeism, and rates of on-the-job injury.

C **Strategies for preventing and controlling adverse effects of psychosocial factors**
  1. Based on the assessment, the specific sources of occupational stress for a worker group and work organization can be targeted for organizational change.
    a. The identified source of stress can guide the intervention; for example,

upper extremity pain and dysfunction might require an ergonomic improvement.

   b. If the stress is related to organizational dysfunction (e.g., ineffective communication), managers and workers should be involved in the design of the intervention.

2. The levels of prevention can be applied to stress control strategies (Baker & Karasek, 1999).

   a. Primary prevention focuses on the reduction of job stressors; for example, making changes within the organization.

   b. Secondary prevention focuses on the development of strategies to deal with stressful conditions; for example, improving the workers' ability to cope with the stressors.

   c. Tertiary prevention focuses on programs that provide treatment and rehabilitation for stress-related conditions; it includes EAPs and counseling services.

3. Preparation for a stress prevention program should include the following (NIOSH, 1999):

   a. Building awareness about job stresses

   b. Securing top management commitment and support

   c. Involving employees in all phases of the program

   d. Obtaining the resources needed to develop an effective program

IX Evaluating Interventions Targeting Adverse Effects of Psychosocial Factors

A Evaluating strategies and programs

1. Because intervention research is relatively recent, published work describing the results of stress-reducing interventions is scant; evaluation is needed to document whether interventions are producing benefits.

2. Studies suggest that interventions that focus on the worker, such as stress management programs, have short-term benefits.

3. A combination of techniques (for example, both stress management programs and organizational interventions) are evidently more effective than a single technique.

4. Evaluations of interventions designed to prevent and control the adverse effect of psychosocial factors should include both short-term and longer-term measures.

B Evaluation serves to inform the occupational and environmental health nurse regarding needed changes in stress reduction programs.

1. Job stress prevention and control are continuous processes.

2. Evaluation serves to appropriately redirect the intervention strategy.

BIBLIOGRAPHY

Baker, D.B. & Karasek, R.A. (1999). "Stress." In B.S. Levy & D.H. Wegman, (Eds.) *Occupational health: Recognizing and preventing work-related disease and injury*, 4th ed. (pp. 419-436). Philadelphia: Lippincott Williams & Wilkins.

Beaton, R. & Murphy, S. (1993). Sources of occupational stress among fire fighters/EMTs and fire fighter/paramedics and correlations with job-related outcomes. *Prehospital and Disaster Medicine, 8,* 140-150.

Beaton, R. (1996). Work related anxiety. In International Labour Office (Ed.), *ILO Encyclopedia of Occupational Health and Safety*, 4th ed. (pp. 5.11-5.22). Geneva, Switzerland: ILO.

Beaton, R., Murphy, S., Pike, K., & Corneil, W. (1997). Social support & network conflict in firefighters and paramedics. *Western Journal of Nursing Research, 19*, 297-313.

Boxer, P. & Wild, D. (1993). Psychological distress and alcohol use among fire fighters. *Scandinavian Journal of Environmental Health, 19*, 121-125.

Bronfenbrenner, U. (1977). Toward and experimental ecology in human development. *American Psychologist, 32(7)*, 513-531.

Cohen, S., Frank, E., Doyle, W., Skoner, D., Rabin, B., & Gwaltney, J. (1998). Types of stressors that increase susceptibility to the common cold in healthy adults. *Health Psychology, 17*, 214-223.

Elisburg, D. (1995). Workplace stress: legal developments, economic pressures, and violence. In J.F. Burton (Ed.), *1995 Workers' Compensation Year Book* (pp. 1217-1222). Horsham, PA: LRP Publications.

Ferrie, J.E., Shipley, M.J., Marmot, M.G., Stansfield, S.A., & Smith, G.D. (1998). An uncertain future: The effects of threats to employment security in white-collar men and women. *American Journal of Public Health. 88(7)*, 1030-1036.

French, J.R., Caplan, R.D., Van Harrison, R. (1982). *The mechanisms of job stress and strain.* Chichester, United Kingdom: John Wiley & Sons.

Freudenheim, M. (1987, May 26). Business and Health. *New York Times.*

Hawley, A.H., (1950). *Human Ecology: A theory of community structure.* New York: Plume Press.

Hurrell, J.J. & McLaney, M.A. (1988). Exposure to job stress—a new psychometric instrument. *Scandinavian Journal of Environmental Health (14):suppl 1*, 27-28.

Jeffress, C. (1998). Protecting the lives of working Americans. Speech to The Engineering and Safety Service of the American Insurance Services Group. San Antonio, TX.

Kahn, R.L. & Boulding, E. (1964). *Power and conflict in organizations.* New York: Basic Books, Inc.

Karasek, R.A., Theorell, T., Schwartz, J.E., Schnall, P.L., Pieper, C.F., & Michela, J.L. (1988). Job characteristics in relation to the prevalence of myocardial infarction. *American Journal of Public Health, 78*, 910-918.

Karasek, R. & Theorell, T. (1990*). Healthy work: stress, productivity, and the reconstruction of working life.* New York: Basic Books, a division of Harper Collins Publishers.

Kendall, N.A. (1999). Psychosocial approaches to the prevention of chronic pain: the low back paradigm. *Baillieres Best Practice Research in Clinical Rheumatology. 13(3)*, 545-554.

Kessler, R.C., Barber, C., Birnbaum, H.G., Frank, R.G., Greenberg, P.E., Rose, R.M., Simon, G.E., & Wang, P. (1999). Depression in the workplace: effects on short-term disability. *Health Affairs, 18(5)*, 163-71.

Levenstein, C., Wooding, J., & Rosenberg, B. (1999). Occupational health: A social perspective. In B.S. Levy & D.H. Wegman, (Eds.) *Occupational health: Recognizing and preventing work-related disease and injury*, 4th ed. (pp. 27-50). Philadelphia: Lippincott Williams & Wilkins.

Levy, B.S. & Wegman, D.H. (1999). *Occupational health: Recognizing and preventing work-related disease and injury*, 4th ed. Philadelphia: Lippincott Williams & Wilkins.

Lowman, R. (1993). *Counseling and psychotherapy of work dysfunctions.* Washington, D.C.: APA Press.

MacCallum, R. & Glaser, R. (1998). Psychological influences on surgical recovery: Perspective from psychoneuroimmunology. *American Psychologist, 53*, 1209-1218.

MacLennan, B.W. (1992) Stressor reduction: An organizational alternative to individual stress management. In J.C. Quick, L.R. Murphy, & J.J. Hurrell (Eds.) *Stress & well-being at work.* Washington DC: American Psychological Association.

Maslach, C. (1993). Burnout: A multidimensional perspective. In W.B. Schaufeli, C.C. Maslach, & T. Marek (Eds.) *Professional burnout: recent developments in theory and research.* New York: Taylor & Francis.

McAbee, R. (1991). Occupational stress and burnout in the nursing profession: A model of prevention. *AAOHN Journal, 39(12)*, 568-575.

Moore, S.Y. (1999). The effect of layoff threat and personal mastery on work performance over a three year period. Paper presented at APSA/NIOSH conference, Washington, DC.

Morin, C., Culbert, J., & Schwartz, S. (1994). Nonpharmacological interventions for insomnia: A meta-analysis of treatment efficacy. *American Journal of Psychiatry, 151(8)*, 1172-1180.

National Institutes of Health. (1988) *Proposed national strategies for the prevention of leading work-related diseases and injuries*, Part 2. Cincinnati, OH: U.S. Department of Health and Human Services.

National Institutes of Health. (1995). Integration of behavioral and relaxation approaches into the treatment of chronic pain and insomnia, *NIH Technology Assessment Conference Statement, October 16-18*, 1-34. Bethesda, MD: NIH.

National Institute for Occupational Safety and Health (1996). *Violence in the workplace: Risk factors and prevention strategies*. Cincinnati, OH: U.S. Department of Health and Human Services.

National Institutes for Occupational Safety and Health. (1997). *Plain language about shiftwork*. Cincinnati, OH: U.S. Department of Health and Human Services.

National Institutes for Occupational Safety and Health. (1999). *Stress . . . at work*. Cincinnati, OH: U.S. Department of Health and Human Services.

Noer, D. (1993). *Healing wounds: Overcoming trauma of layoffs and revitalizing downsized organizations*. San Francisco: Jossey-Bass Publishers.

Occupational Health and Safety Administration. (1999). OSHA Workplace violence summary sheet. http://www.osha.gov/oshinfo/priorities/violence.html

Oldham, G.R. & Gordon, B.I. (1999). Job complexity and employee substance use: the moderating effects of cognitive ability. *Journal of Health and Social Behavior, 40(3)*, 290-306.

Salazar, M.K. & Beaton, R. (2000). Ecological model of occupational stress: Application to urban firefighters. *AAOHN Journal, 48(10)*, 470-479.

Salazar, M.K. & Graham, K.Y. (1999). Evaluation of a case management program: Summary and integration of findings. *AAOHN Journal, 47(9)*, 416-423.

Sauter, S.L., Murphy, L., & Hurrell, J.J. Jr. (1990). Prevention of work-related psychological disorders. *American Psychologist, 45(10)*, 1146-1158.

Sears, S., Urizar, D., & Evans, G. (2000). Examining a stress-coping model of burnout and depression in extension agents. *Journal of Occupational Health Psychology, 5*, 56-62.

Selye, H. (1974). Stress and distress. *Comprehensive Therapeutics, 1(8)*, 9-13.

Spratlen, L.P (1994). Perceived workplace mistreatment in higher education: characteristics and consequences. *AAOHN Journal 42(11)*, 548-54.

Standen, P., Daniels, K., & Lamond, D. (1999). The home is a workplace: Work-family interaction and psychological well-being in telework. *Journal of Occupational Health Psychology, 4(4)*, 368-381.

Stiles, D. (1994). Video display terminal operators: Technology's biophysical stressors. *AAOHN Journal, 42(11)*, 541-547.

U.S. Department of Labor (1998). Dealing with workplace violence: A guide for agency planners. http://www.opm.gov/ehg/workplace/index.htm

Williams, J. (1996). Stress, coping resources and injury risk. *International Journal of Stress Management, 3*, 209-221.

14

Examples of Occupational Health and Safety Programs

Janet deCarteret, Marilyn Hau, and Michelle Kom Gochnour

This chapter describes selected examples of occupational health and safety programs that can be used as models in a variety of work settings. Some of these programs are mandated by law (e.g., hearing loss prevention program, hazard communication, drug and alcohol testing); others may be of interest or importance to specific industries or businesses (international travel health and safety, emergency preparedness/disaster plan, ergonomic programs) The basic template that was used to describe these programs can be applied to most any kind of work-site program.

International travel health and safety program

As the world economy becomes more global, an increasing number of companies are conducting a portion of their business in foreign countries. International business travelers may be exposed to illnesses or threats to personal safety during travel to foreign countries. The travel health and safety program described in this section provides guidelines that can be used by the occupational and environmental health nurse to reduce the risk to the personal health and safety of the traveler.

I Purposes of an International Travel Health and Safety Program

A Prepare workers for travel

B Provide recommendations

C Ensure fitness for work

D Prevent illness and injury

E Provide appropriate vaccinations

F Ensure, to the greatest extent possible, the personal safety of the travelers

II Employer's Responsibilities to Traveling Employees

A Develop travel policies and procedures, including emergency evacuation or escape protocols.

B Allocate sufficient resources for the program.

C Provide appropriate travel agency services and travelers' assistance program vendors.

D Provide health and safety information appropriate to the traveler's destination.

E Request security information from destination hotels or other accommodations (dead bolts and view holes on doors, fire safety, 24-hour security, safety-deposit boxes, etc.).

F Provide the medications, supplies, vaccinations, and counseling necessary for the traveler's health and safety.

G Identify resources at the traveler's destination for health or safety emergencies.

H Communicate the program to employees before it is implemented.

III Occupational and Environmental Health Nurse's Responsibilities

A Obtain a health history.
1. Determine significant illnesses, injuries, or current health problems.
2. Identify health risks that may compromise travel plans, such as diabetes or heart disease.
3. List any scars or permanent identifying marks on the worker's body in case identity of the traveler needs to be confirmed.
4. Review any health problems encountered related to previous travel.
5. List all current medications (prescription and nonprescription).
6. Review current health and dental status and provide appropriate interventions or referrals.
7. List all allergies (medications, food, plants, insects, vaccines, etc.).

B Determine and provide appropriate immunizations.
1. Review employee's immunization status.
2. Determine which vaccines are required or recommended for the traveler's destination.
3. Provide appropriate vaccines or resources to obtain those vaccines.
4. Report adverse vaccine reactions to the local health authorities.

C Conduct a physical examination and, if appropriate, determine any health risks before making the travel assignment.

D Test for the human immunodeficiency virus if required for entry, identify blood type, and perform chest x-ray if traveler will be living abroad.

E Review special considerations for the traveler, such as pregnancy or recent surgery.

F Refer the worker for treatment of travel-related problems and follow up on recommendations.

IV Traveler's Responsibilities

A Maintain a current passport and obtain visa and other necessary documents.

B Ensure that adequate time is available for administration of vaccines before departure, usually 4 to 6 weeks.

C Prepare a travel itinerary and leave a copy with family and office staff.

D Confirm travel arrangements (tickets, hotel accommodations, car rental, etc.)

E Review and follow all safety procedures recommended in the travel policy and procedure manual.

F Prepare a list of phone numbers where the traveler can be contacted and names of people whom the traveler can contact in case of an emergency.

V Health and Safety Education for Travel

A Issues related to the safety of the traveler

1. Because business travelers usually travel alone, discuss personal safety, such as avoiding drawing attention to oneself as a "business traveler"; advise traveling in casual attire and being alert to surrounding activities.
2. Provide current information on the political and social climate of the traveler's destination, such as risk of terrorism, kidnapping, theft, and crime.
3. Encourage the use of travelers' checks or bank cards instead of carrying large sums of currency.
4. Discuss methods to reduce risk of theft of important documents and personal property.
5. Review the traveler's itinerary
   a. Length of stay at each destination
   b. Type of work to be performed (office versus field work)
   c. Specific hazards associated with the work to be done
   d. Type of accommodations (housing, utilities, services)

B Business travel and stress

1. Business travel differs from tourism; the following factors may add to the stress of business travelers:
   a. Job performance requirements
   b. Tight schedules
   c. Sudden departures
   d. Separation from family and home
   e. Fear of the potential for kidnapping and terrorism
2. Considerations that may be appropriate for short-term assignments
   a. Discuss living accommodations and schedules.
   b. Help the traveler understand the culture of the destination country and how to dress appropriately.
   c. Provide the traveler with resources for health care or emergency situations.
   d. Provide information on safe driving in destination country.
3. Considerations that may be appropriate for long term assignments include loneliness, job demands, living in hotels, and traveling alone.
   a. Offer training and country-specific culture programs to those preparing to work abroad.
   b. Provide a copy of the appropriate evacuation procedure and be clear about instructions.
   c. Identify resources for health or psychological concerns for the traveler (e.g., an employee assistance counselor, if available, or insurance for health care).
   d. If the traveler's family will also be living abroad, provide information on

housing accommodations, the lifestyle and culture of the destination country, and schooling options for dependents.

C **Issues related to the health of the traveler**

1. In many countries, illnesses such as "traveler's diarrhea" can be caused by food or water contaminated with bacteria, viruses, or parasites; the following high-risk foods should be avoided:
   a. Undercooked meat, poultry, or seafood, which may contain harmful organisms
   b. Raw fruits or vegetables, which may contain harmful bacteria if not thoroughly washed with a chlorine solution
   c. Tap water (including ice made from tap water), which may be unchlorinated and contaminated with fecal material
   d. Unpasteurized dairy products, which may contain organisms such as the salmonella bacteria
2. Prevention of illness may be further enhanced by the following recommendations:
   a. Give hepatitis A vaccine (for high endemic areas).
   b. Drink bottled water, purify water through boiling for at least 10 minutes, or use water-purification tablets as recommended.
   c. Follow the basic principles for safe handling of foods.
   d. Follow the basic principles of good hygienic practice.
3. Management of traveler's illnesses may include the following:
   a. Oral rehydrating fluids (electrolyte solutions) for diarrhea
   b. Prophylactic antibiotics to prevent certain bacteria-caused illnesses
   c. Good hygienic practices to avoid reinfection (e.g., proper disposal of contaminated items, thorough hand washing)
4. Assemble an appropriate medical emergency kit (Box 14-1).

VI Control of Prevalent Communicable Diseases

A Malaria is a febrile illness caused by the blood parasite plasmodium, of which there are four species (*P. Falciparum* is the species with the greatest potential to kill and is the most important to prevent [Wolfe, 1993]).

1. Symptoms
   a. May include fever, chills, muscle aches, and headache
   b. Will occasionally include vomiting, diarrhea, and coughing
2. Risk
   a. Because malaria is spread by mosquitoes, the risk is greatest in areas where mosquito activity is high.
   b. The highest rate of mosquito activity occurs in Africa, where mosquitoes carry the malaria parasite.
   c. Mosquito activity is highest at night, especially just after dusk.
   d. The risk increases during rainy and hot seasons.
3. Prevention
   a. Use antimosquito measures, such as repellents (permethrin), long-sleeved clothing, long pants, and mosquito netting.
   b. Sleep in screened or air-conditioned rooms if possible.
4. Control
   a. Antimalarial medications (chemoprophylaxis) include mefloquine, doxycycline, and chloroquine.
   b. There is currently no vaccine against malaria.

BOX 14-1

Traveler's medical kit recommendations

- **Essential Items**
An adequate supply of medications for health conditions specific to the traveler
Additional prescriptions (with generic name) as determined by physician
Copies of medical and eyeglasses prescriptions
- **Nonprescription Items**
Analgesic (aspirin, acetaminophen, ibuprofen)
Antibiotic skin ointment (Bacitracin, Betadine, Mycitracin)
Antiseptic (providone iodine)
Anticonstipation (many brands of laxatives are available)
Antidiarrheal (lopermide [Immodium AD], bismuth subsalicylate [Pepto Bismol])
Anti-motion sickness (meclizine [Bonine], dimenhydrinate [Dramamine])

Antihistamines (diphenhydramine [Benadryl])
Adhesive bandages (Band-Aids, Curad)
Antacids (Tums, Rolaids, Maalox)
Oral rehydrating salts (available at sporting goods stores)
Disposable thermometers (Fever Scan)
Water purification tablets
- **Prescription Items**
Altitude sickness prophylactics (acetazolamide [Diamox])
Antibiotics (oral doxycycline, ciprofloxacin, or erythromycin)
Antimalarials (mefloquine, choloquine, or doxycycline)
Sleeping medications (Halcion, Restoril)
- **Additional Medical Supplies**
Disposable syringes and needles
Latex gloves
Skin closures (Steri-Strips)
Suture removal kit

---

5. Treatment
   a. Medications such as sulfadoxine-pyrimethamine (Fansidar) and halofantrine (Halfan) may be taken as self-treatment if fever or flulike symptoms occur.
   b. Self-treatment is only a temporary measure, and prompt health evaluation is imperative.

B Sexually transmitted diseases (STDs): Individuals traveling abroad may be at risk for contracting STDs if they engage in sex while abroad; thus the health care provider must include education specific to STDs.
   1. Individuals assigned to long-term assignments abroad are more likely to engage in casual sex than are short-term travelers.
   2. Discuss the risk of engaging in casual sex abroad.
   3. Encourage the use of condoms and other safe sex practices.
   4. Warn about the effects of alcohol and drugs, which may contribute to careless sexual behavior.

C Discuss cultural attitudes concerning prostitution in the traveler's destination country.
   Note: Table 14-1 provides information regarding other selected physiologic health hazards.

TABLE 14-1

Selected physiological health hazards

Jet lag: Jet lag is the disruption of the traveler's sleep–wake cycle. It usually occurs when traveling over two or more time zones

Symptoms	Prevention
Insomnia	Adjust sleep schedule
Fatigue	Drink extra fluids (preferably water)
Poor concentration	Reduce coffee and alcohol consumption
Irritability	Exposure to light may help in resetting circadian rhythm
Headache	
Myalgia	

Altitude sickness: Altitude sickness is a cluster of symptoms caused by lack of oxygen. The symptoms may include headache, shortness of breath, lightheadedness, fatigue, insomnia, loss of appetite, and nausea. It can be life threatening.

Risk factors	Prevention	Treatment
Ascent over 6000 feet	High carbohydrate diet	Descent and rest
Rapid ascent without acclimation	Extra fluid intake	Aspirin or acetaminophen
Obesity	Reduce strenuous activity	
Strenuous activity at high altitudes	Slow, gradual descent	Diamox
Use of sleeping pills or sedatives	Acetazolamide (250 mg every 8 hours for 3-5 days before ascent	
Previous history of altitude sickness		

VII Post-Travel Evaluation for Long-Term Travelers

This type of evaluation is usually not necessary for short-term travelers; however, it should be performed when indicated.

A **Provide immediate evaluation for signs or symptoms of illness.**

B **Perform the following post-travel assessment:**
1. History and physical examination, including the following:
   a. Urinalysis
   b. Stool for ova and parasites if returning from high-risk area
   c. Tuberculosis skin test
2. Post-travel debriefing
   a. Discussion of problems encountered during travel/stay
   b. Recommendations for future travelers

C **Obtain worker's feedback to assist in the evaluation of the international health and safety program.**
1. Use this information to analyze the program's effectiveness and efficiency.
   a. Analyze the cost/benefit ratio of the program's elements.
   b. Evaluate the *overall* effectiveness and cost of program.
2. Make revisions as appropriate based on this information.

Hearing-loss prevention program

The passage of the Hearing Conservation Amendment to the OSH Act in 1983 provided the thrust for the development of hearing-loss prevention programs in industry. Hearing-loss prevention programs can be conducted either within the work site or contracted to a certified audiology testing service. It is recommended, and in some cases required by law, that individuals performing as audiometric technicians become certified through the Council for Accreditation in Occupational Hearing Conservation. The program outlined in this section can serve as a guide to developing a hearing-loss prevention program. It is advised that the program coordinator review and follow requirements established by OSHA or by states with OSHA-approved state plans.

VIII Noise-Induced Hearing Loss

Noise-induced hearing loss caused by occupational exposure has been a compensable occupational disease since the 1950s.

A 5.5 million American workers are exposed to noise levels of 85 dB and above (U.S. Department of Labor, 1992).

B 9 million American workers are exposed above these levels when all noisy jobs, including military, mining, construction, and transportation, are included in the data.

C Estimates suggest that 1 million workers in the manufacturing industry alone have sustained job-related hearing loss (Suter, 1993).

IX Purposes of a Hearing-Loss Prevention Program

A Prevent noise-induced hearing loss

B Reduce worker exposure to harmful noise

C Identify the progression of hearing loss so preventive measures can be taken

D Identify temporary hearing loss before it becomes permanent

E Comply with federal regulations or OSHA-approved state plans (OSHA Noise Standard CFR 1910.95) (Table 14-2)
   1. OSHA regulations limit work-site noise exposure to 90 dBA time-weighted average (TWA) over an 8-hour work shift. Hearing-loss prevention programs and hearing protection devices (HPDs) are mandatory, as are engineering controls.
   2. Hearing-loss prevention programs (HLPPs) are mandatory in an environment where the daily noise level equals or exceeds 85 dBA over an 8-hour, time-weighted average (TWA); appropriate HPDs are to be provided. (Table 14-2 suggests policies regarding HLLPs based on time-weighted averages.)

F The rationale for and benefits of a work-site HLPP
   1. Better labor-management relations
   2. Decreased likelihood of antisocial behaviors resulting from annoyance
   3. Greater job satisfaction, increased productivity, and better quality of life resulting from reducing noise in the workplace

TABLE 14-2

Developing a hearing conservation program: suggested policies based on time-weighted average ranges

TWA in dB(A)	Workers included in the HCP	HPD utilization	HPD selection options
84 or below	no	voluntary	free choice
85-89	yes	optional*	free choice
90-94	yes	required	free choice
95-99	yes	required	limited choice
100 or above	yes	required	very limited choice

Royster & Royster, 1990. Reprinted with permission from CRC press.

*Use of a hearing protective device (HPD) will be required for any worker who shows a significant hearing change, or of all workers if audiometric database analysis results or group hearing trends indicate inadequate protection.

4. Improved worker efficiency and job performance
5. Reduced accident rates, illnesses, and lost work time
6. Reduced risk of workers' compensation claims
7. Reduced loss of trained and experienced personnel

X Management's Role in an HLPP

A Develop an HLPP policy, including disciplinary action for noncompliance.

B Identify program personnel and define their responsibilities.
   1. Provide a qualified physician, an otolaryngologist, or an audiologist to supervise the program.
   2. Identify the program coordinator and other personnel responsible for the program's components; all participants should be enthusiastic and committed to the HLPP.

C Provide personnel, space, supplies, and funding for the program.

D Provide all elements of the program to workers free of charge.

E Make a good-faith effort to eliminate or reduce sources of noise and to reevaluate the noise level when there are changes in exposure.

F Post appropriate warning signs and ear-protection requirements at entrances to areas with noise levels exceeding 85 dBA.

G Conduct periodic evaluations to ensure the quality and effectiveness of the program.

XI The Role of the Hearing-Loss Prevention Coordinator

The responsibilities of the hearing-loss prevention coordinator may include the following:

A Perform an otoscopic examination and audiometric testing (the coordinator may want to seek in-service training from an occupational audiologist).

B Coordinate the testing schedules and follow-up procedures.

C Keep accurate, clear, and complete testing and counseling records.

D Select, fit, and monitor the wearing of appropriate hearing-protection devices.

E Act as liaison between workers and other members of the team.

F Take a health or aural history on each worker participating in the program.

G Educate and train workers on how to protect themselves from hearing loss.

H Refer workers to appropriate sources for further testing or medical treatment when indicated.

XII The Role of Workers

A Each worker is responsible for complying with the program by wearing appropriate hearing protection.

B It is the responsibility of workers, especially supervisors, to encourage co-workers to wear hearing protection devices.

C Workers should immediately report changes in noise levels on the work floor to their supervisors, safety personnel, or other responsible individuals.

XIII Program Requirements

A successful program requires the following:

A The support, cooperation, and participation of all levels of management

B Support of workers, because they are the most knowledgeable about the work environment

C Cooperation of union leaders, where applicable, and the person responsible for work-site safety

D Review of the OSHA standard (29 CFR 1910.95) or the OSHA-approved state plan, where applicable

XIV Noise Assessment and Control

A If reliable information indicates noise exposure in the work site, conduct noise measurements (to be performed by an acoustical engineer, industrial hygienist, occupational audiologist, or a professional proficient in noise-level measurement); include all continuous, intermittent, and impulse noise within an 80-dB(A) to 130-dB(A) range taken during a typical work situation.
   1. Use only sound-level meters or noise dosimeters that meet the American National Standards Institute (ANSI) specifications (Type II instruments).
   2. Use a sampling strategy that will pick up all continuous, intermittent, and impulse sound levels from 80 to 130 dBA, and include all those sound levels in the total noise measurement.
   3. Permit workers and/or their representatives to observe monitoring.
   4. Notify workers of noise exposure at or above an 8-hour TWA of 85 dBA.

B Purpose and use of sound-survey results
   1. Identify areas of the work site where hazardous noise levels exist.
   2. Identify workers to be included in the HLPP.
   3. Classify workers' noise exposures to define policies for hearing protection devices and prioritize areas for noise-control efforts.

4. Identify safety hazards in terms of interference with speech communication and warning-signal detection.
5. Evaluate noise source for noise-control purposes.
6. Document noise levels for legal purposes.

C Noise-control measures

1. Engineering controls are the most effective and the most desirable long-term solutions and may include any of the following:
   a. Eliminate the source of noise.
   b. Redesign the process to be quieter.
   c. Isolate machinery to prevent vibrations and noise from radiating.
   d. Build an enclosure around noisy machinery.
   e. Use absorptive material on walls and ceilings.
   f. Erect a barrier or noise-reducing curtain around the noisy area.
   g. Add a muffler to noisy tools.
   h. Keep machinery well balanced, oiled, and in good repair.
2. Recommendations related to work practices that will decrease the risk of noise hazards should be developed.
3. Administrative controls are implemented when engineering and work-practice controls are not feasible.
   a. Rotate workers to less noisy areas.
   b. Perform high-noise tasks when fewer workers are present.
4. Personal protective equipment is provided when engineering and administrative controls are not feasible.
   a. Provide appropriate hearing protection devices (ear plugs, muffs, helmets).
   b. Provide a selection of appropriate styles and types at no cost to workers.

XV Worker Training and Education

A Conduct the program initially for new hires and annually for workers who are included in the HLPP.

B Describe the characteristics of sound (complex combination of pure tones found in the environment that result in a vibratory disturbance in the pressure of fluid in the ear and capable of being detected by the organs of hearing).

C Explain where noise is found.

1. Cite occupational, recreational, and environmental sources (Table 14-3), including cumulative effects from multiple sources.
2. Provide examples of different types of noise from actual locations at the work site (where most noise exposure occurs).

D Describe the effects of noise (in addition to hearing loss).

1. Physical problems include effects on the cardiovascular and gastrointestinal systems, headache, stress, and fatigue.
2. Psychologic problems include annoyance, feeling of isolation among workers, masking of warning shouts and signals, and interference with speech communication.

E Provide overview of signs and symptoms of hearing loss.

1. Tinnitus (ringing in the ear) is a sign of an overtaxed auditory system.
2. Awareness of hearing loss usually does not occur until the loss is significant.

TABLE 14-3

Some commonly encountered noise levels

Source	dB(A) level	Effect
Jet plane	140	Acoustic trauma: May cause
Gunshot blast (impulse)	140 (pain threshold)	permanent damage to the
Automobile horn	120	delicate hair cells of the cochlea
Rock band	110	Noise-induced hearing loss:
Chain saw	110	Long exposure over 90
Car racing	110	dB(A) may eventually cause
Motorcycle	100	permanent hearing loss
Subway	90	
Average factory	80-90	
Noisy restaurant	80	Usually will not cause
Busy traffic	75	permanent hearing loss
Conversational speech	65	
Average home	50	
Quiet office	40	
Soft whisper	30	

Sources: Environmental Protection Agency, 1978; Royster & Royster, 1990.

3. Perception that others are "mumbling" is often a sign of hearing loss.
4. Occupational hearing loss is usually bilateral; hearing loss in only one ear may be caused by pathological processes other than occupational exposures or acoustic trauma to that ear.

F **Explain anatomy and physiology of the outer, middle, and inner ear; a diagram or model of the parts of the ear will be helpful (Fig. 14-1).**
1. Outer ear: collects sound waves and funnels them into the ear canal.
2. Middle ear: sound impinges on ear drum and is transmitted mechanically to the bones of the middle ear (hammer, anvil, and stirrup) and transmitted to the fluid-filled cochlea in the inner ear. The hammer, anvil, and stirrup are also known as the malleus, incus, and stapes, respectively.
3. Inner ear: transmits sound waves through hair cells in the cochlea that send electrical impulses to the auditory nerve, which transmits the signals to the brain where the sound is interpreted.

G **Explain types of hearing loss.**
1. Hearing loss from acoustic trauma
   a. Results from a single exposure such as a loud, explosive blast or a blow to the head
   b. May rupture the eardrum and damage the middle and inner ear
2. Sensorineural hearing loss
   a. Results in changes in the receptive cells; occurs from long-term exposure to noise
   b. Is usually bilateral
   c. Is not usually apparent until hearing loss is severe
   d. Can be caused by trauma, use of certain ototoxic drugs, aging, disease, or heredity
   e. Is usually irreversible, its severity depending on the intensity, frequency, and duration of noise exposure

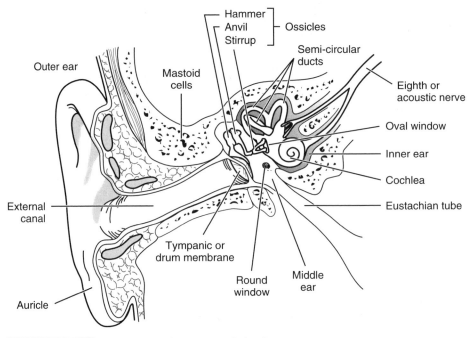

FIGURE 14-1 *Sectional diagram of the human ear*

Courtesy The Sonotone Corporation, Boca Raton, Florida.

3. Conductive hearing loss
   a. Occurs from obstruction of sound through the outer and inner ear
   b. May be caused by wax buildup, presence of a foreign body, ruptured eardrum, infection, otosclerosis, or injury
   c. May be (in most instances) reversed or stabilized by appropriate treatment or surgery

XVI Hearing Protection Devices (HPDs)

A Provide HPDs at no cost, or more-expensive devices at minimal cost, for workers to use when engaged in noisy activities outside the workplace.

1. Ear plugs (aural inserts): formable or molded, made of soft material (many types and styles are available)
   a. Advantages: small, inexpensive, easy to use, comfortable, can be worn for long periods
   b. Disadvantages: need to be kept clean, may become contaminated with dirt and grime, may cause allergic reaction in some individuals, may produce wax buildup, are difficult to monitor at a distance
2. Ear muffs (circumaurals): plastic-foam–filled cuffs that fit snugly against the head and are attached to an adjustable headband
   a. Advantages: easy to fit and easy to monitor from a distance
   b. Disadvantages: expensive, large, and bulky; may be difficult to use with hard hats or respiratory equipment; and may become loose with head movement
3. Canal caps (semiaurals): ear-plug–like tips connected by a lightweight headband
   a. Advantages: suitable for short-duration and off-and-on wearing

  b. Disadvantages: uncomfortable if worn for long periods; not suitable for areas where the noise level is high

 4. Custom-fitted ear plugs: molded to ear, solid or filtered, that allow speech to enter but reduce harmful noise.

  a. Advantages: suitable for very small or hard-to-fit ear canals; can be filtered for special needs.

  b. Disadvantages: the material may shrink; the fit may change if worker gains or loses weight.

B The *noise reduction rating* **(NRR): Hearing-protective devices by law must contain a number that reflects the amount of noise that will be reduced by their use. The formula that is used in the workplace is to subtract the NRR number from the dB level of noise exposure.**

 1. The NRR is determined in laboratories with selected subjects and may not reflect real work situations. OSHA adjusts the NRR by 50% (e.g., 30 dB NRR = 15 dB in the real workplace).

 2. OSHA indicates a dB(C) scale is used in NRR and needs to be corrected to dB(A) by subtracting 7 from the NRR [noise level in dB(A) – [NRR – 7] = estimated exposure in dB(A)]

C Evaluate workers' perceptions and motivations related to the use of HPDs.

 1. Identify barriers to compliance with recommendations.

 2. Develop strategies to address concerns of workers related to the use of HPDs.

D Fitting of HPDs

 1. Offer several style and varying sizes.

 2. Evaluate workers to determine the types of hearing protection best suited to each worker's anatomy and job situation.

 3. Instruct workers on proper placement, limitations, and care of HPDs.

 4. Follow the manufacturers' directions.

XVII Audiometric Testing

A Purpose and procedure

 1. Testing is performed to determine baseline hearing and to monitor the effects of noise exposure.

 2. The test is implemented under the direction and supervision of an audiologist, otolaryngologist, or qualified physician.

 3. Both the test environment and the audiometer must meet criteria set by the American National Standards Institute.

  a. Audiometric testing shall consist of pure-tone, hearing threshold measures at no less than 500, 1000, 2000, 3000, 4000, and 6000 hertz (Hz)

  b. Right and left ears shall be individually tested.

  c. The 8000-Hz threshold should also be tested as an option and as a useful source of information about the etiology of a hearing loss.

 4. The test must be performed by a licensed or certified audiologist, otolaryngologist, or physician; or by a technician who is certified by the Council for Accreditation in Occupational Hearing Conservation.

  a. A worker's baseline audiogram is performed at least 14 hours after noise exposure, or at the time of hire for job placement, or when a worker is transferred from a non-noisy to a noisy work site.

  b. The baseline audiogram is used as a reference against which future audiograms are compared.

  c. An annual (or periodic) audiogram may be performed well into the work shift to provide information on the effectiveness of noise-control measures; it must be taken within one year of the baseline test.

d. An exit, or termination, audiogram is performed when work-site noise exposure ceases; it is not an OSHA requirement, but it may be important in determining the extent of employer liability for workers' compensation determination.

B **Duties of the audiometric technician may include the following:**
1. Calibrating the audiometer at least daily by testing the same individual with stable hearing
2. Taking a health history and noise-exposure history
   a. Performing a visual and otoscopic examination of the ears
   b. Explaining the purpose of the test
   c. Administering a pure-tone audiometric test
   d. Providing immediate feedback and counseling

C **Audiometric evaluation**
1. Normal hearing, in general, falls within hearing threshold levels between 0 and 25 dB; it may vary slightly from left to right ear and may be age dependent (Fig. 14-2).
2. A *standard threshold shift* (STS) (also referred to as *significant threshold shift*) is an average shift in either ear of 10 dB or more at 2000, 3000, and 4000 Hz compared with the baseline audiogram.
   a. An STS may require referral to an audiologist, an otolaryngologist, or a qualified physician.
   b. Depending upon program supervisor protocol, an exposed worker whose test reveals an STS may be retested within 30 days of the annual test before referral.
   c. Workers must be notified in writing within 21 days of determination of the STS.

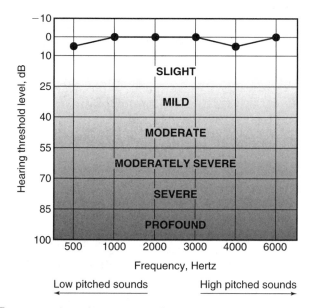

FIGURE 14-2 *Normal audiogram and degrees of hearing loss*

Royster & Royster, 1990. Reprinted with permission from CRC Press.

3. A *temporary threshold shift* (TTS) occurs shortly after exposure and improves gradually if the noise has not been too loud or the exposure too long.
   a. The greatest recovery takes place in 1 to 24 hours if the worker is removed from exposure.
   b. When a TTS occurs, the adequacy of the HPD should be checked.
4. A *permanent threshold shift* occurs when hearing loss persists after removal from exposure; it is associated with damage to the delicate sensory hair cells in the inner ear. If there is no improvement within one week, the loss is usually permanent.

D Criteria for referral to audiologist, otolaryngologist, or a qualified physician
   1. When an infection in the ear is suspected
   2. When hearing loss is unilateral
   3. When the worker complains of pain in the ear
   4. When an STS is evident
   5. Other criteria, as determined by a supervising audiologist or physician

XVIII Recordkeeping

A Audiometric test records must include the worker's name, identification number, duties performed at job location, type of hearing protection worn, date of the test, the examiner's name, date of the last audiometer calibration, and the worker's most recent noise exposure assessment. It is also advisable to document any worker counseling.

B In accordance with 29CFR 1910.20(d), medical monitoring records (audiometric records) shall be retained for at least the duration of the affected employee's employment plus 30 years.

C Noise exposure monitoring records shall be retained for 30 years.

D Background-noise measurements of the room where work is performed should be recorded and maintained.

E Audiometric and noise-exposure records should be accessible upon request to workers, former workers, worker-designated representatives, and others as required by law.

F If the employer ceases to do business, all records must be transferred to the successor employer and kept in accordance with the law.

XIX Program Evaluation

A Assess the completeness and quality of the program components.

B Compare annual audiograms with baseline for individuals and groups to determine the success of control measures; identify areas where further controls are needed.

C Develop a checklist specific to the work environment to ensure that all components of the program are being followed and comply with the appropriate standards.

Hazard communication program

The *hazard communication standard* was promulgated by OSHA in 1983 as a means of reducing risks related to chemical exposure in the American work force. The following *hazard communication program* is provided as a guide to assist in compliance with this standard. Some of the suggested elements may not be required but are included as recommendations to ensure a successful program. It is important that each program coordinator review the standards applicable to his or her jurisdiction. Because no single written program will work for all work sites, programs should be tailored to comply with the law and to protect workers against exposures specific to their work settings.

XX Purposes of a Hazard Communications Program

A Ensure that the hazards of all chemicals produced or imported into the workplace are evaluated and that information concerning these hazards is transmitted to employers and workers.

B Prevent illness, injury, or death from exposure to hazardous chemicals and substances in the workplace.

C Comply with OSHA's Hazard Communication Standard (HCS) 29 CFR 1910.12.

XXI Management's Role

A Provide workers with a company policy statement, which should include the following:
   1. A statement that indicates that Company X is committed to protecting the health and safety of its workers
   2. A statement indicating that all workers will be informed of known hazardous substances that can cause illness, injury, or death
   3. A statement that all workers will be trained at the time of hire, when they move to an area with new hazards, and when a new hazard is introduced into the workplace
   4. The identification of individuals (or their job titles) who will be responsible for implementing and managing the hazard communication (HazCom) program

B Provide a written program (OSHA looks for this first) that includes the following:
   1. A list of hazardous chemicals present in the workplace
   2. The proper labeling of all containers of chemicals in the workplace
   3. The preparation of MSDSs (ANSI Z400.1)
   4. The implementation of worker training programs about the hazards of chemicals and measures that can be taken to protect workers from dangerous exposures

XXII Description of the Program

A The goals and objectives of the HazCom program
   1. Identify and assess all chemical substances in the workplace that may pose physical or health hazards to workers.
   2. Communicate to all workers the presence of potentially hazardous substances in the workplace through training and provision of accessible MSDSs, which must be kept current.
   3. Train all workers in the safe handling of potentially hazardous substances.

4. Properly label all chemical containers with warning notices and the handling and disposal procedures of hazardous substances. All known hazardous chemicals or chemical compounds that are not covered under other federal acts are covered under the OSH Act.

B **Definitions**

1. A *chemical* is any element, chemical compound, or mixture of elements and compounds.
2. A *hazardous chemical* is any chemical that is a health or physical hazard.
   a. *Health hazards* include chemicals that are known carcinogens, toxic or highly toxic agents, agents that damage the reproductive system, irritants, corrosives, sensitizers, hepatotoxins, neurotoxins, agents that act on the hematopoietic system, and agents that damage the lungs, eyes, skin, or mucous membranes.
   b. A *physical hazard* is any chemical for which there is scientifically valid evidence that it is a combustible liquid, compressed gas, or organic peroxide, or that it is explosive, flammable, pyrophoric, unstable (reactive), or water reactive.

XXIII Elements of the HazCom Program

A **Responsibilities of a program coordinator**

1. Keep accurate inventory of all hazardous chemicals and substances used in the workplace. (It may be helpful to work with the purchasing department to identify the chemicals that have been purchased or ordered.)
2. Obtain MSDSs from the manufacturers or suppliers of all chemicals used in the workplace.
3. Provide training programs for workers when any hazardous chemical is used in the workplace and when any new physical or health hazard is introduced into the workplace.
4. Ensure that all chemicals are properly labeled and stored.

B **Elements of worker training programs**

1. The program is communicated to all current and new workers at least annually.
2. The standard is summarized during the training program.
3. The location of the written program is communicated and readily accessible to all workers.
4. The location of the list of hazardous chemical products and the master list and location of MSDSs must be communicated and accessible to all workers. (OSHA interprets "readily accessible" to include the use of electronic means such as computers with printers, microfiche machines, the Internet, CD-ROMs, and fax machines, provided there is an adequate back up system in the event of a power failure.)
5. The program provides mechanisms for understanding its components; for example, the worker should understand the following:
   a. How to read and understand MSDSs
   b. The labeling of hazardous chemicals and products
   c. The health and safety hazards of the chemicals used in the workplace
   d. The safe handling and disposal of hazardous chemicals
   e. The signs and symptoms of overexposure (nausea, vomiting, headache, dizziness, burn, rash, etc.)

       f. Emergency procedures for exposure events

       g. Methods and observations that may be used to detect the presence or release of hazardous chemicals

       h. Controls that are in place to protect workers, such as PPE

       i. Where workers can obtain more information about hazardous chemicals

C Training standards for contract workers

    1. Inform all contract workers of the location of the MSDSs.

    2. Provide workers with personal protective equipment (PPE).

    3. Inform workers of the chemical hazards in their work area.

    4. Explain the labeling system of hazardous chemicals used by the company.

    5. Emphasize emergency procedures in event of exposure.

D Training standards for nonroutine hazardous tasks

    1. Provide training for the specific hazardous chemicals to which the workers will be exposed.

    2. Provide workers with PPE appropriate for those hazardous chemicals.

XXIV Material Safety Data Sheets

MSDSs require the following information:

A All items on the MSDS must be completed, leaving no blank spaces. (Computer generated MSDSs do not have to follow this requirement because of electronic formatting considerations.)

B The generic *and* common names of the chemical

C A description of the chemical's characteristics (e.g., liquid, vapor, solid, flammable, explosive, etc.)

D A list of the chemical characteristics that make it hazardous to health (e.g., carcinogenic, corrosive, highly toxic, irritant)

E The primary routes of entry into the body (e.g., absorption, inhalation, ingestion, injection)

F Permissible exposure limits set by OSHA, and threshold limit values set by the American Congress of Governmental Industrial Hygienists

G Information on the chemical's listing on a hazardous chemical registry, such as the Annual Report of Carcinogens, if applicable.

H Precautions for safe handling, along with the recommended type of PPE

I Measures to control exposure to the chemical, such as engineering, work practices, administrative controls, and PPE

J Emergency and first-aid procedures if an exposure occurs

K Date the MSDS was prepared and the name, address, and phone number of the manufacturer or other responsible party

L The MSDS must be printed in English (and may, in addition, be printed in other languages).

XXV Trade Secrets

A A *trade secret* is any confidential formula, pattern, process, device, information, or compilation of information that is used in an employer's business and that gives the employer an opportunity to obtain an advantage over competitors who do not know or use it.

B A manufacturer may withhold the identity of a certain chemical when knowledge of that chemical by other manufacturers could give the latter a competitive advantage, except in the following situations:

1. A treating physician or occupational and environmental health nurse determines that a medical emergency exists and the identity of that chemical is necessary for emergency first-aid treatment.

2. In a nonemergency situation, when the name of the chemical is requested in writing by a health professional (e.g., physician, occupational and environmental health nurse, industrial hygienist, toxicologist, or epidemiologist) who is providing occupational and environmental health services to exposed workers for valid reasons described in the OSH Act, a signed confidentiality statement may be required by the manufacturer.

XXVI Container Labeling and Warning Requirements

A All chemical containers entering the workplace must be clearly marked with the identity of the chemical, appropriate warnings, and the name of the manufacturer.

B All chemicals transferred to other containers must be marked with the information listed on the original container.

C All unmarked containers must be reported to the program coordinator immediately.

D Generic warning labels are available from U.S. Department of Transportation for such chemicals as flammable gas, flammable solid, oxidizer, or corrosive.

XXVII Recordkeeping

Although not required by OSHA, keeping records of worker training and education, including the content of the training program and the names and signatures of workers, is important.

A Well-maintained records ensure that all workers have been trained in handling and storing products that contain hazardous substances.

B Records document that HazCom training has been provided; this is helpful during an audit of workers' compensation claims.

XXVIII Evaluation

A Observe how chemicals are actually being handled by workers.

B Solicit feedback from workers and management on how the program is working.

C Make a checklist of all elements of the program to ensure that the program is working and complies with appropriate standards (Box 14-2).

Drug and alcohol testing program

It is estimated that substance abuse costs employers billions of dollars each year as a result of increased injuries, fatalities, absenteeism, excessive use of health care benefits, decreased productivity, and theft. Although the workplace is a strategic place for preventing and identifying early substance abuse, many businesses still do not have drug-free workplace programs. The Department of Transportation

---

BOX 14-2

Checklist for a hazard communication program

- Obtained a copy of the rule
- Read and understood the requirements
- Assigned responsibility for tasks
- Prepared an inventory of chemicals used in the workplace
- Ensured that containers are properly labeled
- Obtained an MSDS for each chemical

- Prepared a written program
- Made MSDSs available to workers
- Conducted training for workers
- Established procedure to maintain current program
- Established procedures to evaluate completeness and effectiveness of the program

---

Source: U.S. Department of Labor, 1995.

MSDS, material safety data sheet.

has developed comprehensive federal regulations that mandate drug and alcohol testing for transportation workers. These regulations include an excellent model for employers considering drug and alcohol testing programs; this model serves as the basis of the program described in this chapter.

XXIX Purposes of a Drug and Alcohol Testing Program

The purposes of a *drug and alcohol testing program* are to avoid hiring workers who use illegal drugs, deter workers from abusing drugs and alcohol, and identify and refer to treatment those workers who are presently abusing drugs or alcohol.

A Definitions

1. A *drug* is any chemical substance that produces physical, mental, emotional, or behavioral changes in the user.
2. *Drug and alcohol abuse* is the use of any drug or alcohol in a medically, socially, or legally unacceptable manner.
3. *Substance abuse* occurs whenever an illegal drug is used, when a prescribed drug is misused, when drugs or alcohol are consumed to the point of physical or mental impairment, or when alcohol is used in an amount or at a time prohibited by an employer's policy.

B Drug-free workplace programs may include the following:

1. A company policy
2. An EAP
3. Supervisory training
4. Employee-awareness education
5. Drug and alcohol testing

XXX Preliminary Considerations

A Before establishing a drug and alcohol testing program, employers must review all laws and regulations applicable to their jurisdiction regarding disabilities, rehabilitation, and discrimination.

B The National Labor Relations Act requires bargaining with unions before changing work rules and policies.

C Public employers must consider constitutional rights; unreasonable search and seizure is the most common challenge.

XXXI Program Components

A Components of a company policy for a drug testing program
1. Explain why the program is being implemented.
2. Describe substance abuse–related behaviors that are prohibited.
3. Thoroughly explain the consequences for violations of the policy.
4. Inform workers that their employer is not required under federal regulations to provide rehabilitation, pay for treatment, or reinstate the worker in a safety-sensitive position; these issues may be negotiated with unions.
5. Involve unions in policy development.
6. Include ongoing worker input into policy development.
7. Give workers 30 to 60 days' notice before the testing program starts.

B Recordkeeping recommendations
1. Maintain records that each worker has been notified of the company policy regarding drug testing.
2. Have workers sign a receipt that they received a copy of the policy.
3. Provide information and training to workers well before the program begins.
4. Provide face-to-face training with an opportunity for employees to ask questions (the most effective format).

C Other considerations
1. Administrative issues
   a. Employers should keep detailed records of their drug and alcohol abuse prevention programs; federal agencies will conduct inspections or audits of employers' programs.
   b. Worker's alcohol testing records are confidential; without a release they may be released only to the employer and substance abuse professional (and to the DOT, if applicable).
2. Business analysis
   a. Drug abuse in the United States is a severe problem and a factor in business competitiveness.
      1) 74 percent of adults who use illegal drugs are employed.
      2) Absenteeism is 66 percent higher among drug users than individuals who do not use drugs.
      3) 47 percent of workplace accidents are drug-related.
      4) Employee turnover is significantly higher among drug users than among individuals who do not use drugs.
   b. Comparison analysis of the costs of drug testing with the costs of accidents, injuries, industrial injury time loss, workers' compensation claims, and productivity before and after initiating a drug testing program can provide helpful information.

XXXII Employee Assistance Programs

EAPs provide a support system and counseling services for workers and for management. (Chapter 12 provides additional information about EAPs.)

A EAPs may consist of formal programs, a listing of available resources, or participation in consortia (groups or associations of employers) that provide testing and other related services.

B EAPs must be viewed as a confidential source of help.

C Workers must understand that EAPs will not shield them from disciplinary action if behavior continues.

XXXIII Training and Education

A Supervisors' responsibilities
1. Observe and document unsatisfactory job performance.
2. Confront workers about unsatisfactory job performance according to company procedures.
3. Recognize and manage drug crisis situations.
4. Understand the policy and their role in its implementation.
5. Understand the effects of substance abuse.
6. Feel comfortable with evaluating work performance and understand performance evaluation procedures.
7. Know how to refer to individuals qualified to diagnose and offer assistance for drug and alcohol problems.

B Elements of a comprehensive employee education program
1. Provide information about the dangers and effects of alcohol and drug abuse.
2. Describe the impact of substance abuse on safety, productivity, and the company's bottom line.
3. Describe program components, the EAP, and testing procedures and protocols.
4. Describe the signs and symptoms of drug and alcohol abuse.
5. Describe regulatory requirements and the employer's policy and procedures.
6. Explain how and where workers can get help for drug and alcohol problems.

XXXIV The Drug Free Workplace Act of 1998

A Purposes of the Drug Free Workplace Act
1. Educate small business concerns about the advantages of a drug-free workplace
2. Provide grants and technical assistance in addition to financial incentives to enable small business concerns to create a drug-free workplace
3. Assist working parents in keeping their children drug-free
4. Encourage small business employers and employees alike to participate in drug-free workplace programs

B Elements of a Drug-free workplace programs
1. A written policy, including a clear statement of expectations and prohibitions related to drug and alcohol abuse and the consequences of violating those expectations and prohibitions
2. Drug and alcohol abuse prevention training for a total of not less than 2 hours for each employee, and additional voluntary drug and alcohol abuse prevention training for employees who are parents
3. Employee illegal drug testing, with analysis conducted by a drug testing

laboratory certified by SAMHSA or approved by the College of American Pathologists for forensic drug testing, and a review of each positive test result by a medical review officer

4. Employee access to an employee assistance program, including confidential assessment, referral, and short-term problem resolution
5. Continuing alcohol and drug abuse prevention education

XXXV Elements of a Drug and Alcohol Testing Program

A **A successful testing program must contract with reliable, professional laboratories.**

1. Laboratory certification (and monitoring) by the Substance Abuse and Mental Health Services Administration (SAMHSA) is required for federally mandated testing. (SAMHSA was formerly the National Institute of Drug Abuse.)
2. The testing methodology required by the DOT is a two-stage process, starting with an initial screening test, which, if positive for one or more drugs, is followed by a confirmation test.
   a. The very sensitive initial screening test (immunoassay) looks for the presence or absence of drugs.
   b. The confirmation test is performed for each identified drug using state-of-the-art gas chromatography/mass spectrometry analysis.
3. The testing program must establish testing protocols, such as the specific drugs to be tested and the cutoff levels.
   a. The most common drugs tested for (and required by federal testing) are marijuana, cocaine, amphetamines, opiates (including heroin), and phencyclidine.
   b. Other drugs also abused but less commonly tested include barbiturates (including sedatives and tranquilizers), hallucinogens, inhalants, and "designer drugs."
   c. Cutoff (laboratory reporting) levels are established by SAMHSA.

B **The chain-of-custody procedures ensure that the specimen's security, proper identification, and integrity are not compromised.**

1. The procedures track the handling and storage from initial collection to final disposition.
2. A positive test result must be linked back to the individual whose name appears on the specimen bottle label.
3. All personnel who handle the specimen are documented; no unauthorized access to the specimen is possible, and no adulteration or tampering takes place.

C **The Omnibus Transportation Employee Testing Act of 1991 requires that drug testing procedures for most transportation workers include split-specimen procedures.**

1. Each urine specimen is subdivided into two bottles labeled as *primary* and *split* specimens; both bottles are sent to the laboratory.
2. Only the primary specimen is opened and used for the urinalysis; the split-specimen bottle remains sealed and is stored in the laboratory.
3. If the analysis of the primary specimen confirms the presence of illegal, controlled substances, the worker has 72 hours to request the split specimen be sent to another SAMHSA-certified laboratory for analysis.

D **To protect worker and employer, a medical review officer (MRO) reviews and interprets all drug test results before they are reported to the employer.**
1. Federal regulations require the MRO to contact the worker in person or by telephone and conduct an interview to determine if there is an alternative medical explanation for the drugs found in the worker's urine specimen.
2. If the worker provides appropriate documentation and the MRO determines that it is legitimate medical use of the prohibited drug, the drug test result is reported to the employer as negative.

E **As a quality assurance measure for the testing laboratory, employers are required by federal regulations to perform blind sample testing.**

F **Types of tests**
1. *Preemployment,* or *applicant, testing* is conducted to prevent hiring workers with drug or alcohol problems; it is the most popular type of drug testing because it avoids union problems and potential future problems associated with substance-abusing workers.
2. *Post-accident testing* is used to determine if drug or alcohol abuse was a contributing factor in the accident, identify drug and alcohol abusers, and deter drug and alcohol abuse.
3. *Reasonable suspicion testing* is conducted when an employer suspects that a worker is using alcohol or drugs in violation of the company's policy, based on "specific, contemporaneous, and articulable observations concerning the appearance, behavior, speech, or body odor" of the worker (U.S. Department of Transportation, 1994b).
4. *Random testing* is conducted without suspicion that any particular worker is using drugs, and it identifies workers who are abusing drugs or alcohol but have been able to use the predictable testing schedule to escape detection.
   a. Candidates for random testing should be selected using a simple random sampling method so that all workers eligible for testing are equally likely to be tested.
   b. An excellent deterrent and early intervention tool, random testing is recommended for workers in safety- or security-sensitive positions and for workers in companies in which alcohol and drug abuse problems are common.
   c. Federal regulations require random drug testing of at least 50% and random alcohol testing of at least 25% of safety-sensitive workers (the random testing rate is determined annually based upon the random positive rate for each industry).
   d. Because alcohol is legal, random alcohol testing must be conducted just before, during, or just after a worker's performance of safety-sensitive duties.
5. *Return-to-duty* and *follow-up testing* are conducted when a worker who has tested positive for drugs and been removed from the workplace returns to work or to performing safety-sensitive duties.
   a. Federal regulations require that follow-up tests must be unannounced and that a minimum of six tests must be conducted in the first 12 months after a worker returns to duty; follow-up testing and monitoring may continue for up to 5 years.
   b. The frequency of the follow-up tests should depend on the characteristics of the abused drug and the worker's abuse-related behavior.

G **Federal regulations require that breath testing for alcohol be done with**

evidential breath-testing devices approved by the National Highway Traffic Safety Administration.

H Some federal regulations require certain categories of safety-sensitive workers to report *any* medical use of controlled substances.

I Federal regulations pertaining to alcohol-related conduct mandate that a worker's performance of safety-sensitive functions is prohibited under the following circumstances:
1. If an alcohol breath test indicates an alcohol concentration of 0.04 or greater
2. While using alcohol
3. Within 4 hours after using alcohol
4. When using alcohol within 8 hours after an accident or until tested
5. When refusing to submit to an alcohol test

XXXVI Consequences of Drug and Alcohol Abuse

A The consequences of drug and alcohol misuse must be defined before beginning the program.

B Workers who abuse drugs or alcohol must be immediately removed from safety-sensitive functions. Return to duty requires the following:
1. Evaluation by a substance-abuse professional
2. Compliance with any treatment recommendations
3. A return-to-duty drug or alcohol test (with the result of the alcohol test less than 0.02)
4. The worker to be subject to unannounced follow-up drug or alcohol tests

Emergency preparedness/disaster plan

The following basic emergency plan can serve as a framework to use in development of a site-specific emergency preparedness/disaster plan. Some of the suggested actions may not be necessary, but they should be considered to ensure a comprehensive program. The program should be tailored to establish regulatory compliance for the applicable region or jurisdiction and to protect workers and the community against the emergency conditions that have the greatest potential for occurring in a given facility.

The goal of an emergency-management plan is to predict the unpredictable. So the best that can be done is to continue to audit, review, and identify risks associated with workplace activities. There is no way you can do it too often (Hans, 1995).

XXXVII Purposes of an Emergency Preparedness/ Disaster Plan

A Prevent, or at least control, harm to people (highest priority) and property (secondary priority) in event of an emergency or disaster.

B Contain the extent of property loss, only when the safety of all staff and neighbors at risk has been clearly established.

C Prevent harm to the environment and the surrounding community.

D Facilitate automatic disaster response by avoiding delays caused by decision making.

E Identify previously unrecognized hazardous conditions that would aggravate an emergency and take steps to eliminate them.

F Identify deficiencies, such as lack of resource coordination to handle an emergency.

G Raise safety awareness.

H Demonstrate the company's commitment to the safety of its workers.

I Establish regulatory compliance with OSHA's 29 CFR 1910.38 plans for emergency action and fire response; 29 CFR 1910.119 for process safety management; 29 CFR 1910.120 for hazardous waste operations; and 29 CFR 1910.151 for medical services and first aid.

J Provide consistency with and support for local emergency plans and response agencies.

XXXIII The Scope of the Plan

A The emergency preparedness/disaster plan is site-specific; it is governed by the following factors:
1. Nature of work performed
2. Number of workers and contractors at site
3. Hours of operation

B The plan applies to all persons on site, including workers, contractors, and visitors.

C Steps in developing the plan
1. A vulnerability assessment, which includes a consideration of required responses and necessary resources
2. Input from community agencies with responsibilities for emergency response

D The plan should include regular planning meetings and drills.

E Cost considerations: Because major emergencies are low-probability events, they compete with other company financial allocations.

F A written plan should be available for inspection and copying by workers, their representatives, community emergency-response agencies, and OSHA personnel.

XXXIX Program Responsibilities

A Disaster planning committee
1. Disaster planning requires the expertise of many people; planners may include representatives of company management, occupational health and safety personnel, human resources, risk managers, accounting, security, and union representatives.
2. The number of people and their functions will depend on the size and complexity of the workplace.
3. Hazard control, emergency-response, legal requirements, and administrative concerns must be addressed in the plan.

B Safety director
1. Performs the function of emergency-response team coordinator for planning and training

2. Provides and maintains the inventory of hazard monitoring equipment and personal protective clothing and equipment used for hazardous materials response
3. In an emergency response, acts as the safety officer
4. Conducts post-emergency investigations

C **Management**
   1. Encourages and supports emergency-response plans, activities, and training
   2. Ensures that workers are familiar with and follow the procedures of the plan
   3. Informs the disaster planning committee of any new conditions or potential problems that warrant planning for emergency responses
   4. Reviews and approves revisions to the plan
   5. Ensures adequate resources for implementation and maintenance of the plan
   6. Supports coordination with local community emergency-response programs

D **Supervisors**
   1. Encourage and support worker emergency-response activities and training
   2. Ensure that workers are familiar with and follow the plan's procedures
   3. Inform the disaster planning committee of any new conditions or potential problems that warrant planning for emergency responses

E **Human resources director**
   1. Acts as public relations officer in an emergency by maintaining communication to the news media
   2. Provides communications between upper management (site and corporate) and the emergency-response team
   3. Communicates with families that may be affected by the emergency

F **Environmental protection manager**
   1. Ensures proper reporting of environmental contamination as required by law and corporate policy
   2. Ensures proper disposal of hazardous and medical waste in an emergency

G **Health center manager**
   1. Acts as medical officer, as defined in the National Fire Academy Incident Command System, during an emergency
   2. Provides and maintains an inventory of emergency medical equipment and supplies
   3. Supervises on-site medical emergency-response team members in caring for victims during an emergency response
   4. Directs or provides emergency victim triage, treatment, and transportation
   5. Communicates with community rescue and medical emergency responders and with hospital emergency department staff
   6. Ensures that current emergency patient care protocols are signed by the appropriate health care professionals and updated regularly
   7. Ensures that the on-site training of the medical emergency-response team in first aid and cardiopulmonary resuscitation (CPR) is provided and kept current according to criteria of the certifying agency
   8. Schedules and arranges physical examinations for respirator users and emergency responders according to company protocol and regulatory

requirements, such as for hazardous materials (HazMat) technicians outlined in OSHA 29 CFR 1910.120

H **Emergency-response personnel and first-aid team members, hazardous materials response team members, and fire brigade members**
1. Provide rapid emergency services within the property boundaries in accordance with the assigned response team
2. Maintain knowledge and skills through participation in on-site training programs and drill exercises
3. Refrain from response activities that are beyond the level of their training and equipment
4. Keep emergency-response routine activities from interfering with their normal job responsibilities

I **Information technology manager**
1. Ensures creation and maintenance of computer data backup files.
2. Maintains off-site contingency data storage
3. Ensures capability of reinstallation and restoration of computer hardware and software

J **Workers**
1. Know the facility evacuation plans and evacuate as instructed during actual and practice alarms
2. Report all emergencies, including health, fire, chemical, and intrusion, by calling a designated phone number
3. Follow instructions of the evacuation team leaders, emergency-response team members, and community emergency-response personnel

K **Security personnel**
1. During an emergency, rope off the predesignated section of parking lot for emergency-response vehicles
2. Prevent curiosity seekers from entering the site
3. Prevent removal of company documents and property during the disruptions of a site emergency
4. Escort arrivals to meet with the appropriate company representative (e.g., the news media to the Human Resources Director) at a predesignated meeting location

L **Switchboard operator**
1. Properly handles emergency calls by determining the nature of the emergency and the details outlined on the emergency call form
2. Notifies the on-site emergency-response personnel when an employee emergency call is received
3. Summons community emergency-response agencies at the direction of the emergency-response manager in charge
4. Activates the site alarm system when directed by the emergency-response manager in charge
5. Receives and documents all bomb threats telephoned to the switchboard, and reports them immediately to management

M **Maintenance supervisor**
1. Provides, maintains, and ensures monthly inspections of all fire-response equipment and supplies, self-contained breathing apparatus equipment and tanks, and rescue hardware and tools stored for emergency response
2. Maintains emergency power-generating capability

3. Directs shutdown, repair, and start-up of utilities involved in site emergencies
4. Provides post-incident assessment of hazards and damage to property and equipment
5. Makes regular rounds, being alert to fire potentials, chemical leaks, and utility failures

N **Technical consultants**
1. Respond to the incident command operations center, when requested, to interpret and advise on the status and potential escalation of a chemical incident
2. Attend annual training on hazardous materials emergency response

XL General Emergency Procedures

A **Communication strategies**
1. Notification phone list: Compose a list of names, site phone extensions, home phone numbers, and pager numbers of everyone whose support your company might need.
2. Community-response phone list: Compose a list of agencies with names, phone numbers, and pager numbers of every agency whose support your company might need; possibly include security companies, insurance companies, photographers, attorneys, and public relations firms.
3. Throughout the facility, install bright red, manual, fire-alarm pull stations that are linked to the local fire department alarm console.
4. Locate evacuation alarms throughout the facility that can be activated by the switchboard operator.
5. Set up an internal communication system consisting of a designated emergency telephone number and a pager system.
6. Establish family notification procedures, to be conducted as necessary by the human resources director or other company official.
7. Utility companies will be contacted as necessary by the maintenance supervisor.
8. Regulatory agencies requiring reporting of hazardous materials release will be notified by the environmental protection manager; the local OSHA office will be notified by the safety director in accordance with OSHA requirements in event of a work-related fatality or hospitalization of workers.

B **Organization: Personnel in command will be established according to the nature of the emergency, as follows:**
1. Medical emergencies: the occupational health physician or the occupational and environmental health nurse is in command.
2. Fire emergencies: the fire brigade captain is in command in incipient level fires; in major structural fires, the local fire department is in command.
3. Hazardous materials releases: the HazMat team captain is in command; in major releases involving the community, the local fire department's HazMat technician team is in command.
4. Natural disasters, intrusions, and bomb threats: the human resources and safety directors share command in coordination with security; in events of immediate threat involving bomb threats, violence, and intrusions, the local police authority is in command.
5. Overall coordination of plan development and implementation is under the direction of the emergency-response team coordinator.

6. Design and annual review of this plan are under the direction of the disaster planning committee chairman.

C Evacuation procedures

1. Assign individuals to assist handicapped workers in emergencies.
2. Identify evacuation routes and alternate means of escape; make these known to all persons at site.
3. Keep the routes unobstructed through regular safety inspections.
4. Evacuation routes should be clearly posted.
5. Evacuation and fire drills should be held at least annually to practice the documented plans; every drill or actual emergency incident should be followed by an in-depth evaluation to include all levels of responders.

D Personnel accountability during an evacuation

1. Specify safe locations for staff to gather for head-counts to ensure that everyone has left the danger zone.
2. Each department must assume responsibility for its workers and its visitors.
3. Reenter the building only after being advised to do so by the senior management.
4. Have a designated and an alternate head-counter—one for every 20 workers.
5. Notify the incident command of the results of the count and of any missing persons.
6. Designate sufficient inside locations when sheltering-in-place (workers are moved to a designated safe location within the building) is preferred over evacuation, as in tornadoes, hurricanes, earthquakes, or hazardous materials vapor clouds.

E Information dissemination

1. Insurers will be notified by the human resources department or site management.
2. Community and media will be advised by the human resources director; a preselected site should be designated for media and press releases.

F Authority notification and reporting

1. The local emergency planning committee will be notified by the local fire department as required by regulations.
2. The national response center will be notified by the safety director when mandated by regulatory requirements.
3. The local environmental protection agency will be notified, when mandated, by the environmental protection manager.
4. Other notifications may be necessary for your region; company policy may require certain company representative notifications.

G Recordkeeping

1. All health records will be established and maintained by the occupational and environmental health nurse.
2. All fire maintenance and repair records will be maintained by the maintenance supervisor.
3. Boiler records and emergency generator testing records will be maintained by the maintenance supervisor.
4. Incident response records will be established and maintained by an appropriate designee.

5. Hazardous materials release reports will be established and maintained by the environmental protection manager.
6. All other records will be established and maintained by the human resources director and by the safety director, based on the nature of the record and the incident.

XLI Specific Emergency Procedures

The procedures outlined in this section can be applied to numerous emergency scenarios, including hurricane, flood, major blizzard, bomb threat, fire, medical emergency, and hostile events.

A A tornado is imminent
   1. Description: A tornado is imminent, and you have no time to report to the designated tornado shelter.
   2. Action plan: Seek safety under a table, desk, or heavy piece of equipment that offers protection from falling debris; use a coat or similar item to protect your face and eyes; put on safety equipment such as safety glasses and hard hat.
   3. Post-threat plan: Call the designated numbers for help (if phones are operational); inspect your work area for damage; follow evacuation, cleanup, or other recovery activities as directed.

B A tornado warning has been issued
   1. Description: A tornado warning has been issued, and time permits additional preparation.
   2. Action plan: Seek shelter immediately in interior rooms without windows, such as bathrooms, closets, and so forth; shut off utilities and processes that will not become hazardous when interrupted; wear any personal safety equipment.
   3. Post-threat plan: Call the designated numbers for help if needed (if phones are operational); inspect your work area for damage; follow evacuation, cleanup, or other recovery activities as directed.

C Hazardous material—a small spill or release has occurred
   1. Description: A small spill that poses no safety, environmental, or health danger and can be handled safely without additional assistance or equipment beyond standard personal safety equipment
   2. Action plan: Close valves and right drums or bottles according to your training and the MSDS; prevent the chemical from entering a drain; add neutralizing agents, adsorbents, or pillow.
   3. Post-threat plan: Dispose of material according to site hazardous waste procedures. Fill out an accident form.

D Hazardous material—a large spill or release has occurred
   1. Description: A significant threat to health and safety from vapors or fume inhalation, skin contact, flammability, environmental contamination, rapid spill proliferation, and loss of site safety control
   2. Action plan
      a. Get yourself and others out of the danger zone. Rope off the area to prevent entry, call the designated number immediately and advise on the nature of the spill, the chemicals involved, and the exact location; do not attempt to rescue co-workers.

b. The on-site HazMat team will respond to the incident according to their training and equipment capabilities or will request help from the local fire department's HazMat technician team.

c. Occupational health providers will respond to provide emergency victim care and monitor the HazMat team members.

d. Exposure victims will be decontaminated as necessary by the HazMat team before being released to community emergency-response providers. The hospital will be notified.

3. Post-threat plan: The size of the release may necessitate a report to governmental authorities. Cleanup operations will be arranged according to the nature of the spill, such as via commercial chemical cleanup companies.

XLII Recovery Procedures

A **Critical incident stress debriefing (CISD): "Reactions to trauma/crisis in the workplace may have far-reaching repercussions on the emotional and financial status of an organization. It is imperative to address these issues and situations as they occur" (Lewis, 1993).**

1. CISD will be offered to all affected employees in event of an emotionally traumatic emergency response, which can precipitate critical incident stress similar to post-traumatic stress disorder.

2. This debriefing will be offered between 24 to 48 hours after the event, the time when debriefing is most effective.

3. Trained CISD leaders will be obtained from the local fire department's CISD resources.

B **Post-incident evaluation**

1. Incident investigation

   a. Its chief purpose is to prevent similar future losses by identifying and evaluating present losses, reporting to OSHA, and assessing insurance claim needs.

   b. Conduct the investigation at the scene of the incident, keeping the site as undisturbed as possible.

   c. Take photos, make drawings, and take measurements, as appropriate.

   d. Interview all witnesses one at a time and privately.

   e. Seek the root causes.

2. Reports

   a. Provide regulatory reports as required.

   b. Provide internal reports according to company policy.

   c. Provide press releases as needed.

C **Damage assessment**

1. Each worker is expected to evaluate the worksite for damages, make a report to supervisors, and complete a maintenance work order.

2. The occupational health department will provide a report of injuries, fatalities, and hospitalizations to the safety and human resources departments and establish follow-up case-management procedures.

3. Maintenance will evaluate utilities, building structure, and major processing equipment for damages and report to the safety department and upper management.

4. Section supervisors will evaluate worker reports and departmental damages, including lost records, lost or damaged equipment, and any damages that pose a safety hazard or delay the return to normal operations, and will report these to the maintenance and safety departments and management.

D Cleanup and restoration

1. The company's employee assistance program (EAP) will be contacted for services if applicable.
2. Cleanup operations will be supervised by the maintenance department, which will use outside contractors as needed, after approval from management.
3. Accounting will quantify financial losses and restoration costs for management.
4. Management will establish a priority list for restoration processes to return to normal operations.
5. Professional services such as legal assistance will be arranged by management as applicable.
6. Information technology will provide smooth and rapid restoration of computer services.

XLIII Program Maintenance

A Location and upkeep of the emergency plan document

1. Distribution: plant manager, shift supervisors, emergency-response team coordinator, safety, occupational health services, human resources, maintenance, switchboard, local fire department, local emergency planning committee
2. The plan will be reviewed and updated annually by the disaster planning committee, with changes being implemented by the chairman.

B Testing and drills

1. Evacuation drills will be conducted at least annually.
2. Emergency-response team drills will be conducted monthly, using methods such as table-top drills, skills practice, and mock drills.
3. A mock disaster drill will be conducted annually and should include community emergency-response agencies.
4. Emergency responders will be required to pass annual performance tests of procedures such as CPR, according to their area of response.
5. Follow-up assessment will include identifying processes that proceeded as planned, areas requiring improvement, and equipment and operating procedures that need to be added, deleted, or modified. Participants will be advised of the findings.

C Training

1. The HazMat team will be trained by a recognized, qualified training firm that is able to provide awareness, operations, and technician levels of training in accordance with the requirements of 29 CFR 1910.120. Training will be provided for appropriately designated workers, who will also receive annual refresher training.
2. Fire brigade members will be trained to the level of incipient fire response in accordance with NFPA (National Fire Protection Association) 600 and OSHA Standard Subpart L by the local fire department, with refresher training annually.

3. First-aid and CPR training will be provided by the occupational and environmental health nurse with monthly training sessions and annual refresher programs; training curriculum will be in accordance with the standard of the American Heart Association or National Red Cross and with the OSHA Compliance Guideline 2-2.53C, promulgated in October, 1990.

D Equipment

1. Each emergency-response team will maintain its own equipment, with the exception of the fire and self-contained breathing apparatus equipment, which will be maintained by the maintenance department.
2. Equipment inspections will be conducted and recorded monthly; deficiencies will be reported to the emergency-response coordinator.
3. The emergency-response coordinator will provide annual updated lists of on-site equipment to the disaster planning committee chairman for inclusion in the appendices of this plan as labeled.
4. Medical and first-aid equipment will be located at the occupational health service center, and additional first-aid kits, stocked by the occupational and environmental health nurse, will be located at the entrance of each department.

E Facilities

1. The occupational health service will be the site for client care, if it is not conducted at the scene.
2. A designated meeting location will serve as the media center and will contain a site plot plan, photographs of emergency-response drills for reference, telephones, fax machine, podium, and extra tables and chairs.
3. A predesignated location will serve as the incident command post to conduct centralized emergency operations management. This facility will contain two-way radios, site plot plans, telephone, fax machine, set of MSDSs, a copy of this plan, and emergency lanterns.

XLIV Appendices to Include in a Written Plan

A Appendix A: Hazardous Materials Inventory with Location. Provide a complete list of all the hazardous substances on site and the department and building where they are located.

B Appendix B: Facility/Site Plot Plan. Provide a current map of the entire site. If appropriate, provide building plans for each building on site, including locations of fire equipment, emergency exits, evacuation routes, alarm locations, first-aid equipment locations, and other sites as needed.

C Appendix C: List of Fire Protection Equipment. Provide a comprehensive list of all fire alarm and response equipment, including fire-fighting foam, fire coats and other protective equipment, fire hoses, etc.

D Appendix D: List of Plant Emergency Safety and Rescue Equipment. Provide a comprehensive list of all plant safety and rescue equipment, such as tripods and confined-space harnesses, chemical neutralizers, spill blankets, shovels, respirators, etc.

E Appendix E: List of Plant Emergency Medical Equipment. Provide a list of all on-site first-aid and professional medical equipment, such as stethoscopes, antidotes, stretchers, splints, etc.

> ### BOX 14-3
> *Impact and costs related to WMSDs*
>
> - WMSDs account for greater than one third of all occupational injuries and illnesses reported to the Bureau of Labor Statistics each year.
> - More than 600,000 employees suffer lost-workday WMSDs each year in the United States.
> - WMSPs result in $15 to $20 billion in workers' compensation costs each year
> - WMSPs result in estimated costs of $45 to $54 billion for time and manpower to conduct accident investigations, decreased productivity and quality, job retraining costs, replacement hiring costs, increased absenteeism, decreased worker morale, and litigation costs
> - Not included in these numbers are the musculoskeletal disorders that are not recognized as work related, but are treated under the employee's general medical insurance.
> - Pain and suffering to workers and their families are not included either.

Source: http://www.osha-slc.gov/ergonomics-standard/overview.html.

Ergonomics programs

Work-related musculoskeletal disorders (WMSDs) are among the most costly injuries in terms of the pain and suffering of workers and direct and indirect costs to employers (Box 14-3). An increasing number of employers are recognizing the value and importance of implementing ergonomics strategies and programs in their workplaces. Successful prevention of WMSDs requires a multifaceted approach that focuses on prevention and is tailored to the specific needs of the organization. This section describes the elements of a comprehensive ergonomics program.

XLV Overview of Ergonomics

A Ergonomics "is the science and practice of designing jobs or workplaces to match the capabilities and limitations of the human body" (Washington State Department of Labor and Industries [WSDOLI], 1993, 1999).

B Ergonomics is concerned with the interaction of the worker with the job.

C Ergonomics is a multidisciplinary science that considers knowledge from four areas (Rom, 1998).

1. Human factors engineering, which focuses on the "information processing requirements of the interaction between people, machines and the environment."

2. Anthropometry, which is "the science of measurement and the art of application that establishes the physical geometry, mass properties, and strength capabilities of the human body."

3. Occupational biomechanics, which applies the laws of physics and engineering to the physical interaction of workers with their work environments.

4. Work physiology, which is concerned with the responses of the body (e.g., respiratory, cardiovascular, and musculoskeletal systems) to the metabolic demands of work.

XLVI Work-Related Musculoskeletal Disorders

A *Ergonomic injuries*, also called *work-related musculoskeletal disorders* (WMSDs), typically include soft tissue injuries to the muscles, tendons, ligaments, joints, blood vessels, and nerves; they exclude injuries from slips, trips, falls, motor vehicle accidents, or being struck by objects.

B WMSDs may result from the following conditions:
1. Awkward postures, such as working with hands above head
2. High hand force, such as gripping an unsupported object
3. Highly repetitive motions, such as performing intensive keying
4. Repeated impact, such as using the hand as a "hammer"
5. Heavy, frequent, awkward lifting
6. Moderate to high hand-arm vibration caused by using equipment such as grinders or sanders
7. Whole body vibration, such as occurs when driving heavy equipment
8. Combinations of any of these conditions

C Examples of injuries are muscle strains and tears, ligament sprains, joint and tendon inflammation, pinched nerves, degeneration of spinal discs, carpal tunnel syndrome, tendonitis, and rotator cuff syndrome.

D Studies suggest that the greater the intensity, duration, and frequency of exposure to physical risk factors, the more likely it is that a worker will sustain a WMSD.

E Several studies provide evidence that WMSDs are associated with various work-related conditions.
1. A NIOSH report concluded that there is "strong evidence of an association between WMSDs and certain work-related physical factors when there are high levels of exposure and especially in combination with exposure to more than one physical factor" (USDHHS, 1997a).
2. The National Academy of Science (NAS) concluded that there is evidence that workers in occupations with high exposures to ergonomic hazards are more likely to report pain, injury, loss of work, and disability than are workers in low-risk jobs. (WSDOLI, 1999)
3. NAS also noted that there is "compelling evidence" that reducing biomechanic stress on the job reduces the risk of injuries (Jeffress, 1999).

F Virtually any worker is potentially at risk of exposure to WMSD.

XLVII Ergonomic Regulation

A Workers are protected from ergonomic hazards by the OSHA general duty clause (Chapter 3).

B In 1990, OSHA developed ergonomics program-management guidelines for meat-packing plants.

C The ADA of 1990 and workers' compensation laws also provide a legal framework for ergonomic concerns.

D Some states, OSHA, and some international agencies have developed or are in process of promulgating regulations requiring workplaces to implement ergonomics programs to reduce the incidence of WMSDs.

XLVIII Purposes of an Ergonomics Program

A Identify potential ergonomic hazards in the work setting.

B Provide a framework for the development of strategies to prevent and control work-related hazards.

C Reduce workers' exposures to workplace conditions or hazards that can cause or aggravate WMSDs.

D Limit the costs related to WMSDs, for both the company and the worker.

E Help the company comply with health and safety regulations.

XLIX Program Components

Successful ergonomics programs require management leadership and commitment and worker involvement. The program includes identifying hazards, developing prevention and control strategies, implementing health management techniques, training and educating employees, and conducting a thorough program evaluation.

A The role of management; the manager
1. Is visibly involved in planning, developing, and implementing the company's ergonomic program.
2. Demonstrates commitment of time and resources.
3. Delineates responsibility for the various components of the program.
   a. Assignment of resources
   b. Delegation of authority and responsibility for program components
   c. Implementation of workplace policies that value health and safety as important as productivity and quality
   d. Demonstration of concern for workers' well being
   e. Inclusion of workers in all aspects of the ergonomics program
   f. Training of workers and encouraging their involvement on committees to identify hazards and to offer suggestions for abatement
   g. Providing all workers access to the written ergonomic program

B The role of the worker; the worker
1. Reports hazards found in the workplace.
2. Reports any symptoms of WMSDs without fear of retribution.
3. Participates in training.
4. Participates on ergonomic teams and joint management/labor safety committees.

C *Work-site analysis* is a health and safety review to identify hazards that cause WMSDs, the risk factors that pose the hazards, and the causes of the risk factors (Chapter 9).
1. *Hazards* are the physical stressors and workplace conditions that pose a risk of WMSDs (Table 14-4).
2. *Risk factors* are the elements of the job that increase the likelihood that a hazard will cause WMSDs.

TABLE 14-4

Hazard definitions

Force	The amount of physical effort required by the worker to perform a task or operate tools and equipment (Putz-Anderson, in Zabel & McGrew, 1997). Effort is affected by type of grip, weight of the object, dimensions of the object, temperature, pinching, vibration, duration, and repetition (Washington State Department of Labor and Industries, 1993).
Repetition	Number of movements that occur in a given amount of time to complete a task, or performing the same motions repeatedly (Washington State Department of Labor and Industries, 1993)
Awkward postures	Any deviation from a relaxed, neutral body posture; any body segment positioned outside the neutral range. Causes decreased muscle strength and fatigue of muscles and supporting tissues (Zabel & McGrew, 1997).
Extreme environmental conditions	Cold or heat, noise, lighting, vibration, and air quality (Zabel & McGrew, 1997)
Vibration	Whole body or segmental
Static postures or sustained exertions	Body postures requiring a fixed position, requiring muscle contraction for a period of time (Washington State Department of Labor and Industries, 1993; Zabel & McGrew, 1997).
Contact stress	Contact of a part of the body with a hard surface or edge, resulting in crushing or pinching of tissue (Washington State Department of Labor and Industries, 1993)
Psychosocial and work organizational issues	Excessive work rates, external pacing of work, excessive work duration, shift work, imbalance of work-to-rest ratios, restriction of movement, inadequate relief periods, lack of task variety, business culture and attitudes, social support, job security, job satisfaction, management/supervisor support, work load, electronic monitoring, demanding incentive pay or work standards (Washington State Department of Labor and Industries, 1993; Zabel & McGrew, 1997; (http://www.cdc.gov/niosh/pdfs/95-119.pdf).

Chapter 9 provides additional information about hazards. NOTE: Risk increases when several hazards are coupled in a single job.

3. The duration of exposure to the risk factor and combinations of risk factors may increase the likelihood of WMSDs.

D **Surveillance can be active or passive.**
1. *Passive surveillance* is the "collection and analysis of data obtained from existing record sources" that identifies the patterns of injuries and illnesses or potential WMSDs (NIOSH, 1995).
    a. Review of company records provides data to target work areas and work processes for further evaluation, and to prioritize the jobs to investigate for hazards.
    b. Data gathered may be used as baseline information to evaluate efforts of prevention.
    c. Passive surveillance includes multiple data sources.
        1) Workers' compensation records
        2) OSHA 200 log and supplemental records (OSHA Form 101)
        3) Accident/incident reports

4) Safety meeting minutes or reports
5) Equipment and tool evaluation records,
6) Costs related to short-term and long-term disability
7) Group health insurance utilization reports
8) Absentee and lost workday data, job turnover data
9) Restricted-work and job-transfer information
10) Nurse's daily log

2. *Active surveillance* is the proactive development of methods to collect data to determine trends in WMSDs or identify symptoms that indicate risk for WMSDs.

   a. Symptom surveys, worker questionnaires, and symptom diaries allow workers to track the symptoms they encounter during and after work, relating it to the tasks of their job. Examples include the following:
      1) Discomfort rating scales
      2) Body part maps

   b. These methods depend upon worker self-report, which may limit the validity of the information.

   c. The advantage of worker reports is the ability to identify jobs with potential risk factors for WMSDs before full-blown injuries or illness occurs.

   d. The data gathered may be useful in evaluating ergonomic interventions.

E **Work-site hazard evaluation examines both job demands and human capacities.**

1. The purposes of a work-site hazard evaluation include:
   a. Identify hazards that may be risk factors for WMSDs.
   b. Identify and correct the causes of the hazards.
   c. Examine the interaction of the worker with the job demands.

2. The job demand evaluation examines the components of the work environment which include:
   a. Tools, machines, and materials
   b. Workstation and the physical environment
   c. Job tasks, including the organization environment in which it is performed

3. Job hazard analysis encompasses the methods used to analyze job tasks and the performance demands of jobs.
   a. These methods include direct observation or videotaping of workers and work processes, job function lists, and site surveys.
   b. Tools to assist in the job hazard analysis include videotape, ergonomic checklists, and forms. Examples can be found on the NIOSH web site (http://www.cdc.gov/niosh/pdfs/95-119.pdf), and Chapter 9 presents additional information.
   c. Checklists are used to identify common hazard sources in a timely manner, while ensuring that systematic and standardized procedures are followed.
   d. Videotaping allows time-and-motion analysis, to identify risks, such as repetition or awkward and static postures, or to describe regular and irregular activities that are part of the job.

4. Human capacities are an integral part of ergonomics; however, for most job demands, there aren't well-defined limits.
   a. Design of workstations can be complimented by use of anthropometric tables.

BOX 14-4

Human capacities guidelines and performance measures

Human capacities guidelines
- NIOSH Lifting Equation (http://www.cdc.gov/niosh/ 94-110.html)
- Liberty Mutual Manual Handling Tables
- ANSI S3.34-1986 (R1997) Hand Arm Vibration Standards (http://web.ansi.org/default.htm.)
- Job Strain Index (http://sgwww. satx.disa.mil/hscoemo/tools/ strain.htm)
- Physiological measures, such as heart rate, blood pressure, oxygen consumption, and body temperature are sometimes used to assess the effects of work demands on the body (http:// www.cdc.gov/niosh/pdfs/ 95-119.pdf.)
- Subjective assessments, such as perceived exertion ratings and scales, collect information used to determine human capacity. Normally they are combined with physiologic measures (http:// www.cdc.gov/niosh/pdfs/ 95-119.pdf).

Performance measures
- Time
- Accuracy
- Frequency
- Amount achieved or accomplished
- Consumption or quantity used

---

    b. Several guidelines for determining human capacities coupled with the human requirements of the job that will minimize the risk of injury have been researched and published (Box 14-4).

    c. When worker's capacities are exceeded by the demands of the job, performance is affected.

F **Hazard prevention and control components focus on ways to reduce or eliminate the hazards associated with risk factors for WMSDs.**

    1. The most widely accepted hierarchy for controlling workplace hazards is as follows:

        a. Engineering controls aim to remove the hazard or limit its risk in the work process by altering the physical work area, work tools, or work process. (See Box 14-5)

        b. Administrative controls (policies and procedures implemented and supported by management) aim to reduce the worker's exposure to risk factors or hazards; administrative controls also include work-practice

---

BOX 14-5

Considerations for engineering controls

Tool and Equipment Design

Tools and equipment should be:
- Sized to fit the individual user
- Counterweighted to minimize the force necessary to use the tool
- Balanced so the grip is at the center of gravity
- Designed without sharp edges
- Designed to minimize vibration and minimal rotational forces
- Designed to minimize tension on finger-triggers

Controls and Displays
- Location of controls and displays depends on:
  - Importance, frequency, and sequence of use
  - Height of user
- Controls and displays should be visible and accessible
- Controls and displays should be spaced to accomodate personal protective equipment

Workstation and Work Environment Design

Design of workstations should consider:
- Workspace layout
- Work surfaces
- Standing and walking surfaces
- Seating
- Work fixtures
- Materials handling
- Storage
- Lighting
- Noise levels
- Temperature regulation

Work Methods and Process

Work methods and process should consider:
- Work rates
- Sequence of actions
- Job steps

---

controls (strategies for the manner in which work is performed). Examples include the following:

1) Scheduling strategies to limit time of exposure to specific hazards
   a) Job rotation—alternating a worker between two or more jobs within a single workday to minimize the exposure to hazards. The jobs or tasks should consist of significantly varied risk factors.
   b) Job enlargement—this form of job rotation varies the type of risk factors the worker is exposed to in different work tasks.
2) Rest breaks or recovery pauses
3) Training
4) Tools and equipment maintenance schedules
5) Scheduled housekeeping for work areas
6) Providing for worker control over job pace and processes

2. Personal protective equipment (PPE) provides a barrier between the worker and the hazard source. Examples of accepted PPE for ergonomic exposures include the following:
   a. Vibration attenuation gloves
   b. Ear plugs or noise reduction devices
   c. Antifatigue insoles
   d. Knee pads
   e. Temperature control clothing

f. Eye protection
g. Wrist supports or splints and back belts are not considered PPE.
  1) Wrist supports or splints are considered immobilization devices; they may be included in medical treatment as part of the health management program.
  2) NIOSH believes that "evidence for the effectiveness of back belts is inconclusive" (http://www.cdc.gov/niosh/ergoscil.html).

L Training and Education

Training and education are an integral part of an ergonomics program.

A Ergonomic awareness provides the basic education on ergonomics and WMSDs (Box 14-6).

B Job-specific training provides education in the hazards specific to particular job tasks and the methods to avoid the risk factors for WMSDs (Box 14-6).

C Supervisors and managers also need to have training to properly ensure safe work practices and implement ergonomic controls.

D Videotaping of hazardous jobs and risk factors can be useful as a training tool (e.g., demonstrating proper and improper work processes and techniques).

E Training should be conducted:
1. In the primary language of the workers
2. At the appropriate education level of the workers
3. On paid time
4. In a method and style appropriate to the workers and workplace

---

BOX 14-6

Contents of ergonomics training

Awareness training
- Types of WMSDs associated with jobs
- Symptoms of WMSDs
- Recognition and reporting of symptoms
- Hazards
- Risk factors for WMSDs
- Principles of ergonomics (such as neutral postures)
- Workplace analysis methods
- Prevention and control methods
- Workplace policies and procedures for reporting
- Content of the ergonomic program
- Worker's role
- Responsibility for components of program
- Reporting procedures

Job specific training
- Job specific hazards
- Tool and equipment maintenance
- Hands-on training for a new job
- New employee safe work practices
- New work processes
- Proper lifting techniques
- Correct body postures and motions
- Use of PPE, if any

LI Health Care Management

A *Health care management* is the effective use of available health care resources to ensure early detection, evaluation, and treatment and prevent impairment and disability related to WMSDs.

B Health care management encompasses a wide range of activities (Box 14-7).

C Preplacement physical examinations may be used to identify existing conditions, but are not considered useful in screening workers for risk.

D Components of health care management may be done within the company, or contracted out to other service providers.

E The health care management team should include the occupational and environmental health nurse, company physician or other licensed health care providers, physical or occupational therapist, nurse case manager, and the safety/industrial hygiene department.

LII Documentation and Recordkeeping

A Develop a written program that provides the following:
1. The basis for documentation of plans
2. Historical record of activities
3. Data to use in evaluating the program.

B Maintain and store all training and education records.

C Documentation of the following data is advised:
1. Risk factors and hazards
2. Worker aggregate and individual symptoms records
3. Injury and illness records
4. Treatment records
5. Hazard prevention and control measures

BOX 14-7

Components of health care management

- Health surveillance
- Occupational health history taking
- Early recognition and reporting of symptoms of WMSDs
- Access to evaluation and appropriate conservative treatment, including referral
- Alternative duty or transitional work programs—placing workers into temporary positions to accommodate their functional capacity limitations while recovering from WMSDs
- Job evaluations and periodic workplace walk-throughs
- Education for health care providers on workplace hazards
- Rehabilitation and work hardening—work hardening involves gradually introducing the full workload over time, enabling the worker to build up endurance for the job
- Injury and illness case management
- Recordkeeping and confidentiality

D Keep personal health data, such as occupational health histories, treatments, and symptom questionnaires and surveys that contain information that may identify workers, in confidential health files. The information released to other company employees should be aggregate data only.

LIII Program Evaluation

A Ergonomic evaluation can be accomplished using the quality assessment (i.e., structure, process, outcome) framework developed by Donabedian (1966) (Chapter 8, Section V).

1. Examples of structural elements to be considered in an ergonomic evaluation
   a. Evidence of management support and commitment to the program
   b. Adequate human, financial, and training resources to implement and evaluate the program
   c. Policies and procedures that are supportive of the program
   d. Evidence of employee participation
   e. Support of health and safety identified in the company's mission statement
2. Examples of basics to include in the process evaluation include tracking the actions taken to implement the program and the dates the activities were accomplished:
   a. Establishment of the ergonomic team completed by stated date
   b. Number of employees afforded ergonomic training
   c. Number of requests for ergonomic evaluations of workstations or tools
   d. Number of ergonomic evaluations completed
   e. Number and type of ergonomic solutions implemented
3. Outcome evaluation elements cover the effects achieved or the goal achieved by the ergonomics program or specified components of the program.
   a. Worker outcomes that should be examined
      1) Incidence of reported WMSDs
      2) Description of the severity of the WMSD
      3) Completeness of incident reporting by workers
      4) Worker morale
      5) Worker's quality of life
   b. Organizational outcomes that should be examined
      1) Affects of WMSDs on productivity and quality of product or service
      2) Workers' compensation costs related to WMSDs
      3) Number of restricted duty days or days away from work
      4) Turnover and absenteeism data

B Training and education evaluation must examine both knowledge and skills.

C Videotaping before and after ergonomic interventions provides objective demonstration of ergonomic controls and hazard reduction.

BIBLIOGRAPHY

American Association of Occupational Health Nurses. (1995). Accident investigation. *AAOHN Advisory*. Atlanta, GA: AAOHN.

American Public Health Association. (1990). *Control of communicable diseases in man* (15th ed.). Washington, DC: American Public Health Association.

Auf der Heide, E. (1989). *Disaster response principles of preparation and coordination.* St. Louis, MO: C.V. Mosby.

Bernardo, M.A. (1988). *Drug abuse in the workplace: An employer's guide for prevention.* (2nd ed.). Tustin, CA: Substance Abuse Training Systems (Substance Abuse Awareness Program, Employee Handbook, DPS).

Bezruchka, S.A. (1992). *The pocket doctor: Your ticket to good health while traveling* (2nd ed.). Seattle, WA: The Mountaineers.

Daugherty, J. (1995). Hazard communication for small plants. *Occupational Hazards, 57*(2), 37.

Dawood, R. (1994). *Traveler's health: How to stay healthy all over the world.* New York: Random House.

Donabedian, A. (1966). Evaluating the quality of medical care. *Milbank Fund Quarterly, 44(3),* 166-206.

Environmental Protection Agency (1978). Protective noise levels, EPA 550/ 9-70-100. Washington DC: Environmental Protection Agency.

Fagel, M.J. (1994). Drilling for disaster. *Occupational Hazards, 56*(7), 23–25.

Gasaway, D.C. (1987, Feb. 26). Thirteen steps to developing an effective hearing conservation program. *Plant Engineering,* 51–53.

Hans, M., (1995). Are you prepared for a crisis? *Safety + Health, 151*(6), 38.

Hau, M. (1995). Emergency action plans: Is yours just an illusion? *Safety + Health, 151*(9), 156.

Jeffress, C. (1999). Ergonomics in the Workplace. Presented to Massachusetts Ergonomics Fair in Firchburg, MA.

Jong, E.C. (1995). *The travel tropical medicine manual.* Philadelphia: W. B. Saunders Co.

Kelly, R.B. (1989). *Industrial emergency preparedness.* New York: Van Nostrand Reinhold.

LaBar, G. (1992). Hazard communication: A performing art. *Occupational Hazards, 55(20),* 35–38.

Levy, B.S. & Wegman, D. H. (Eds.). (1999). *Occupational health: Recognizing and preventing work-related disease* (4th ed.). Boston: Little, Brown & Company.

Lewis, G.W. (1993). Managing crises and trauma in the workplace: How to respond and intervene. *AAOHN Journal, 41*(3), 124-130.

Machles, D. (1999). Travel health information on the internet. *AAOHN Journal. 47(7),* 337-338.

McGill, L.D. (1989, Autumn). OSHA's hazard communication standard: Guidelines for compliance. *Employment Relations Today,* 181–187.

Meyer, M.U. & Graeter, C. J. (1995). Health professional's role in disaster planning: A strategic management approach. *AAOHN Journal, 43(7),* 251-262.

National Institute for Occupational Safety and Health. (1995). Cumulative trauma disorders in the workplace: Bibliography. (http://www.cdc.gov/niosh/pdfs/95-119.pdf)

Ostendorf, J.S., Rogers, B., & Bertsche, P. K. (2000). Ergonomics: CTD management evaluation tool. *AAOHN Journal 48(1),* 17-24.

Rom, W.N. (1998). *Environmental & occupational medicine* (3rd ed.). Philadelphia: Lippincott-Raven Publishers.

Royster, J.D. & Royster, L. H. (1990). *Hearing conservation programs: Practical guidelines for success.* Chelsea, MI: Lewis Publishers.

Russell, G., (1994). *The revised NIOSH lifting equation* [On-line]. Available: http:// www.industrialhygiene.com/calc/lift.html.

Saphire, L.S. & Doran, B. (1996). International travel preparedness—A guideline for occupational health professionals. *AAOHN Journal. 44(3),* 123-128.

Sarkus, D.J. (1992). A complete written disaster plan helps maintain business as usual. *Occupational Health and Safety, 61(9),* 34-36.

Schneider, S. (1999). National Academy of Sciences workshop and report on the science of ergonomics. *Applied Occupational and Environmental Hygiene, 14(2),* 75-7.

Snook, S.H. & Ciriello, V. M. (1991). The design of manual handling tasks: revised tables of maximum acceptable weights and forces. Ergonomics *34(9)*, 1197-213.

Suter, A.H. (1993). *Hearing conservation manual* (3rd ed.). Milwaukee, WI: Council for Accreditation in Occupational Hearing Conservation.

Thompson, M.C., Holihan, E., & MacNeal, B. (1996). Health on the road: Developing a program for international travelers. *AAOHN Journal, 40(6),* 300-309.

Travers, P.H. & McDougall, C. (1995). *Guidelines for an Occupational Health & Safety Service.* Atlanta, GA: AAOHN Publications.

U.S. Department of Health and Human Services. (1990). *A practical guide to effective hearing conservation programs in the workplace* (DHHS [NIOSH] publication No. 90-120). Washington, DC: U.S. Government Printing Office.

U.S. Department of Health and Human Services. (1997a). *Musculoskeletal disorders and workplace factors: a critical review of epidemiological evidence for work-related musculoskeletal disorder of the neck, upper extremity, and low back* [On-line]. Available: http://www.cdc.gov/niosh/ergoscil.html.

U.S. Department of Health and Human Services. (1997b). *Elements of ergonomics programs: a primer based on workplace evaluations of musculoskeletal disorders* [On-line]. Available: http://www.cdc.gov/niosh/ephome2.html.

U.S. Department of Health and Human Services. (1997c). *Worker protection: Private sector ergonomics programs yield positive results* (Letter Report, 08/27/97, GAO/HEHS-97-163 [On-line]). Available: http://www.cdc.gov/niosh/gaoergo.html.

U.S. Department of Health and Human Services. (1997d). Comments by R. Niemeier to DOL on the Occupational Safety and Health Administration Proposed Rule on Ergonomic Safety and Health Management, February 1 and August 24, 1993 [On-line]. Available: http://www.cdc.gob/niosh/pdfs/95-119.pdf.

U.S. Department of Labor, Occupational Safety and Health Administration. (1983). Final rule. Rules and regulations: OSHA noise standard. 29 CFR 1910.95. *Federal Register, 48(46).*

U.S. Department of Labor, Occupational Safety and Health Administration. (1989). *OSHA's expanded hazard communication standard* (Fact Sheet No. OSHA 89-26) 1989-242-368/08071. Washington, DC: U.S. Government Printing Office.

U.S. Department of Labor, Occupational Safety and Health Administration. (1991). *Occupational noise exposure compliance assistance guideline,* 1991-519-701-20406, Washington, DC: U.S. Government Printing Office.

U.S. Department of Labor, Occupational Safety and Health Administration. (1992). *Hearing conservation.* OSHA Publication No. 3074 (Revised).

U.S. Department of Labor, Occupational Safety and Health Administration. (1994). *Chemical hazard communication.* (OSHA Publication No. 3084, revised). Washington, DC: U.S. Government Printing Office.

U.S. Department of Labor, Occupational Safety and Health Administration. (February 9, 1994). Final Rule. Hazard communication. 29 CFR Part 1910, 1200, *Federal Register, 45(27).*

U.S. Department of Labor, Occupational Safety and Health Administration. (1995). *Hazard communication guidelines for compliance* (OSHA Publication No. 3111, revised). Washington DC: U.S. Government Printing Office.

U.S. Department of Labor. (1991). *Ergonomics program management guidelines for meatpacking plants* [On-line]. Available: http://www.osha-slc.gov/Publications/Osha3123.pdf\.

U.S. Department of Labor. (1998). OSH Act, section5, 1970, amended July 1998 [On-line]. Available: http://www.osha-slc.gov/OshAct_toc/OshAct_toc_by_sect.html.

U.S. Department of Labor. (2000). *Ergonomics standard proposal* [On-line]. Available: http://www.osha-slc.gov/ergonomics-standard/overview.html.

U.S. Department of Transportation. (1994a, February). *Alcohol and drug rules: An overview.* (P.L. 100-690, 41 USF & 701 et seq.).

U.S. Department of Transportation. (1994b, February). *Alcohol and drug rules.* 49 CFR 382 et. al., 49 CFR Part 40, *Federal Register.*

Washington State Department of Labor and Industries, Industrial Safety and Health Division. (1993). *Understanding "Right to Know."* P413-000 (3/93). Olympia, WA: Washington State Department of Labor and Industries, Industrial Safety and Health Division.

Washington State Department of Labor and Industries (WSDOLI). (1993). *Fitting the job to the worker: an ergonomics program guideline.* Olympia, WA: WSDOLI.

Washington State Department of Labor and Industries (WSDOLI). (1999). Ergonomics Web site [On-line]. Available: http://www.lni.wa.gov/wisha/ergo/default.htm.

Washington State Industrial Safety and Health Act, RCW 49.17, Department of Labor, WAC 296.24.073.

Weinstock, M.P. (1993). Hazard communication: Clearing up the confusion. *Occupational Hazards, 54(7),* 35-39.

Wolfe, M. S. (Ed.). (1993). *Health hints for the tropics* (11th ed.). Northbrook, IL: American Society of Tropical Medicine and Hygiene.

Wuorinen, V. (1986). *Emergency planning.* Hamilton, Ontario, Canada: Canadian Centre for Occupational Health and Safety.

Zabel, A.M. & McGrew, A.B. (1997). Ergonomics: A key component in a CTD control program. *AAOHN Journal 45(7),* 350-358.

SECTION THREE

Advancing Professionalism in Occupational and Environmental Health Nursing

~

CHAPTER

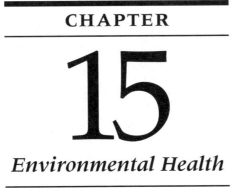

15

Environmental Health

JANE LIPSCOMB AND BARBARA SATTLER

The environment is one of the primary determinants of individual and community health. Nurses must understand the mechanisms and pathways of exposure to environmental health hazards, basic prevention and control strategies, the interdisciplinary nature of effective interventions, and the role of research and advocacy. Environmental-protection standards in the United States are intended to be health-based and therefore health-protective.

Environmental health comprises those aspects of human health, including quality of life, that are determined by physical, chemical, biological, and social and psychological problems in the environment. It also refers to the theory and practice of assessing, correcting, controlling, and preventing those factors in the environment that can potentially affect adversely the health of present and future generations. (WHO, 1993)

I Introduction

A The environment of the 21st century

1. Tens of thousands of synthetic chemicals that did not exist before the 1940s have been introduced to the environment.
2. Synthetic chemicals can be found in food, air, soil, and water—in workplaces, schools, homes, and communities.
3. Synthetic chemicals can be found within human bodies (including breast milk) in measurable amounts.
4. To date, there is limited information regarding the human health effects associated with many of the synthetic chemicals in our environments (EPA, 1998).
5. Publicly accessible toxicity data are *not* available for 71% of the 3,000 high-production industrial chemicals (EPA, 1998).

B Magnitude of environmental health issues

1. Chemical exposures
   a. Of the top 20 environmental pollutants that were reported to the Environmental Protection Agency (EPA) in 1997, nearly 75% were known or suspected neurotoxins; this accounted for more than a billion pounds of neurotoxins being released into the air, water, and land.
   b. 1.2 billion pounds of pesticide products are intentionally and legally released each year in the United States.

c. More than 50% of Americans live in an area which exceeds current national ambient air quality standards for ozone, nitrous oxide, sulfuric oxide, and particulates.

d. Forty states have issued one or more health advisories for mercury in their waterways; ten states have issued advisories for *every* lake and river within their borders.

e. Mobile sources (motor vehicles) are the number one cause of air pollution in the United States.

f. Antibiotics, 17b-estradiol (estrogen-like chemical), caffeine, and acetaminophen have been found in measurable quantities in the nation's streams.

g. *Consumer Reports* (1998) tested leading-brand beef baby food and measured dioxin levels that exceeded the EPA allowable quantities by 100 times.

h. Thirty million Americans drink water that exceeds one or more of the EPA safe drinking-water standards. Contaminants include lead, other heavy metals, nitrites, dioxin, hydrocarbons, pesticides, radon, and cyanide. (Some of the contaminants are naturally occurring.)

2. Human health concerns associated with environmental exposures

a. Combinations of commonly used agricultural chemicals, in levels typically found in groundwater, can significantly influence the immune and endocrine systems and neurological function in laboratory animals.

b. Thirty-seven pesticides registered for use on food are neurotoxic organophosphates.

c. It has been estimated that radon may be responsible for about 20% of lung cancers among nonsmokers (Zenz, 1994).

d. Several pesticides and herbicides have been linked to leukemia.

e. Endocrine disrupters are a diverse group of compounds that include plasticizers, polychlorinated biphenyls, many pesticides, and dioxins.

1) These compounds are so pervasive that studies have shown them to appear in 95% of the population.

2) When exposure to these chemicals occurs very early in life, these compounds have the potential to disrupt critical endocrine pathways with potential to disrupt effects on the reproductive, neurologic, and immunologic systems.

3) Dioxin mimics estrogen.

f. Poor indoor and outdoor air quality increases asthma's severity.

g. The environment has a principle role in causing cancer.

C **Chemical, biologic, and radiologic risks in the environments in which people live, work, play, and learn**

1. The relationship between environment and health is determined by host factors such as age, gender, genetic makeup, underlying diseases, dose-response factors, and the length of time exposed. (Chapter 5 provides additional information about toxicology.)

2. Chemical and radiological exposures can be cumulative. Occupational and environmental health nurses must assess a person's total exposure to environmental risks in order to understand and address potential health threats.

3. As in occupational health, environmental health is based upon a public health model with an emphasis on prevention. Preventive interventions in

environmental health include pollution prevention, product design, engineering controls, purchasing choices, and education.

4. Although U.S. environmental standards (e.g., EPA, OSHA) are "health-based," they often are not sufficiently protective of our most vulnerable populations.

   a. Standards are often based on the health risks to an otherwise healthy, 70 kilogram (154 pound), white male.

   b. The standards may not provide sufficient protection to pregnant women and fetuses, young children, the frail and the elderly, or the immuno-compromised.

II Environmental Health Assessment

A **Potential environmental exposures and environmentally related diseases can be assessed individually or on a community-wide basis.**

1. Individual environmental health assessments should take into account all of the potential exposures that a person may have in the home, work place, school, and community.

   a. The Agency for Toxic Substances and Disease Registry (ATSDR) has developed a general assessment tool (ATSDR, 1992) and an assessment tool specifically for pesticide exposures in agricultural settings.

   b. The Children's Environmental Health Network has developed a health assessment tool for children (http://www.cehn.org).

2. Community environmental health assessments identify potential exposures in water (including drinking water), air (including indoor air), dust (including lead-based paint particles), soil (including exposures from current and previous land use), and radiation (ionizing and nonionizing).

   a. There is no single source for environmental assessment information and often there will be no community-specific information.

   b. Assessments may depend on extrapolating down from aggregate national, statewide, county, or metropolitan exposure data.

3. A geographic information system (GIS) is a method for assessing community risks to environmental exposures and potential health problems.

   a. A GIS consists of computerized mapping of graphically related data that may be specific to environmental exposures and health outcomes.

   b. More information on GIS may be obtained from http://www.gisportal.com, the Agency for Toxic Substances and Disease Registry or geography departments in universities.

4. An essential competency for environmental health assessments is knowledge of the federal, state, and local health and environmental statutes, regulations, and practices regarding what data are collected and how they are accessed.

B **Epidemiology and toxicology are the principle sciences used to determine the relationship between environmental exposures and health outcomes. (Chapter 5 provides an overview of these sciences.)**

1. Environmental epidemiology

   a. Analytical studies (cohort and case control) are often the design of choice in environmental health; experimental studies are rarely done because it is unethical to intentionally expose individuals or communities to environmental hazards.

   b. Cluster investigations are often used to respond to community concerns about an excess of cancer or birth defects.
      1) These investigations usually render negative or equivocal results.
      2) Cluster investigations are most convincing when the disease in question is rare and very specific for the putative etiologic exposure, as is the case in asbestos causing mesothelioma.
   c. Limitations are inherent in environmental epidemiology.
      1) Exposures are often poorly defined and measured.
      2) A very limited understanding of the health effects of mixed exposures makes studying the most common type of environmental exposure situations particularly challenging.
      3) Often a relatively small number of individuals (e.g., a community) constitute the study populations, yielding limited statistical power to detect an association between exposures of concern and health effects.
      4) A lack of understanding about variability in the susceptibility of segments of the populations (e.g., the poor, children, elderly) limits the ability to compare findings across studies.
      5) The long latency between many environmental exposures and the evidence of chronic disease, in particular cancer, creates additional challenges to exposure assessment.

2. Environmental toxicology
   a. Toxicology, which is the science that investigates the adverse affects of chemicals on health, is similar to pharmacology (Table 15-1).
   b. The effects of drugs and hazardous chemicals can be immediate (acute), long-term, or can present after a latency period often associated with cancer outcomes.
   c. Host factors must be considered when looking at therapeutic drugs or hazardous chemicals. Such factors as age, sex, genetics, weight, drugs that the person may be taking, and pregnancy status may effect the therapeutic or toxic effect of a drug or a chemical.
   d. Drugs are taken voluntarily and often under the supervision of a licensed health care provider. Hazardous chemical exposures are often involuntary.
   e. The regulatory process by which a drug comes to the market includes several stages of animal and human testing. The regulatory process for hazardous chemicals that are not food, drug, cosmetic, or pesticide in nature does not require *any* original testing.

III Children and Environmental Health

A **Children have unique risks related to environmental exposures.**
   1. The metabolic and physiologic processes of children differ dramatically from those of adults. Their skin, respiratory, and gastrointestinal absorption of toxic materials is greater than that of adults.
   2. Children's normal exploratory behavior (e.g., hand-to-mouth activity and crawling) increases opportunities to ingest toxicants such as lead-based paint.
   3. Children spend most of their time indoors and therefore come into contact with a large number of household chemicals and pollutants used for cleaning, personal care, and hobbies.

TABLE 15-1

Comparison of pharmacology and toxicology

Pharmacology	Toxicology
Pharmacology is the scientific study of the origin, nature, chemistry, effects, and use of drugs.	*Toxicology* is the science that investigates the adverse effects of chemicals on health.
Dose refers to the amount of a drug absorbed from an administration.	*Dose* refers to the amount of a chemical absorbed into the body from a chemical exposure.
A drug can be administered one time, short-term, or long-term.	*Exposure* is the actual contact that a person has with a chemical. Exposure can be one-time , short-term or long-term.
A *dose-response curve* graphically represents the relationship between the dose of a drug and the response elicited.	A *dose-response curve* describes the relationship of the body's response to different amounts of an agent such as a drug or toxin.
Routes of administration are oral, IM, IV, dermal, topical, etc.	*Routes of entry* are ingestion, inhalation, dermal absorption.
With drugs there are therapeutic responses (desirable) and side effects (undesirable). Beyond the therapeutic dose, a drug may become toxic.	In toxicology, only the toxic effects are of concern. *Toxicity* is the ability of a chemical to damage an organ system, disrupt a biochemical process, or disturb an enzyme system.
Potency refers to the relative amount of drug required to produce the desired response.	The *potency* of a toxic chemical refers to the relative amount it takes to elicit a toxic effect compared with other chemicals.
Biological monitoring is done for some drugs: clotting time is monitored in patients on anticoagulants like warfarin. Actual drug levels are measured for some drugs like digoxin.	*Biological monitoring* is done for some toxic exposures, such as blood lead levels or metabolites of chemicals such as cotinines for environmental tobacco smoke.

Sattler, 1998.

IM, intramuscular; *IV,* intravenous.

4. Children born today will cumulatively have more exposures throughout their lifetime than children born in earlier times.
5. Exposure to environmental toxins may disrupt and cause permanent damage to the developing nervous, immune, and respiratory systems of young children.

B **Children have not routinely been included in risk assessment and most environmental health regulations are based on studies of adult males.**

C **There is increasing evidence that a wide range of reproductive disorders, including male and female infertility, menstrual irregularities, spontaneous abortion or fetal loss, major and minor birth defects, and developmental abnormalities, may result from human exposure to any of a number of toxic substances.**

D Environmental hazards affecting children
  1. Ten million U.S. children live within four miles of a toxic waste dump.
  2. One million children in the United States exceed currently acceptable levels of lead in their blood (10 µg/dl); this exposure may be associated with a

range of health effects, including behavioral (e.g., violent behavior) and cognitive effects.

3. Environmental tobacco smoke is responsible for 7 million lost school days by children.

4. Epidemiologic studies suggest a relationship between nitrates in drinking water and juvenile diabetes.

5. Many children are exposed to toxins from manufacturing plants in their neighborhoods; for example, 20% of the children in Arkansas who live near an herbicide manufacturing plant, had herbicide residues in their urine.

6. Asthma is the number one reason that children miss school and are hospitalized in the United States.

IV Environmental Justice and Advocacy

A *Environmental justice* refers to the "fair treatment for people of all races, cultures, and incomes, regarding the development of environmental laws, regulations, and policies" (http://www.epa.gov/swerosps/ej/index.html).

1. The environmental health status that poor communities experience is subject to the compounding effects of poor housing, poor nutrition, poor access to health care, unemployment, underemployment, and employment in the most hazardous jobs.

2. The environmental risk burden is generally greater for minorities and those who are economically disadvantaged because they are exposed to a greater number and intensity of environmental pollutants in food, air, water, homes, and workplaces.

3. Information sharing may be inadequate or less effective in economically disadvantaged communities as a function of language and literacy issues, in addition to the challenge of understanding technical language in warning signs and other right-to-know materials.

4. Indicators of increased risk include:
   a. Proximity to hazardous waste sites, polluting industries, and incinerators
   b. Substandard housing that may have friable asbestos, deteriorating lead paint, and yards with contaminated soil

5. Federal mandates to address environmental justice include:
   a. Environmental Justice Act (1993)
   b. Executive Order 12898 (1994): Federal Actions to Address Environmental Justice in Minority Populations

6. The passage of federal legislation resulted in the development of policies to more comprehensively reduce the incidence of environmental inequity by mandating that every federal agency act in a manner to address and prevent environmental illnesses and injuries.

7. In 1994, the National Environmental Justice Advisory Council was created as a federal advisory committee to the EPA to convene community, governmental, and business constituents to assess environmental justice issues and make recommendations to the Administrator of the EPA.

B *Advocacy* and *environmental justice* are interrelated concepts of critical importance to the field of environmental health.

1. *Case advocacy* refers to the process of advocating for individual patients and families to solve problems and secure needed services.

2. *Class advocacy* is aimed at changing policy, institutional systems, and norms, laws, or patterns of resource allocation to improve the health of the group or community.
   a. *Collaborative approaches* (e.g., membership on planning and advisory committees) are characterized as citizens and authorities working collaboratively to reach an agreed upon goal.
   b. *Campaigning approaches* (e.g., lobbying) require that citizens or professionals work singly or collectively to persuade authorities that new problem definitions and solutions are needed.
   c. *Contest strategies* (e.g., protest marches) involve citizen organizing to force attention to community problems that they feel are being ignored or mishandled by authorities.
3. Nurses are often the primary health care providers in poor and disenfranchised communities; advocacy on behalf of these communities is critical to improving the health of these communities.

V Risk Assessment, Risk Management, and Risk Communication

Risk is the probability of undesirable effects (or unhealthy outcomes) arising from exposure to a hazard. Risk assessment, risk management, and risk communication are critical strategies for dealing with environmental risks.

A *Risk assessment* **refers to the use of available information to evaluate and estimate exposure to a substance and the resulting adverse health effects.**
   1. Risk assessment includes the following four steps:
      a. *Hazard identification* relies on toxicologic and epidemiologic studies of the potential of a substance to cause harm.
      b. *Dose-response evaluation* measures whether the harm increases with increasing doses of the substances.
      c. *Exposure assessment* involves measuring the amount of the chemical or other harmful substances to which a population is exposed with a goal of estimating the dose.
      d. *Risk characterization* involves estimating the public or environmental impact or problem.
   2. Risk assessment, in public health terms, has a much broader definition; it includes individual and community assessment.
   3. An assessment of a community's resources, including their cohesiveness and leadership, should be included as part of a risk assessment.

B *Risk management* **is the process of evaluating alternative strategies for reducing risk and prioritizing or selecting among them.**
   1. Risk management strategies often involve policy development; this may include regulatory, legislative, and voluntary options and may be targeted at the local, state , national, or international level.
   2. Environmental engineering is a critical tool in risk management.
   3. Engineering strategies to control exposure to environmental hazards are similar to the industrial hygiene "hierarchy of controls"; they include the following:
      a. Reduction of pollution at its source (source reduction)
      b. Waste minimization
      c. Reuse, recycling

      d. Emissions control

      e. Waste cleanup

4. Risk-management strategies should always include education of all involved parties regarding the nature of risk and the costs and benefits of proposed risk-management strategies.

5. Coalition building and community action are vehicles to successful risk management.

6. Legal remedies may be used to manage risk in combination with the above strategies.

7. Community members should always be "at the table" when decisions are being made about risk management.

8. The *Precautionary Principle* assumes that where there are possible threats of serious or irreversible damage, lack of scientific certainty shall not be used as a reason for postponing cost-effective measures to prevent environmental degradation.

C *Risk communication,* **in the context of environmental health, is the art of communicating about the potential health risks associated with environmental exposures.**

1. There are four elements to consider in risk communication: the message, the messenger, the audience, and the context.

      a. Considerations related to the *message*

         1) Environmental health risks are often difficult to define.

         2) Exposures may be difficult to characterize.

         3) The exposed population may be very diverse in age and many other important variables.

         4) Exposures will always include multiple chemicals because it is the nature of "environments" (whereas most scientific investigation is primarily about individual chemicals and rarely chemical mixtures).

         5) Sometimes scientific evidence is inconclusive or nonexistent.

      b. Characteristics of the successful *messenger*

         1) The messenger must be perceived as trusted and credible. Nurses are considered highly credible and trustworthy sources of information within the community.

         2) The messenger must be prepared to communicate with empathy and care when the message evokes hostile emotions.

      c. Characteristics of the *audience*

         1) Audiences bring individual biases to any forum in which environmental health risks might be discussed.

         2) Audience's distrust of the messenger may be based on their feelings about who the messenger represents (e.g., government, industry, or an environmental organization).

         3) An audience may trust or distrust a messenger based on his or her age, race, sex, etc.

      d. Considerations related to *context*

         1) Risk communication does not occur in a vacuum; it often occurs when there has been a perceived environmental health threat such as a potentially contaminated water supply, an accidental release of a hazardous chemical, or a newly identified hazardous waste site adjacent to a daycare center.

         2) The conditions and context will influence the audiences' ability to listen and trust.

TABLE 15-2

Factors that affect perceptions of risk

Risks may be *perceived* as "less" or "more" risky based on the following attributes:

Less risky	More risky
Voluntary	Involuntary
Familiar	Unfamiliar
Controllable	Uncontrollable
Controlled by self	Controlled by others
Not memorable	Memorable
Not dread	Dread
Chronic	Acute
Diffuse in time and space	Focused in time and space
Not fatal	Fatal
Immediate	Delayed
Natural	Artificial
Individual mitigation possible	Individual mitigation impossible
Detectable	Undetectable

Source: Sandman, 1993.

      3) The media can play an important part in a community's understandings and biases regarding environmental risk.

2. Risk communication is affected by risk perception. Table 15-2 lists factors that affect the perceptions of risk.

3. The Environmental Protection Agency has created a list of *7 Cardinal Rules for Risk Communication:*

    a. Accept and involve the public as a legitimate partner.

    b. Plan carefully and evaluate your efforts.

    c. Listen to your audience.

    d. Be honest, frank, and open.

    e. Coordinate and collaborate with other credible sources.

    f. Meet the needs of the press.

    g. Speak clearly and with compassion.

VI Federal Agencies

A Numerous federal agencies deal with issues related to the environment, including safety and health in the workplace. (Appendix I provides addresses of agencies.)

1. Federal agencies have become increasingly involved in examining and monitoring the impact of the environment on the health of the public. Examples of this involvement include the following:

    a. The Department of Transportation, which regulates hazardous materials transportation

    b. The Food and Drug Administration, which regulates food safety

    c. The ATSDR (within USDHHS), which is responsible for environmental health-related issues associated with actual or potential exposure to hazardous substances from waste sites, unplanned releases, and other sources of pollution in the environment (ATSDR, 1992).

2. Environmental statutes and regulations may be promulgated and implemented on a federal, state, or even local level.

3. Most environmental statutes are media-specific, such as air, water, soil, and food.

4. As with occupational health statutes, states must adhere to the federal environmental statutes. States may promulgate more stringent, but not less stringent, statutes and regulations.

B **The EPA and its state counterparts are the primary regulatory agencies responsible for environmental protection and the protection of health from environmental risks.**

1. The EPA was established by Congress through the 1970 National Environmental Policy Act to permit coordinated and effective governmental action on behalf of the environment.

2. The EPA endeavors to abate and control pollution systematically by properly integrating a variety of research, monitoring, standard setting, and enforcement activities.

3. The EPA coordinates and supports research and antipollution activities by state and local governments, private and public groups, individuals, and educational institutions.

4. The EPA also reinforces efforts among other federal agencies to monitor and control the impact of their operations on the environment.

5. Each state has a designated agency that is responsible for regulatory oversight of all environmental regulations and standards.

6. The EPA has 10 regional offices around the country.

7. Most environmental-protection laws are reauthorized by Congress every 5 years.

C **The U.S. Department of Health and Human Services is the department of the federal executive branch most concerned with the nation's human health concerns. Within USDHHS, the following subagencies focus on environmental health:**

1. The National Institute of Environmental Health Sciences is the principle federal agency for biomedical research on the effects of chemical, physical, and biologic agents on human health and well-being.
   a. The Institute supports research and training focused on harmful agents in the environment.
   b. Research forms the basis for preventive programs for environmentally related diseases and for action by regulatory agencies.

2. The ATSDR was created by Superfund legislation in 1980.
   a. ATSDR's mission is to prevent or mitigate adverse human health effects and diminished quality of life resulting from exposure to hazardous substances in the environment.
   b. ATSDR's activities include public health assessments, health investigations, exposure and disease registry, emergency response, toxicologic profiles, health education, and applied research.

3. The Centers for Disease Control and Prevention is charged with protecting the nation's public health.
   a. Within the CDC, the National Center for Environmental Health (NCEH) focuses on environmental health issues.
   b. The mission of the NCEH is to promote health and quality of life by preventing or controlling disease, injury, and disability related to the

interactions between people and their environment outside the work place.

4. The Consumer Product Safety Commission provides information on health and safety effects related to consumer products, including chemical hazards in consumer products.

D **The Department of Energy (DOE) regulates industry involved in energy research and production, and manages many national energy research facilities. It is responsible for providing a framework for a balanced, comprehensive national energy plan.**

1. The Office of Environment, Safety and Health of the DOE provides independent oversight of departmental execution of environmental and occupational safety and health, nuclear and non-nuclear safety, and environmental restoration.

2. The Office of Environmental Management provides program policy development and guidance for the assessment and cleanup of inactive waste sites and facilities and for waste management operations.

E **The U.S. Department of Agriculture (USDA), as part of its food safety administration, regulates pesticides, hormones, and antibiotics used in food supply.**

1. The mission of the USDA's Food, Nutrition and Consumer Services is to ensure access to nutritious, healthful diets for all Americans, through food assistance and nutrition education for consumers.

2. The Food and Drug Administration (FDA) inspects food and drug manufacturing plants and warehouses; collects and analyzes samples of foods, drugs, cosmetics, and therapeutic devices for adulteration and misbranding; and enforces the Radiation Control Act as related to consumer products. With the USDA, the FDA collects information about food required by a number of regulations (U.S. Department of Agriculture, 1998).

F **The Nuclear Regulatory Commission licenses, inspects, and regulates civilian use of nuclear energy to protect health and safety and the environment. This is achieved by licensing persons and companies to build and operate nuclear reactors and other facilities and to own and use nuclear materials.**

G **The Occupational Safety and Health Administration was created within the Department of Labor under the Occupation Safety and Health Act (OSH Act) of 1970 to promulgate and enforce national occupational health and safety standards (Chapter 3).**

H **The National Institute for Occupational Safety and Health was established by the OSH Act to conduct research on occupational diseases and injuries, respond to requests for assistance by investigating problems of health and safety in the workplace, and recommend standards to OSHA.**

VII Accessing Information and the "Right to Know"

A **Access to information about environmental risks in our food, water, and soil is provided through a variety of agencies via an array of federal and state statutes.**

1. A range of environmental right-to-know statutes and regulations exist; the

mandatory labeling of store-bought foods is an example of a consumer right-to-know requirement.
   a. Access to information about food is provided by a number of regulations, implemented by the USDA and FDA.
   b. This information includes the ingredients, nutritional content, and in some instances health-related information, such as the designation that a food is *organic*.
2. Access to information about water is provided under two statutes: the Clean Water Act and the Safe Drinking Water Act.
   a. The Clean Water Act was promulgated to protect the nation's waterways, whereas the Safe Drinking Water Act protects drinking water from its source to the tap.
   b. Through the Safe Drinking Water Act, residents who purchase water from a water provider have the right to know what is in their drinking water.
   c. Annually, as part of the drinking water right-to-know regulations, the water utility must provide a "consumer confidence" or "right-to-know" report listing the contaminants (chemical, biologic, and radiologic) that have exceeded EPA standards within the last year and their probable sources.
   d. Information regarding the source of surface drinking water can be obtained from the EPA web site.
3. Industrial contaminants that are released into the air or water are reportable, based on the chemical and its quantity, under the right-to-know component of the Superfund Amendments and Reauthorization Act of 1986 (SARA).
   a. SARA requires polluters to report certain effluents and emissions.
   b. Two sources of information about SARA are the EPA web site and http://www.scorecard.org (an excellent source for community environmental assessments).
4. Employees have the right to know under the Hazard Communication Standard, an occupational safety and health standard regulated by OSHA (Chapter 14 provides additional information about this standard).
5. States may establish additional rights to know.
6. The 1966 Freedom of Information Act provides that any person can make requests for government information.
   a. Citizens are not required to identify themselves or why they want the information.
   b. Certain restrictions exist on work in progress, enforcement confidential information, classified documents, and national security information

Environmental health risks across settings

Individual environmental health assessment should take into account all of the potential exposures that a person may have in their homes, workplace, schools, and community.

VIII Environmental Health Risks in the Home
A Home environments can be affected by the following:
1. Building products (e.g., urea formaldehyde insulation, asbestos, lead-based paint, lead pipes, lead solder)

2. Heating, ventilation, and air conditioning (carbon monoxide)
3. Consumer products (e.g., aerosols, nail polish remover [acetone], air fresheners, and dry-cleaned clothes)
4. Cleaning products (e.g., ammonia, chlorine)
5. Arts/hobby activities (e.g., glues, paints, leaded stained glass)
6. Pesticides
7. Furnishings, including carpets
8. Renovation and rehabilitation activities (e.g, paint removers, adhesives)
9. Contaminants that are taken home from workplaces
10. Inappropriately handled, stored, and disposed household hazardous materials

B **Lead in homes poses a serious hazard to family members.**
1. Dust emanating from lead-based paint poses a major threat to our nation's children.
2. Lead poisoning is the most preventable of the environmentally related diseases that children suffer.
3. There are a wide array of state and federal statutes and regulations regarding lead-based paint poisoning from both the housing inspection/ remediation perspective and the health screening/treatment perspective.
4. Lead-based paint was banned from indoor use in 1978.
5. The symptoms of lead poisoning are varied; they include neurological deficits (affecting both the peripheral and central nervous systems), renal damage, hypertension, and reproductive problems (in both males and females).

C **Pesticides are associated with multiple health effects.**
1. Regular indoor or outdoor use of pesticides increases the risk of leukemia to children who reside in the home.
2. Pesticide "foggers" often have persistent active ingredients that take up residence in textiles such as stuffed animals, pillows, and other items with which children may have close contact.
3. Pesticides applied to produce may pose a threat to health.
4. The Food Quality Protection Act addresses health risks associated with pesticides in food (Appendix VII).

D **Many indoor air contaminants (chemical and biologic) can trigger asthmatic events; biologic contaminants include bacteria, mold and mildew, mites, animal hair and dander, and pollen.**

E **Because of high risk associated with radon, all homes should be tested for radon and, if indicated, remediated.**

F **Environmental tobacco smoke is associated with a wide array of health problems. Smokers should smoke outside, especially if children reside in the home.**

G **Drinking water derived from private wells should be analyzed regularly to determine its fitness for drinking.**

H **Much of the meat and poultry in the United States is treated with hormones (including bovine growth hormone) and antibiotics (more than 50% of the antibiotics sold in the United States are used in animal feed to improve animal growth).**

I In 1990, the Organic Foods Production Act was passed to establish national standards governing the marketing of certain agricultural products as organically produced products, assure consumers that organically produced products meet a consistent standard, and facilitate commerce in organically produced fresh and processed food.

IX Environmental Risks in Schools

A On any given school day, one sixth of the U.S. population can be found in a school building.

B School environments provide many of the same risks as home environments from indoor air contaminants.

1. Schools are more likely to use industrial-strength cleaners and pest control measures that may create health risks for children.
2. Safe and adequate drinking water and sanitary facilities are an issue in some schools.

C Many schools, including those that are expressly vocational training schools, mimic workplaces; automotive programs, arts and science rooms, cosmetology programs, construction shops, and photography darkrooms present risks similar to their industrial counterparts.

1. As such, the industrial hygiene hierarchy of controls should be applied to protect students, teachers, and school staff members from unhealthy exposures.
2. It should be recognized that children may be even more vulnerable to exposures.

D Carpeting can be the source of chemical and biological contaminants. It is advisable to either have easily cleaned surfaces, such as tile flooring, or to have a rigorous cleaning program for carpeting to minimize unhealthy exposures.

X Environmental Risks in the Community

A Environmental health risks in the community may derive from unhealthy air, water, or soil.

1. The Clean Air Act regulates air pollution from fixed sites and non-point sources.
2. Air pollution encompasses anthropogenic chemical emissions (e.g., combustion products, volatile chemicals, aerosols [particulate]), their atmospheric reaction products, and heavy metals.
3. The burning of fossil fuel (e.g., in diesels, industrial boilers, and power plants) and waste incineration are two other major contributors.
4. Health effects associated with air pollution include asthma and other respiratory diseases, cardiovascular diseases (including hypertension), cancer, immunologic effects, reproductive health problems (including birth defects), and neurologic problems.
5. Dioxins and furans are products of combustion from chlorinated compounds resulting from waste incineration.
   a. Incinerated hospital waste is a major source of dioxin in the United States because of the heavy reliance on polyvinyl chlorides in the health care industry.

b. These probable carcinogens are also endocrine disrupters, and are considered by the EPA to be reproductive toxicants.

B **Industrial sites (old and current) are sources of air, water, and soil contamination.**

1. Such sites may be designated Brownfield or Superfund sites.
   a. *Brownfields* are abandoned, idled, or underused industrial and commercial facilities where expansion or redevelopment is complicated by real or perceived environmental contamination (EPA definition).
   b. *Superfund* hazardous waste sites are sites that have been identified by the EPA as the most seriously contaminated in the nation.
      1) The Superfund is also known as the Comprehensive Environmental Response, Compensation, and Liability Act, enacted by Congress on December 11, 1980.
      2) The National Priorities List is a compilation of sites targeted for cleanup under Superfund.
2. These designations (Superfund and Brownfield) are derived from federal and state environmental statutes and are applied when a site is environmentally compromised and creating a health risk.

C **Safe and reliable drinking water is a basic requirement.**

1. Approximately half of the country derives its drinking water from groundwater (via wells) and the other half from surface water (via wells, reservoirs, lakes, and rivers).
2. Public water suppliers must test their final water product for approximately 80 EPA-designated contaminants.
   a. The results of testing must be reported to consumers annually.
   b. There is no regulation requiring residents to test wells from which they derive their drinking water.
3. Our drinking water sources (both ground and surface) may be contaminated by industrial waste streams, pesticides, or fertilizer run-off. Superfund sites often cause groundwater contamination. The most common groundwater contaminant from Superfund sites is trichloroethylene, a carcinogen.
4. Each state must have a plan for protecting their sources of drinking water.
5. The U.S. Geologic Service has measured acetaminophen, caffeine, codeine, and 17-b estradiol in our nation's streams.
   a. These are derived from human waste.
   b. In addition, antibiotics have been measured in aquifers near hog "factories" and concentrated animal feed organizations (factory farms or intensive livestock production operations that are owned by large corporations).
6. Some drinking water contaminants are naturally occurring, such as radon and arsenic.
7. Some drinking water contaminants occur cyclically with the use of agricultural chemicals, such as atrazine-contaminated groundwater during the growing season.
8. Leaking chemical storage tanks (above ground and underground) pose hazards to the soil and groundwater, almost always associated with human health risks.

XI Environmental Risks at Work

A Occupational exposures of concern to surrounding communities include industrial chemicals that may be a source of much environmental degradation within a community.

B Occupational and environmental health nurses can serve a vital role in communities that house industrial sites.
1. Communicating the community's planning efforts for anticipated and accidental chemical releases will help protect the community's health.
2. Occupational and environmental health nurses should establish relationships with public health and other nurses in the community to promote communication regarding industrial activities that may pose a health risk to the surrounding community.
3. Occupational and environmental health nurses can serve on local emergency planning committees, state source-water protection planning boards, and other public forums regarding environmental health protection.

C Information regarding chemical releases from industrial sites is available via the Environmental Defense web site: http://www.*scorecard.org*.

D The EPA provides information collected by its Toxic Release Inventory database via the EPA web site: http://www.epa.gov.

Nurses' roles in environmental health

The following section describes findings and recommendations from the Institute of Medicine report, *Nursing, Health and the Environment* (IOM, 1995).

XII General Environmental Health Competency for Nurses

All nurses should have the following competencies (IOM, 1995):

A Understand the scientific principles and underpinnings of the relationship between individuals or populations and the environment, including the following:
1. The basic mechanisms and pathways of exposure to environmental health hazards
2. Basic prevention and control strategies
3. The interdisciplinary nature of effective interventions
4. The role of research

B Assess and refer, using the following strategies:
1. Successfully completing an environmental health history
2. Recognizing potential environmental hazards and sentinel illnesses
3. Making appropriate referrals for conditions with probable environmental etiologies
4. Accessing and providing information to patients and communities, and locating referral sources

C Demonstrate knowledge of the role of advocacy (case and class), ethics, and risk communication in patient care and community intervention with respect to the potential adverse effects of the environment on health.

D Understand the policy framework and major pieces of legislation and regulations related to environmental health.

XIII The Institute of Medicine's Recommendations on Nursing Practice, Education, Research, and Advocacy

A Environmental health should be reemphasized in the scope of responsibilities for nursing practice.

1. Resources to support environmental health content in nursing practice should be identified and made available.
2. Nurses should participate as members and leaders in interdisciplinary teams that address environmental health problems.
3. Communication should extend beyond counseling individual patients and families to facilitating the exchange of information on environmental hazards and community responses.
4. The concept of advocacy in nursing should be expanded to include advocacy on behalf of groups and communities, in addition to advocacy on behalf of individual patients and their families.
5. Research regarding the ethical implications of occupational and environmental health hazards should be conducted and findings incorporated into curricula and practice.

B Environmental health concepts should be incorporated into all levels of nursing education.

1. Environmental health content should be included in nursing licensure and certification examinations.
2. Expertise in various environmental health disciplines should be included in the education of nurses.
3. Environmental health content should be an integral part of lifelong learning and continuing education for nurses.
4. Professional associations, public agencies, and private organizations should provide more resources and educational opportunities to enhance environmental health awareness in nursing practice.

C Multidisciplinary and interdisciplinary research endeavors should be developed and implemented to build the knowledge base for nursing practice in environmental health.

1. The number of nurse researchers should be increased to build the knowledge base in environmental health as it relates to the practice of nursing.
2. Research priorities for environmental health nursing should be established and used by funding agencies for resource allocation decisions and to give direction to nurse researchers.
3. Current efforts to disseminate research findings to nurses, other health care providers, and the public should be strengthened and expanded.

D Nurses should have the skills to work with the community, environmental groups, and local government, including the following activities:

1. Legislative lobbying
2. Reporting community hazards
3. Advocating for safer environments
4. Policy implementation

E Nurses can be involved with environmental health in other ways, such as the following:

1. Generating data systems for environmental assessment and outcomes

2. Designing "critical paths" that include environmental assessment
3. Conducting impact studies (e.g., consumer goods, land use)
4. Increasing the visibility of nurses in environmental health policy development and implementation
5. Educating, of course, but also petitioning the political system for change. Law changes behavior more effectively than public education (e.g., bike helmet and seat belt laws).
6. Revolutionizing nursing education to focus more on social justice and critical thinking.
7. Serving as role models, and developing role expectations such that attention to environmental health is routine.

BIBLIOGRAPHY

Agency for Toxic Substances and Disease Registry. (1992). *Taking an exposure history, Case studies in environmental health*, No. 26. Atlanta, GA: U.S. Department of Health and Human Services.

Consumer Reports. (1998). Hormone mimics hit home: Tests of plastic wraps, baby foods. *Consumer Report Online*, http://www.consumerreports.org/Special/ConsumerInterest/Reports.

Environmental Health Perspectives: *Journal of the National Institute of Environmental Health Sciences* (including Special Supplements on Children, Cancer, and Asthma)

Environmental Protection Agency. (January, 1998). *Parent's guide to school indoor air quality.* Washington, DC: EPA.

Environmental Protection Agency. (1998). *Chemical hazard data availability study: what do we really know about the safety of high production volume chemicals?* Washington, DC: Office of Prevention, Pesticides and Toxic Substances, http://www.epa.gov/opptintr/chemtest/hazchem.htm

Etzel, R.E., Balk, S.J., & the Committee on Environmental Health of the American Academy of Pediatricians. (1999). *Handbook of pediatric environmental health.* Elk Grove Village, IL: American Academy of Pediatrics.

Greater Boston Physicians for Social Responsibility and the Massachusetts Public Interest Research Group Education Fund (Greater Boston PSR and MASSPIRG). (1996). *Generations at risk: How environmental toxics may affect reproductive health in Massachusetts.* Cambridge, MA: PSR.

Institute of Medicine. (1995). *Nursing, health and the environment: Strengthening the relationship to improve the public's health.* Washington, DC: National Academy Press

Lichtenstein, P., Holm, N.V., Kerkasalo, P.K., Iliadou, A., Kaprio, J., Koskenvuo, M., Pukkala, E., Skytthe, A., & Hemminki, K. (2000). Environmental and heritable factors in the causation of cancer, *New England Journal of Medicine. 343*, 78-84.

Sandman, P. (1993*). Responding to community outrage: Strategies for effective risk communication.* Fairfax, VA: AIHA Publications.

Schettler, T., Solomon, G., Valenti, M., & Huddle, A. (1999). *Generations at risk: Reproductive health and the environment.* Boston, MA: Massachusetts Institute of Technology.

Schettler, T., Stein, J., Reich, F., & Valenti, M. (2000). *In harm's way: Toxic threats to development,* a Report by Greater Boston Physicians for Social Responsibility (PSR), prepared for a joint project with Clean Water. Cambridge, MA: PSR.

Steingraber, S. (1997). *Living downstream: A scientist's personal investigation of cancer and the environment.* NY: Random House.

U.S. Department of Agriculture. (1998). *Agriculture fact book.* Washington DC: Office of Communications.

Zenz, C. (1994). *Occupational medicine* (3rd ed.). St. Louis, MO: Mosby.

16

Research

BONNIE ROGERS

Research is essential to support and expand the knowledge base for occupational and environmental health nursing practice. Through research, occupational and environmental health nurses can improve the health and safety of the workplace, and, ultimately, the quality of workers' lives. This chapter focuses on basic elements in the research process, research priorities, funding sources, evaluation criteria, communication of research findings, and the use of research findings, which are critical to advancing this specialty practice.

I Professional Mandates for Research

A **According to AAOHN's Standards of Occupational and Environmental Health Nursing (Standard X, Research), the occupational and environmental health nurse contributes to the scientific base in occupational and environmental health nursing through research, as appropriate, and uses research findings in practice (AAOHN, 1999).**

　　1. AAOHN supports occupational and environmental health nursing research by encouraging participation and providing resources (through the AAOHN Foundation) to conduct research, and by publishing research in the AAOHN Journal.

　　2. The occupational and environmental health nurse engages in research through activities such as identifying researchable problems; designing and conducting research; disseminating research findings; writing research grant proposals; and collaborating with other disciplines on research studies.

B **The American Nurses Association (ANA) Standards of Clinical Nursing Practice (Standard VII, Research) says, "The nurse uses research findings in practice" (ANA, 1998).**

　　1. The nurse uses research data to develop the plan of care and interventions.

　　2. The nurse participates in research activities as appropriate to the individual's education and position.

II Research Roles of Occupational and Environmental Health Nurses by Education Level

A **Associate Degree/Diploma: The occupational and environmental health nurse identifies clinical problems for research, assists in the development of the research and data collection activities, and uses research as a basis for clinical practice.**

B Baccalaureate Degree: The occupational and environmental health nurse evaluates research for applicability to practice, works with skilled researchers to develop research projects, uses research to refine and extend the practice, and discusses research findings with colleagues.

C Master's Degree: The occupational and environmental health nurse provides expertise related to the research problem, care delivery, and the research process; analyzes the practice problems within the context of the scientific process; contributes to an environment supportive of nursing research; supports the conduct of research; disseminates research findings; collaborates with other disciplines in scientific investigations; and encourages the integration of research into practice.

D Doctoral Degree: The occupational and environmental health nurse develops and conducts independent and collaborative investigations with other scientists; develops methodologies for scientific inquiry into phenomena relevant to the practice of occupational and environmental health and safety; uses analytical methods and integrates findings to explain and extend scientific knowledge to nursing practice; develops and tests interventions to improve worker health and safety; acquires research grant support; disseminates findings; and provides leadership for integrating research findings into practices.

III Purposes of Research

Purposes of research in occupational and environmental health (Polit & Hungler, 1999):

A Help identify and solve problems relevant to nursing practice.

B Improve the effectiveness of nursing care through scientific inquiry using a systematic process.

C Advance the body of knowledge in the occupational and environmental health nursing discipline.

IV Ethics in Research

A To protect all study participants' rights, the investigator must provide subjects with the following:
1. Description of study purpose
2. Discussion of risks and benefits
3. Assurance of confidentiality (and of anonymity, where appropriate)
4. Specification of a contact person

B *Consent* to participate in the research must be obtained from each study subject.
1. Consent usually covers an explanation of the study, procedures used, risks, invasion of privacy, and methods used to protect the identity of the subjects (i.e., anonymity or confidentiality).
   a. *Anonymity:* Protection of participants in a study such that even the researcher cannot link the subjects with the information collected.
   b. *Confidentiality:* Protection of participants in a study such that their identities will not be linked to the information they provide and that individually identifiable information collected will not be divulged.

2. Consent is usually obtained with a written statement from subjects, or it may be described by the researcher in a cover letter notifying subjects to voluntarily return survey forms; in these cases, return of the survey implies consent.

3. Special circumstances may be related to informed consent, such as literacy or non–English speaking workers. The researcher must ensure that study participants have a full understanding of research procedures, which may include reading the consent statements or interpreting information for the participant.

C Research is usually approved by an ethics committee commonly referred to as an Institutional Review Board. This committee oversees the ethical treatment of study participants and assesses the study's impact on them.

V Research Development

This section outlines the scientific process for the conduct of research and the logical steps needed to develop a research proposal. Box 16-1 lists the steps in the research process.

A Identification of the problem
1. The problem that is identified should consist of a situation that needs a solution and that will contribute to improving practice.
2. The problem is relevant to contemporary nursing practice and is stated clearly and precisely.
3. Research of the problem will contribute to the body of nursing knowledge.
4. Research of the problem will explain, describe, and predict behaviors, and will test strategies or interventions to modify or improve outcomes.

B Significance of the Study
1. The research problem needs to address the "so what?" question.
2. The importance of the problem should be explained by describing its critical characteristics, pointing out gaps in the literature, and presenting possible solutions.

C Literature review
1. The literature is discussed to help the researcher critically evaluate existing research and provide a context or frame of reference for the study.
2. Literature sources may include previous studies relevant to clinical or

---

BOX 16-1

Steps in the research process

- Formulate the problem
- Review the literature
- Develop a theoretical framework
- Formulate hypothesis/question(s)
- Identify research variables
- Operationalize variables
- Select research design
- Specify population
- Conduct pilot studies
- Select sample
- Collect data
- Organize data for analysis
- Analyze data
- Interpret results
- Communicate findings

NOTE: There may be some variation in the conduct of pilot studies.

substantive articles, conceptual or theoretical understanding, and method-
ological readings.
3. Material for review and inclusion should be current but also capture
long-standing issues and classical articles.
4. When conducting a literature search, the researcher can use several
resources, such as print indexes or electronic databases (Box 16-2), or
consult with a reference librarian. In any search, key words, text words, or
subject headings can be used to identify articles that may be valuable.
5. When critiquing a research study, the following should be considered:
    a. Clarity, logic, and understandability of the study
    b. Currency of the study and its applicability to practice
    c. Strength of the questions and hypotheses and that they are addressed in
       the analysis
    d. Theoretical framework, if used
    e. Appropriate design, sample, and interpretation of findings
    f. Protection of subjects' rights
    g. Limitations
6. Literature should be analyzed and synthesized.

D **Problem statement/formulation**
1. The problem statement introduces the topic, explains the importance of the
problem, and states what the research intends to study.
2. The problem statements may be grounded within a theoretical framework
(links and explains the relationships among different theories) or conceptual framework (building blocks of theories). However, not all research
studies may be sufficiently developed to have these frameworks (e.g.,
descriptive studies).
3. Types of questions (Brink & Wood, 1988)
    a. Type I research question: Expression of a single concept with the stem
       beginning with "what." Little or no knowledge about the topic exists.
       Example: What are occupational and environmental health nurses'
       attitudes about managed care?
    b. Type II research question: Examines relationships between two or more
       concepts or variables. Example: What is the relationship between stress
       and cholesterol?

BOX 16-2

*Common electronic databases used in occupational and environmental
health*

- **CINAHL:** Cumulative index
  to nursing and allied health
  literature
- **MEDLINE:** Medical literature
  on-line
- **TOXNET:** Toxicology database
- **EMBASE:** Exerpta medica

- **NIOSH TIC:** NIOSH database
- **TOXLINE:** Toxicology
- **HSDB:** Hazardous substance
  database
- **RTECS:** Registry of toxic effects
  of chemical substances

NOTE: Search home pages of federal and state agencies (e.g., OSHA, EPA, NIOSH) for links to other
sources of databases.

   c. Type III research question: Builds on type I and II questions and examines a causal relationship using an experimental design. Asks why. Example: Why does an increase in stress result in increased musculoskeletal disorders?

E **Formulation of hypothesis, if appropriate**
1. Hypotheses require a theoretic basis and are used to test an idea.
2. A hypothesis suggests a relationship among two or more variables and is used when the researchers can predict an outcome. Example: Stress reduction programs are likely to reduce musculoskeletal disorders.

F **Definition of terms**
1. *Conceptual definitions* explain interrelationships among concepts (e.g., self-esteem and eating disorders).
2. *Operational definitions* guide the implementation of the study (e.g., an occupational and environmental health nurse can be defined as a registered nurse whose primary focus is workers and worker populations).

G **Methodology**
1. Designs: There are many types of designs which can be used to answer research questions. Designs fall into two major categories (Polit & Hungler, 1999).
   a. *Experimental designs* are used to test research hypotheses and infer causal relationships.
     1) A true experiment requires random assignment of subjects, a control group, and manipulation of a treatment or intervention (independent variable) for the experimental group. Example: Randomly assign subjects to two groups; administer treatment to one group, and measure the outcome or effect in both groups.
     2) *Quasi-experimental* designs include manipulation of the treatment or intervention; however, this design lacks either a control group or random assignment of subjects.
     3) *Preexperimental designs* manipulate the variable or treatment in only one group (i.e., no comparison group or randomization), and measure the effect.
   b. *Nonexperimental designs* are used when the research does not support an experiment (e.g., survey). Two broad categories are included:
     1) *Descriptive studies* are designed to observe and describe the phenomenon under investigation and are not concerned with relational variables.
     2) *Ex post facto* (sometimes called *correlational*) research examines relationships between variables (that have already occurred) and *implies* a correlation (e.g., smoking and lung cancer).
2. Variables
   a. Dependent variable: This is the study variable under investigation (i.e., the outcome variable).
   b. Independent variable: This is the variable that is presumed to have an effect or influence on the dependent variable. In an experimental design, it is the treatment or intervention.
   c. Example: Is absenteeism higher among workers who work straight or rotating shifts?
     1) Dependent variable: absenteeism
     2) Independent variable: shift work

3. Research instruments/measurements
   a. Instrumentation
      1) Existing instruments or tools are often available for the researcher to use. The researcher should search the literature carefully for available instruments which can be used or modified to answer the research questions.
      2) If no instruments or tools are available, the researcher may need to develop and pilot test a new tool.
   b. Reliability and validity of the instrument
      1) The *reliability* of an instrument is its degree of consistency in measuring responses of the attribute under study. Types of reliability measurements include the following:
         a) *Stability,* which refers to the extent to which the same results are obtained on repeated administrations of the instrument (also referred to as *test-retest*).
         b) *Internal consistency,* wherein all of items included measure a certain attribute, not some other tangential attribute.
         c) *Equivalence,* wherein the instrument produces the same (or equivalent) results when administered by two different observers or raters.
      2) *Validity* refers to the degree to which an instrument measures what it is supposed to measure. Examples include the following:
         a) Content validity, which is concerned with the sampling adequacy of the content area being measured.
         b) Criterion-related validity, which focuses on the relationship or correlations between the instrument and some outside criterion (e.g., an instrument to measure self-performance would be validated by manager ratings).
4. Population and sample
   a. The target population includes all persons who fit the characteristics the researcher wants to study and to whom the results can be generalized. Not all members of a population can be included in a study, so a sample may be used.
   b. The sample size needs to be adequate within the context of the design and problem under investigation.
   c. Depending on subject availability, time, and resources, different types of samples may be used.
      1) Probability sampling: All elements or subjects have an equal chance of being included. Types of samples include random, stratified random, systematic random, and clusters.
      2) Nonprobability sampling: Subject selection is not based on chance (e.g., the subjects are volunteers). Types of samples include convenience, quota, purposive, and snowball.
      3) Probability sampling is more representative of the population; the results of studies that rely on probability sampling are less subject to bias and can be generalized more easily.
5. Data collection: This is the phase of the study wherein the researcher gathers the data specific to the purpose and questions. Several methods can be used, depending on what types of data are needed.
   a. Interview: A generally structured approach with specific questions that can be asked face to face or via the telephone

  b. Questionnaire: A written response to survey items, using a structured format or open-ended questions
  c. Observation: Systematic observation of subjects and recording of data for later analysis
  d. Physiologic: Methods for measuring bio-physiologic data, such as blood and urine samples, electrocardiograms, etc.
  e. Record review: Gathering data from charts related to specific indices or criteria under investigation
  f. Focus group: A group interview with participants assembled to answer questions on a given topic

6. Data analysis: During this phase, the researcher examines the data using statistical approaches, analyzes relationships between the data and the research questions, and forms conclusions and recommendations.

  a. *Quantitative data* provide descriptive statistics and comparative analysis about phenomena measured at the nominal, ordinal, interval, or ratio levels. The higher the level of measurement, the more powerful the results.

    1) *Nominal level* measurement (lowest level) is simply the assignment of numbers to classify data into mutually exclusive categories (e.g., 1 = male, 2 = female).
    2) *Ordinal level* measurement involves the sorting of elements on the basis of their relative standing to each other, yielding a ranking (e.g., 1 = completely independent to 5 = completely dependent).
    3) *Interval level* measurement yields equivalent distance between numerical values on scales (e.g., temperature scale).
    4) *Ratio level* measurement (highest level) permits numerical calculations or operations and has an absolute zero.

  b. *Qualitative data* provide descriptions about phenomena and help generate hypotheses.

  c. *Descriptive analysis* discusses what was found in the study. Common descriptions include the following:

    1) Frequency distributions (i.e., counts of the number of times a value was obtained) presented in tables or graphs that report the overall summary of group characteristics
    2) Summary of a group's characteristics when describing ages, educational levels, etc. (i.e., mean [average], range [highest score minus the lowest score in a given distribution]), and the standard deviation [degree to which scores deviate from each other])

  d. *Inferential analysis* begins to specify relationships between variables.

7. Interpretation of findings

  a. Clearly state the answers to research questions, which hypotheses were supported or not supported, and formulate conclusions and recommendations.
  b. Discuss findings within the context of the practice discipline and suggest future research.
  c. The researcher must be careful in stating to whom the findings are generalized, paying attention to how the sample was selected.

NOTE: For purposes of developing research proposals, the researcher should explain the data analysis plans in detail based on the scientific design of the study.

VI Research Dissemination

A It is essential to disseminate research findings to build knowledge, improve practice, and share results with colleagues (D'Antonio, 1997).

B Most original research is published in peer-reviewed journals, such as the AAOHN Journal.
1. Articles generally provide an abstract, background information, methodology, findings, and discussion sections.
2. Although providing scientific information is critical, research reports should also be reader friendly and applied to practice.

C Research is also disseminated through presentations at scientific meetings and may be discussed in work settings where the research work was conducted.

VII Research Utilization

A Practice application: Implementation of research into nursing practice is guided by its significance, the degree to which results can be generalized to populations, and the feasibility of implementation, including an analysis of cost-benefit issues.

B Evaluation: Several factors should be considered before implementing findings into practice, including critical review of the literature, sample representativeness, adequate study design, ethicality, reliability and validity of instruments, consistency with other studies, and cost-effectiveness.

VIII Research Priorities

A Based on guidance from the membership about important research topics to advance the profession and improve the practice, updated occupational and environmental health nursing research priorities have been published (Box 16-3) (Rogers et al., 2000).

B The National Institute for Occupational Safety and Health has published National Occupational Research Priorities, grouped into three categories (NIOSH, 1996):
1. Disease and injury
   a. Allergic and irritant dermatitis
   b. Asthma and chronic obstructive pulmonary disease
   c. Fertility and pregnancy abnormalities
   d. Hearing loss
   e. Infectious diseases
   f. Low back disorders
   g. Musculoskeletal disorders of the upper extremities
   h. Traumatic injuries
2. Work environment and work force
   a. Emerging technologies
   b. Indoor environment
   c. Mixed exposures
   d. Organization of work
   e. Special populations at risk

BOX 16-3

Research priorities in occupational and environmental health nursing

1. Effectiveness of primary health care delivery at the work site
2. Effectiveness of health promotion nursing intervention strategies
3. Methods for handling complex ethical issues related to occupational and environmental health
4. Strategies that minimize work-related health outcomes (e.g., respiratory disease)
5. Health effects resulting from chemical exposures in the workplace
6. Occupational hazards of health care workers (e.g., latex allergy, blood-borne pathogens)
7. Factors that influence workers' rehabilitation and return to work
8. Effectiveness of ergonomic strategies to reduce worker injury and illness
9. Effectiveness of case-management approaches in occupational illness and injury
10. Evaluation of critical pathways to effectively improve worker health and safety and enhance maximum recovery and safe return to work
11. Effects of shift work on worker health and safety.
12. Strategies for increasing compliance with or motivating workers to use personal protective equipment.

---

3. Research tools and approaches
   a. Cancer research methods
   b. Control technology and personal protective equipment
   c. Exposure assessment methods
   d. Health services research
   e. Intervention effectiveness research
   f. Risk assessment methods
   g. Social and economic consequences of workplace illness and injury
   h. Surveillance research methods

IX Evaluating Research

The following elements should be considered when critically evaluating research reports (Rogers, 1995).

A **Title: Indicates clearly to the reader the intent and topic of the investigation.**

B **Abstract**
   1. Provides a clear but concise statement of purpose
   2. Summarizes the data analysis
   3. Describes important findings

C **Problem statement and purpose**
   1. Provides an introduction to the study topic, including the importance and need for the study.

   2. Identifies variables, basic design, population studied, and data collection methods.

D **Theoretic foundation**
1. The selected framework is relevant to the research and is understandable.
2. There is a clear link between the problem and the framework.

E **Literature review**
1. The literature specific to the problem was reviewed primarily from primary (original) sources in scientific, peer-reviewed journals.
2. Recent and past empirical studies are progressively presented and provide the context and scope of the problem.
3. The research reviewed is critically analyzed, gaps identified, and synopsis with implications for the rationale for the study is provided.
4. The review is clear, concise, and understandable.

F **Methodology**
1. Research questions are clearly stated and hypotheses show a relationship between variables.
2. Variables are conceptually and operationally stated and are amenable to measurement.
3. The research design is clearly indicated, providing the overall statement for the conduct of the research.
   a. Experimental
     1) Subjects are randomly assigned, the control group is identified and adequate, and the intervention is clear and measurable.
     2) Threats to validity of the design are controlled.
   b. Nonexperimental
     1) The best design method to address the research questions is selected and variables are controlled for in the design.
     2) Comparison groups, if used, are equivalent and representative.
4. Subjects and sample
   a. The target population is defined and subjects ascertained.
   b. The sample should be representative of the population and the sample size adequate for the statistical analysis and scientific rigor.
5. Instrumentation
   a. Instruments or tools used should be clearly described and should ask questions pertinent to the research questions or hypotheses.
   b. Validity and reliability data are provided.
   c. Newly developed instruments or tools should be adequately tested and described.
6. Data collection procedures
   a. Methods used to collect the data (e.g., reviews, questionnaires, physiologic measurements) are clearly described.
   b. Data collection procedures are internally consistent.
   c. The setting for data collection is described.
   d. Subject rights are protected.
7. Data analysis
   a. Demographics of the sample are provided and described.
   b. A description of statistical procedures used for data analysis, including levels of measurement appropriate to the questions, is provided.
   c. Research questions or hypotheses are addressed with appropriate descriptive and inferential statistics.

    d. Results are reported and interpreted correctly.

    e. Tables and graphs are used to clarify results and are reported in a way that allows the reader to evaluate the results.

  8. Interpretation and conclusions

    a. Findings that address the research questions are discussed along with their statistical significance and what that means.

    b. Findings are discussed within the context of existing knowledge and gaps are identified.

    c. Application of the findings to nursing practice and a discussion of practical strategies are given.

    d. Methodological problems and limitations are discussed.

    e. The degree to which the findings can be generalized is addressed.

    f. Suggestions for further research are made.

X Funding Research

Good research is not feasible if it cannot find funding.

A There are many sources of support for the conduct of research. (Table 16-1 lists selected sources of funding.)

  1. Professional societies (e.g., AAOHN, ANA)

  2. Government agencies (e.g., NIOSH, DOE, OSHA)

TABLE 16-1

Selected organizations for research funding for health related projects

Organization	Application deadline
Agency for Healthcare Research and Quality (AHRQ). Rockville, MD Phone: 301-594-1844　http://www.ahcpr.gov	February 1, June 1, October 1; January 15, May 15, September 15, for small grants
American Association of Occupational Health Nurses Foundation Atlanta, GA Phone: 770-455-7757　http://www.aaohn.org	December 1
American Cancer Society New York, NY Phone: 404-320-3333　http://www.cancer.org	April 1, October 15
American Federation on Aging Research New York, NY Phone: 212-570-2090　http://www.afar.org	December 15
American Lung Association New York, NY Phone: 212-315-8700　http://www.lungusa.org	October 1 November 1
American Nurses' Foundation Washington, DC Phone: 202-651-7227　http://www.ana.org	June 1
March of Dimes Foundation White Plains, NY Phone: 914-428-7100　http://www.modimes.org/	Varies

Continued

TABLE 16-1

Selected organizations for research funding for health related projects—cont'd

Organization	Application deadline
Metropolitan Life Foundation New York, NY Phone: 212-578-7049 http://www.enterprisefoundation.org	None
Ruth Mott Fund Flint, MI Phone: 810-232-3180 http://www.oneworld.org	March, July, November
National Institute for Nursing Research Bethesda, MD Phone: 301-496-0207 http://www.nih.gov/ninr	February 1, June 1, October 1
National Institute for Occupational Safety and Health Atlanta, GA Phone: 404-262-6575 http://www.cdc.gov/niosh/	February 1, June 1, October 1
National Institutes of Health (Cancer; Eye; Heart, Lung & Blood; Allergy/Infectious Diseases; Arthritis/ Musculoskeletal/Skin; Child Health; Diabetes/Digestive/ Kidney; Environmental Health; General Medical; Drug Abuse; Mental Health; Alcohol; Neuro/Communicative Disorders) Bethesda, MD: Phone: 301-496-7441 http://www.nih.gov Inquire for contact for individual institute	February 1, June 1, October 1
National Science Foundation Arlington, VA Phone: 703-375-7880 http://www.nsf.gov	None
PPG Industries Foundation Pittsburgh, PA Phone: 412-434-2453 http://www.ppg.com	September
Prudential Foundation Newark, NJ Phone: 973-802-7354 http://www.prudential.com	None
Robert Wood Johnson Foundation Princeton, NJ Phone: 609-452-8701 http://www.rwjf.org	None
Sigma Theta Tau International Indianapolis, IN Phone: 317-634-8171 http://www.nursingsociety.org	March 1

3. Foundations (e.g., Macy Foundation, Robert Wood Johnson)
4. Voluntary agencies (e.g., American Cancer Society, American Heart Association)
5. Corporations

B The AAOHN Foundation, established in 1998, has several research awards available to fund competitive applicants for researchable topics.

C The researcher should consider the research topic as it relates to the mission of the funding source before applying (Rogers, 1996 & 1992).

BIBLIOGRAPHY

American Association of Occupational Health Nurses. (1999). *Standards of occupational and environmental health nursing.* Atlanta: AAOHN.

American Nurses Association. (1998). *Standards of clinical nursing practice* (2nd ed). Washington, DC: ANA.

Brink, P.J. & Wood, M.J. (1988). *Basic steps in planning nursing research.* Boston: Jones and Bartlett.

D'Antonio, P. (1997). Toward a history of research in occupational health nursing. *Nursing Research, 46,* 105-110.

National Institute for Occupational Safety and Health. (1996). *National occupational research agenda.* Cincinnati, OH: USDHHS, CDC, NIOSH

Polit, D. & Hungler, B. (1999). *Nursing research: principles and methods.* Philadelphia: J.B. Lippincott.

Rogers, B. (1992). Research funding. *AAOHN Journal, 39,* 485-486.

Rogers, B. (1995). Critically evaluating research studies. *AAOHN Journal, 43,* 54-55.

Rogers, B. (1996). Researchability and feasibility issues in conducting research. *AAOHN Journal, 44,* 58-59.

Rogers, B., Agnew, J., & Pompeii, L. (2000). Research priorities in occupational health nursing. *AAOHN Journal, 48,* 9-16.

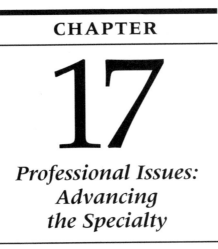

CHAPTER

17

Professional Issues: Advancing the Specialty

ELEANOR McCARTHY CHAMBERLIN AND ELIZABETH LAWHORN

Professional development is the process by which the occupational and environmental health nurse maintains professional competency and contributes to the professional growth of self and others. The purpose of this chapter is to provide an overview of issues and activities that are related to professionalism in occupational and environmental health nursing.

I Professional Associations

A **The American Association of Occupational Health Nurses is the professional association of nurses engaged in the practice of occupational and environmental health nursing.**

1. Major roles and responsibilities of AAOHN
   a. Defines the scope of practice and sets standards for occupational and environmental health nursing practice (AAOHN, 1999).
   b. Develops standards of professional conduct for the occupational and environmental health nurse as described in the AAOHN Code of Ethics (AAOHN, 1998) (Appendix VI).
   c. Promotes the health and safety of workers.
   d. Promotes and provides continuing education for occupational and environmental health nurses and professionals.
   e. Advances the profession by encouraging and facilitating research.
   f. Advocates for occupational and environmental health nursing in business, government, and other professional areas.
   g. Responds to issues critical to the practice of occupational and environmental health nursing.
      1) Governmental affairs action alerts
      2) Position statements and advisories, such as "Entry into Professional Practice", "Occupational Health Surveillance"
      3) Delineation of competencies and performance criteria in occupational and environmental health nursing practice
2. The *AAOHN Journal* is the official Journal of AAOHN. It provides information related to occupational and environmental health nursing practice, advisories, continuing education modules, and research literature.

425

B **AAOHN is guided by its vision and mission statements.**

1. AAOHN's vision statement is to "advance the profession of occupational and environmental health nursing as the authority on health, safety, productivity, and disability management for worker populations." (http://www.aaohn.org/mission.htm)

2. AAOHN's mission is to "advance the profession of occupational and environmental health nursing. AAOHN's mission is fulfilled through:

    a. Promoting professional excellence and opportunities through education and research

    b. Establishing professional standards of practice and code of ethics

    c. Influencing legislative, regulatory, and policy issues

    d. Promoting internal and external communications

    e. Establishing strategic alliances and partnerships" (Smith & Cox, 1997)

C **Contact information for AAOHN**

Address: 2920 Brandywine Road, Suite 100, Atlanta, GA 30341

Telephone: (770) 455-7757   Web site: http://www.aaohn.org

II Professional Credentialing in Nursing

Obtaining and maintaining high-quality nursing care for the public good is the basis of any process used in credentialing nurses, nursing education, and nursing services (ANA, 1979); credentialing is a complex process intended to define levels of practice and associated knowledge, skills, abilities, and competencies.

A **Major credentialing processes**

1. *Accreditation* is the process by which an agency or organization evaluates and recognizes an institution or program of study as meeting certain predetermined criteria or standards (Joel & Young, 1995).

2. An *academic degree* is awarded to an individual who has successfully taken an officially recognized, predetermined series of steps in a particular branch of learning.

    a. The designation of the academic degree signifies the level of education and indicates an arts or sciences area.

    b. The professional degree is similar, but the designation is an indication of the specific field of study (ANA, 1979).

3. *Licensure* is the process by which an agency of government grants permission to persons to engage in a given profession or occupation by certifying that those licensed have attained the minimal degree of competency.

    a. This process is intended to ensure that the public health, safety, and welfare will be reasonably well protected (Joel & Young, 1995).

    b. Licensure also authorizes the use of a particular title.

4. *Certification* is a voluntary process that demonstrates the achievement of mastery in the specialty area.

B **The American Board for Occupational Health Nurses (ABOHN) is an independent, autonomous, nursing-specialty certification board recognized in the United States for certifying individuals in the specialty of occupational and environmental health nursing. ABOHN's role in the certification process includes the following activities:**

1. Setting criteria and standards for certification

2. Setting policies and procedures for conducting certification
3. Using the definitions and standards of occupational and environmental health nursing practice set by AAOHN
4. Providing a peer review certification that attests that certified occupational and environmental health nurses have met standards for knowledge, experience, and education in the specialty
5. Basing the content of examinations on independent research regarding the practice patterns of occupational and environmental health nurses

C **Three certifications in occupational and environmental health nursing are currently available.**
1. COHN: The Certified Occupational Health Nurse credential is offered to registered nurses with associate, diploma, or higher degrees or their international equivalent. The focus of the credential is on the nurse's role as clinician, advisor, and coordinator.
2. COHN-S: The Certified Occupational Health Nurse Specialist credential is offered to nurses with a baccalaureate or higher degree and focuses on the nurse's role as educator, manager, clinician, and consultant.
3. COHN/Case Manager (CM) or COHN-S/CM: The COHN or COHN-S certification is required as a prerequisite for this occupational health case management credential. Therefore, it is understood that the roles validated by those credentials form the basis of occupational health nursing case management (ABOHN, 1999).

III Competency in Occupational and Environmental Health Nursing

The code of ethics, standards of practice, core curriculum, and competencies provide the basis for the scope of practice, knowledge, skill, and the legal and ethical framework in occupational and environmental health nursing.

A *AAOHN Code of Ethics and Interpretive Statements* **(AAOHN, 1998): Provides a guiding ethical framework for decision making and evaluation of nursing actions as occupational and environmental health nurses fulfill their professional responsibilities to society and the profession.**

B *Standards of Occupational and Environmental Health Nursing* **(AAOHN, 1999): Provide guidance for professional practice and serve as a means to ensure accountability to the profession.**

C *AAOHN Core Curriculum for Occupational Health Nursing, first edition* **(1997): Developed and published in 1997; delineated concepts and principals to support the knowledge base for occupational and environmental health nursing.** *The Core Curriculum for Occupational and Environmental Health Nursing* **(this text) has updated and expanded this AAOHN publication.**

D *Competencies and Performance Criteria in Occupational and Environmental Health Nursing:* **Provides guidelines that address the continuum of practice experience and are applicable to every occupational and environmental health nurse in every practice role; performance criteria were developed for each competency (White, Cox, & Williamson, 1999).**
1. The AAOHN defines competency as an outcome-oriented statement of mastery of a particular skill or ability; it has defined the following nine

categories of competency in occupational and environmental health nursing (White, Cox, & Williamson, 1999):
   a. Clinical and Primary Care
   b. Case Management
   c. Work Force, Workplace, and Environmental Issues
   d. Regulatory/Legislative
   e. Management
   f. Health Promotion and Disease Prevention
   g. Occupational and Environmental Health and Safety Education and Training
   h. Research
   i. Professionalism
2. Within each category, three levels of achievement or competence are identified.
   a. *Competent:* Core level for practice in the specialty
   b. *Proficient:* Increased ability to perceive client situations as a whole based on past experiences, focusing on the relevant aspects of the situation
   c. *Expert:* Extensive experience, a broad knowledge base and ability to grasp a situation quickly and initiate appropriate action
3. The full text describing these competencies can be obtained from AAOHN.

IV Strategies for Advancing the Discipline and Practice

The AAOHN Standards of Occupational and Environmental Health Nursing (1999), Standard VIII: Professional Development, states: "The occupational and environmental health nurse assumes accountability for professional development to enhance professional growth and maintain competency." (AAOHN, 1999) Occupational and environmental health nursing is advanced through education, research, continuing education, practice, and other professional activities. (AAOHN, 1999).

A Academic education in safety and health
   1. Occupational Safety and Health Education and Research Centers (ERCs), funded by the National Institute for Occupational Safety and Health, are the primary vehicles for training and educating occupational health and safety professionals, including occupational and environmental health nurses, industrial hygienists, occupational physicians, and occupational safety professionals (Table 17-1).
   2. These ERCs provide academic, research, continuing education, and outreach programs.
   3. Other schools of nursing offer academic degrees and coursework related to occupational health and safety.

B Research (Chapter 16)
   1. The occupational and environmental health nurse participates in research activities at levels appropriate to the individual's education and experience, which may include problem identification, critical analysis of reported research, research project participation, acting as a resource person, and collaborating with colleagues.
   2. The occupational and environmental health nurse develops grant proposals commensurate with education and experience.

TABLE 17-1

Occupational health nursing programs: NIOSH Education and Research Centers (ERCs) and NIOSH-funded project

Continued

Organization/address	Phone/fax/e-mail	Degrees	Program type
University of Alabama at Birmingham School of Nursing, Room 230 1530 3rd Avenue South Birmingham, AL 35294-1210	(W): (205) 934-6858 (F): (205) 975-6142	M.S.N. Ph.D.	Nurse practitioner Researcher
University of California, San Francisco School of Nursing Box 0608 San Francisco, CA 94143-0608	(W): (415) 476-3221 (F): (415) 476-6042 http://nurseweb.ucsf.edu/www/coeh.htm	M.S.	Nurse practitioner Administrator/manager Ph.D. Researcher
University of California, Los Angeles School of Nursing Box 956919 Los Angeles, CA 90095-6919	(W): (310) 825-8999 (F): (310) 206-3241	M.S.N. M.S.N./M.B.A.	Nurse practitioner Administrator/manager Dual-degree option
University of Cincinnati College of Nursing Post Office Box 210038 Cincinnati, OH 45221-0038	(W): (513) 558-5280 (F): (513) 558-7523 or (513) 588-2142	M.S.N.	Nurse practitioner Administrator/manager Ph.D. Researcher
Harvard School of Public Health (HSPH) and Simmons College Graduate School of Health Studies 300 The Fenway Boston, MA 02115	HSPH: (W): (617) 432-3327 (F): (617) 432-0219 Simmons College (W): (617) 521-2135 (F): (617) 521-3045	M.S.N. M.S.N./S.M.	Nurse practitioner Dual-degree option
University of Illinois at Chicago College of Nursing (M/C 802) 845 South Damen Avenue, Room 942 Chicago, IL 60612	(W): (312) 996-7974 (F): (312) 996-7725	M.S. Post-Masters Certificate Ph.D.	Nurse practitioner Administrator/manager Researcher

TABLE 17-1

Occupational health nursing programs: NIOSH Education and Research Centers (ERCs) and NIOSH-funded project—cont'd

Organization/address	Phone/fax/e-mail	Degrees	Program type
University of Iowa College of Nursing 411 Nursing Building Iowa City, IA 52242	(W): (319) 335-7060 (F): (319) 335-7106	M.S.N.	Administrator/manager
Johns Hopkins School of Hygiene and Public Health Room 7503 615 North Wolfe Street Baltimore, MD 21205	(W): (410) 955-4037 (F): (410) 955-1811	M.P.H. M.S.N./M.P.H. Ph.D. Dr.P.H.	Administrator/manager Dual-degree option Researcher
University of Michigan School of Nursing Division of Health Promotion and Risk Reduction 400 N. Ingalls, Room 3182 Ann Arbor, MI 48109-0482	(W): (734) 647-0347 (F): (734) 647-0351	M.S. Ph.D.	Administrator/manager Researcher
University of Minnesota School of Public Health Mayo Building, Box 807 Minneapolis, MN 55455	(W): (612) 625-7429 (F): (612) 626-0650	M.P.H. M.P.H./M.S.N. Ph.D.	Administrator/manager Dual-degree option Researcher
University of Medicine and Dentistry of New Jersey EOHSI 170 Frelinghuysen Road Piscataway, NJ 08854	(W): (732) 445-0126 (F): (732) 445-0130	M.S.N. M.P.H.	Nurse practitioner Administrator/manager
University of North Carolina at Chapel Hill School of Public Health Rosenau Hall: CB 7400 Chapel Hill, NC 27599-7400	(W): (919) 966-1030 (F): (919) 966-0981	M.P.H. M.S. Ph.D.	Administrator/manager Program planner Researcher (epidemiology)

Institution	Phone	Degree	Role/Option
University of South Florida College of Nursing Health Sciences Center: MDC 22 12901 Bruce B. Downs Boulevard Tampa, FL 33612-4700	(W): (813) 974-9160 (F): (813) 974-5418	M.S./M.P.H.	Nurse practitioner Dual-degree option
University of Texas, Houston Health Science Center 7000 Fannin, Suite 1620 Houston, TX 77030	(W): (713) 500-3250 (F): (713) 500-3263	M.P.H. M.S.N./M.P.H.	Nurse practitioner Administrator/manager Dual-degree option
University of Utah RMCOEH Building 512 Salt Lake City, UT 84112	(W): (801) 585-9532 (F): (801) 587-9838	M.S. Post-Masters Certificate	Nurse practitioner Administrator/manager
University of Washington School of Nursing Box 357263 Seattle, WA 98195	(W): (206) 685-0857 (F): (206) 685-9551	M.N. MN/MPH	Administrator/manager Dual-degree option Ph.D. Researcher
University of Pennsylvania School of Nursing 420 Guardian Drive Philadelphia, PA 19104	(W): (215) 898-2194 (F): (215) 573-7381	M.S.N. M.S.N./M.B.A. Post-Masters Certificate	Nurse practitioner Administrator/manager

3. The occupational and environmental health nurse uses research findings in the development of policies, procedures, and guidelines.

C **Continuing education**

1. The occupational and environmental health nurse assumes accountability for professional development to enhance professional growth and maintain competency.

   a. Exercising responsibility in the profession requires learning, applying, and assessing knowledge pertaining to occupational and environmental sciences, technology, information systems, and research; this is a required commitment throughout the occupational and environmental health nurse's professional career.

   b. As nurses in occupational and environmental health assume increased responsibility, there is an obligation to take steps to maintain and increase competency. It is generally accepted that professionals are well prepared and qualified for the functions they perform.

2. The occupational and environmental health nurse determines continuing education needs, initiates independent learning opportunities, seeks additional academic/continuing education, and evaluates learning for effectiveness.

3. Organizational resources are allocated for professional growth activities.

4. The occupational and environmental health nurse acts as role model and student mentor.

5. The occupational and environmental health nurse facilitates learning of colleagues through discussion, demonstration, and quality improvement techniques; the occupational and environmental health nurse incorporates new knowledge into practice, based on scientific research.

6. The occupational and environmental health nurse meets continuing education requirements for certification, licensure, etc.

D **Practice**

1. Occupational health nursing practice is characterized by professionalism and professional commitment.

   a. *Professionalism* describes the conduct or qualities that characterize a practitioner in a particular field or occupation.

   b. *Professional commitment* is carried out in accordance with occupational health nursing standards, scope of nursing practice, and an ethical code.

   c. The occupational and environmental health nurse maintains a professional image and exhibits a high level of respect and dignity for the profession.

2. All nurses are accountable to the client and society for actions taken in nursing practice.

3. The occupational and environmental health nurse demonstrates practice accountability by validating desired outcomes.

4. The occupational and environmental health nurse facilitates the leadership role by recognizing the value of and using professional resources.

5. The occupational and environmental health nurse is guided by standards of practice, which are criteria-based and measurable and ensure accountability to the profession (AAOHN, 1999).

6. The occupational and environmental health nurse practices within an ethical framework to makes ethical judgements for decision making in practice (AAOHN, 1998).

E Growth of the profession

1. Key elements to advancing occupational and environmental health nursing practice
   a. Creating and communicating a vision statement (Section I.B.1.)
   b. Creating and communicating a mission statement (Section I.B.2.)
   c. Developing and communicating a strategic plan
2. The implementation of these elements is carried out by the AAOHN Board of Directors and the members of the association.
   a. The AAOHN Board of Directors is responsible for creating/developing and communicating these changing elements.
   b. The current level of success in advancing occupational and environmental health nursing practice will be possible only with the continuing and complete participation of each member (Smith, 1997).
3. The occupational and environmental health nurse supports the growth of the profession through the following activities:
   a. Membership in professional associations
   b. Serving on association committees and boards
   c. Assuming leadership positions in elected capacity
   d. Coordinating and expanding services into the occupational health/managed care area to meet the challenges of the current health care environment.
4. The occupational and environmental health nurse acts as a role model in the following ways:
   a. Applies concepts of autonomy, influence, fairness, and risk taking to the professional role
   b. Supports education to increase knowledge and expertise
   c. Supports research as the foundation for professional practice
   d. Precepts students regarding the professional role and knowledge enhancement

V Role Expansion

The role of the occupational and environmental health nurse will continue to expand. In collaboration with other professionals, the occupational and environmental health nurse will assume new responsibilities.

A *Case management* **responsibilities/opportunities will require conducting job analyses and functional-capacity job assessments and working with community agencies to provide the most appropriate and cost-effective services for employees and family members with complex illnesses and injuries.**

B *Environmental health* **responsibilities/opportunities will include analyzing aggregate data related to incidence/prevalence, epidemiologic trends and patterns, and work practices related to injury/illness events (O'Brien, 1995; Rogers, 1994).**

C *Management* **responsibilities/opportunities will include conducting cost-benefit analyses of available internal and external health care services, participating in the selection and design of benefits and benefit programs, and providing expertise in program design, implementation, and management and outcome measurement.**

D *Primary care* **responsibilities/opportunities will be in consumer education**

related to health promotion, disease prevention, self-care, and appropriate access to a reformed health care system; nurse-managed primary care delivery at the work site for employees and their families; and provision of international health care services to traveling employees (O'Brien, 1995; Rogers, 1994).

E *Consulting* opportunities will be to provide expertise in occupational and environmental health to colleagues, government, and private sector for the purpose of improving workers' health.

F *Presenter/speaker* responsibilities/opportunities will be increasingly available and will serve as an excellent forum not only for professional development within our specialty, but for enhancing collaborative efforts with other colleagues, organizations, agencies, and disciplines.

VI Partnerships in Occupational and Environmental Health

A Collaboration: The occupational and environmental health nurse collaborates with a multidisciplinary team in assessing, diagnosing, planning, implementing, and evaluating care of workers.

1. Collaboration often occurs with physicians, industrial hygienists, toxicologists, safety professionals, and ergonomists to identify, monitor, and control workplace hazards and promote a healthy workplace.
2. Collaboration among professionals and others is essential to providing appropriate interventions and treatments of high quality.
3. Collaboration with external agencies supports a safe and healthful work environment.
   a. Governmental agencies and programs (e.g., Occupational Safety and Health Administration, National Institute for Occupational Safety and Health, Environmental Protection Agency, Agency for Toxic Substance and Disease Registry)
   b. Voluntary agencies (e.g., American Heart Association, American Cancer Society, American Diabetes Association)
   c. Nursing organizations (e.g., American Nurses' Association)
   d. Other specialty organizations (e.g., National Safety Council)and professional associations (e.g., American Industrial Hygiene Association)

B Advocacy: The occupational and environmental health nurse has a responsibility to be an advocate for occupational and environmental health nursing practice and the work-force and community populations served.

1. The following activities help the nurse fulfill this responsibility within occupational and environmental health nursing.
   a. Active involvement in professional associations at all levels
   b. Participation on AAOHN committees and task forces charged with developing practice guidelines, vision, mission, strategic plan, etc.
   c. Assuming a leadership role and serving as a mentor and role model for the professional development of peers, colleagues, and others.
2. The following activities help the nurse fulfill this responsibility outside occupational and environmental health nursing.
   a. Increasing awareness of the scope of occupational and environmental health practice among other organizations, associations, agencies, specialty practices, and health care professionals

   b. Getting involved and encouraging and empowering peers to participate in discussions with their state and federal legislators
   1) State legislators need to be knowledgeable and informed about issues that are relevant to occupational and environmental health.
   2) Occupational and environmental health nurses should be alert to new legislation, and to changes and challenges to existing legislation, that affects the health and safety of workers and worker populations.

BIBLIOGRAPHY

American Association of Occupational Health Nurses. (1998). *AAOHN code of ethics and interpretative statements.* Atlanta, GA: AAOHN.

American Association of Occupational Health Nurses. (1999). *Standards of occupational and environmental health nursing.* Atlanta, GA: AAOHN.

American Board for Occupational Health Nurses, Inc. (ABOHN). (1999) *1999-2000 Directory of certified occupational health nurses.* Hinsdale, Illinois: ABOHN.

American Nurses Association. (1979). *The study of credentialing in nursing: A new approach.* VI(12) 82–92.

American Nurses Association (ANA). (1995). *By-laws* (Article 1, Section 2). Washington DC: ANA.

Burgel, B. (1993). *Innovations at the worksite: Delivery of nurse-managed primary health care services.* Washington, DC: American Nurses Publishing.

Joel, L.A. & Young, L.K. (1995). *Dimensions of professional nursing.* McGraw-Hill Inc., *20:* 457–490.

O'Brien, S. (1995). Occupational health nursing roles: Future challenges and opportunities. *AAOHN Journal, 43(3),* 148–152.

Rogers, B. (1994). *Occupational health nursing: Concepts and practice.* Philadelphia: W.B. Saunders Co.

Salazar, M.K. (1997). *AAOHN core curriculum for occupational health nursing.* Philadelphia: W.B. Saunders Co.

Smith, S & Cox, A.R. (1997). Beyond today—Strategic planning for the future of the profession. *AAOHN Journal, 45,* 427-430.

White, K., Cox, A., Williamson, G. (1999).Competencies in occupational and environmental health nursing., *AAOHN Journal, 47(12),* 552-568.

APPENDIX

I

Occupational and Environmental Health and Safety Resources

Professional Associations

American Association of Occupational Health Nurses, Inc. (AAOHN), Suite 100, 2920 Brandywine Road, Atlanta, GA 30341, phone (770) 455-7757, fax (770) 455-7271.

American College of Occupational and Environmental Medicine (ACOEM), 1114 N. Arlington Heights Road, Arlington Heights, IL 60004, phone (847) 818-1800, fax (847) 818-9266.

American Conference of Governmental Industrial Hygienists, Inc. (ACGIH), 1330 Kemper Meadow Dr., Suite 600, Cincinnati, OH 45240, phone (513) 742-2020, fax (513) 742-3355.

American Industrial Hygiene Association (AIHA), 2700 Prosperity Avenue, Suite 250, Fairfax, VA 22031, phone (703) 849-8888, fax (703) 207-3561.

American Public Health Association (APHA), 100 I Street NW, Washington, DC 2000-3710, phone (202) 777-APHA, fax (202) 777-2534.

American Society for Safety Engineers (ASSE), 1800 East Oakton, Des Plaines, IL 60018-2187, phone (847) 699-2929, fax (847) 768-3434.

Human Factors and Ergonomics Society, P.O. Box 1369, Santa Monica, CA 90406, phone (310) 394-1811, fax (310) 394-2410.

National Safety Council (NSC), 1121 Spring Lake Drive, Itasca, IL 60143-3201, phone (630) 285-1121, fax (630) 285-1315.

Certifying Organization

American Board for Occupational Health Nurses, Inc. (ABOHN), 201 East Ogden Road, Suite 114, Hinsdale, IL 60521-3652, phone (630) 789-5799, fax (630) 789-8901.

Publications

Journals

AAOHN Journal, the official journal of the American Association of Occupational Health Nurses, published monthly by SLACK, Inc., 6900 Grove Road, Thorofare, NJ 08086-9447.

American Industrial Hygiene Association Journal, the official journal of the American Hygiene Association, published monthly by the American Industrial Hygiene Association, 2700 Prosperity Avenue, Suite 250, Fairfax, VA 22031.

Applied Occupational and Environmental Hygiene, an international journal published monthly by Applied Industrial Hygiene, Inc., a wholly owned subsidary of ACGIH (American Conference of Governmental Industrial Hygienists, Inc.), 1330 Kemper Meadow Dr., Cincinnati, OH 45240.

Journal of Occupational and Environmental Medicine, the official journal of the American College of Occupational and Environmental Medicine, published monthly by Williams & Wilkins, 351 West Camden Street, Baltimore, MD 21201-2436.

Journal of Occupational Health Psychology, published quarterly by the Educational Publishing Foundation, 750 First Street NE, Washington, DC 20002-4242.

Safety and Health, published monthly by the National Safety Council, 1121 Spring Lake Drive, Itasca, IL 60143.

Books

DiBenedetto, D.V., Harris, J.S., & McCunney, R.S. (1996). *OEM Occupational Health and Safety Manual.* Beverly, MA: OEM Press.

Fleming, L.E., Herzstein, J.A., & Bunn, W.B. (1997). *Issues in international occupational and environmental medicine.* Beverly, MA: OEM Press.

Harris, J.S., Belk, H.D., & Wood, L.W. (1992). *Managing employee health care costs: Assuring quality and value.* Boston: OEM Press.

Levy, B.S. & Wegman, D.H. (2000). *Occupational Health: Recognizing and Preventing Work-Related Disease and Injury* (4th ed.). Philadelphia: Lippincott Williams & Wilkins.

Menzel. N.N. (1998). *Workers' comp management from A to Z: A "how to" guide with forms* (2nd ed.). Beverly, MA: OEM Press.

Moser, R. (1999). *Effective management of occupational and environmental health and safety programs* (2nd ed.). Beverly Farms, MA: OEM Press.

Rogers, B. (1994). *Occupational health nursing: Concepts and practice.* Philadelphia: WB Saunders (NOTE: At this writing, a second edition is in process.).

Other

American Association of Occupational Health Nurses, *SuccessTools: Strategies for Thriving & Surviving in Business.* Module One: Measuring and articulating value; Module Two: Developing business expertise.

Sources of Internet/Computer Information

AAOHN Home Page, http://www.aaohn.org provides information on association products and services and links to practice resources, including topic discussion forums.

Computers in Nursing Journal, Lippincott Company Publishing, 12107 Insurance Way, Suite 114, Hagerstown, MD 21740. Can be accessed through http://www.nursingcenter.com.

Directory of Occupational Health and Safety Software, Computers in Occupational Medicine (section of ACOEM), 1114 N. Arlington Heights Road, Arlington Heights, IL 60004.

Informatics Issues and Strategies for the 21st Century Health Care Executive, American Organization of Nurse Executives, AHA Services, Inc., P.O. Box 92683, Chicago, IL 60675-2683.

The Nurse Executive Guide to Directing and Managing Information Systems, The Center for Health Care Information Management (CHIM), 900 Victors Way, Suite 124, Ann Arbor, MI 48108.

OSHA ComputerLed Information System (OCIS), U.S. Government Printing Office, Washington, DC 20402-9325, phone (202) 783-3238. Contains agency documents, technical information, and training materials on CD-ROM.

Sources of Technical Information

CHEMTREC: 24-hour hotline to provide information about chemicals. To obtain information call (800) 262-8200 or (703) 741-5501.

TOXNET: Comprehensive database that provides toxicity data on chemicals, available though Melars Management Section, National Library of Medicine, Building 38, Room 4N421, 8600 Rockville Pike, Bethesda, MD 20894, phone (800) 638-8480.

Poison Control Centers: These centers are located in every state. Each has a 24-hour hotline to provide emergency information and referrals. Information about centers can be found on the inside covers of local phone directories.

National Pesticide Telecommunications Network: A cooperative effort of Oregon State University and the U.S. Environmental Protection Agency that provides objective, science-based information about a wide variety of pesticide-related subjects. To obtain information call (800) 858-7378.

Government Resources

Agency for Toxic Substances and Disease Registry (ATSDR), ATSDR, 1600 Clifton Road, NE, Atlanta, GA 30033.

Clearinghouse on Health Indexes, U.S. Department of Health and Human Services, Center for Disease Control and Prevention, National Center for Health Statistics, Division of Data, Hyattsville, MD 20782, phone (301) 458-4636.

Environmental Protection Agency (EPA), Public Information Center, PM-211B, 401 M Street SW, Washington, DC 20460.

National Institute of Environmental Health Sciences (NIEHS), National Institutes of Health, Public Health Service, U.S. Department of Health and Human Services, P.O. Box 12233, Research Triangle Park, NC 27709.

National Institute of Nursing Research, National Institutes of Health, Public Health Service, U.S. Department of Health and Human Services, Building 45, Room AN-12, 45 Center Drive MSC 6300, Bethesda, MD 20892-6300.

National Institute for Occupational Safety and Health (NIOSH) *Headquarters*, 200 Independence Ave. SW, Washington, DC 20201, phone (800) 35-NIOSH or (800) 356-4674.

Occupational Safety and Health Administration (OSHA), U.S. Department of Labor, 200 Constitution Avenue NW, Washington, DC 20210. Films and printed material available through regional OSHA offices, or through OSHA Publications Office, 200 Constitution Avenue NW, Washington, DC 20210, phone (202) 219-4667, fax (202) 219-9266.

Office of Occupational Health Nursing, Occupational Safety and Health Administration, Directorate of Technical Support, Room 4618, 200 Constitution Avenue NW, Washington, DC 20210, phone (202) 693-2120.

International Agencies, Organizations, and References

International Labour Office Occupational Safety and Health Branch (ILO-SHB), Bureau International de Travail-Service de la securité et de l'hygiéne du travail (BIT-Sec-Hyg), and Information Safety and Health Information Center, 4 route des Morillons, CH-1211 Geneva 22 (Switzerland).

International Labour Office (ILO). (1997). *Encyclopedia of occupational health and safety* (4th ed.). Geneva, Swizterland: International Labour Organization.

International Occupational Safety and Health Information Centre, Centre international & information de securité et d'hygiene du travail (CIS). IL0, 4 route des Morillons, CH-121 Geneva 22 (Switzerland).

International Organization for Standardization (ISO), Organization internationale de normalization. 1 rue de Varembe, CH-1211 Geneva 20 (Switzerland).

Lehtinen, S. & Mikheev, M. (1994). *WHO worker's health programme and collaborating centers in occupational health.* Geneva: World Health Organization.

Pan American Health Organization and Regional Office for the Americas of the World Health Organization (PAHO), 525 Twenty-third Street NW, Washington, DC 20037.

Regional Office for Europe of the World Health Organization (WHO-EURO-Environmental Health Service), Scherfigvej 8, DK-2100 Copenhagen (Denmark).

World Health Organization-Office of Occupational Health (WHO-OCH). Organization Mondials de la Sante—Office de la medicine du travail (OMS-OCH). 20 rue Appia, CH-1211 Geneva 27 (Switzerland).

International Travel Safety and Health Program Resources

American Society of Tropical Medicine and Hygiene, 60 Revere Drive, Suite 500, Northbrook, IL 60062, phone (708) 480-9592, fax (708) 480-9282.

Centers for Disease Control and Prevention, Atlanta, GA 30333

- CDC Hot Line (recorded messages 24 hours a day), phone (404) 332-4559
- http://www.cdc.gov/travel.html

Chin, J. (Ed.). (2000). *Control of communicable diseases in man* (17th ed.). Washington, DC: American Public Health Association.

International Society of Travel Medicine, P.O. Box 871089, Stone Mountain, GA 30087-0028, phone (770) 736-7060, fax (770) 736-6732, e-mail: bcbistm@aol.com.

International Travel Safety and Health Program (TRAVAX). Travel Health Information Services, phone (608) 831-2331, fax (414) 774-4060.

Jong, E.C. (1995). *The travel tropical medicine manual.* Philadelphia: WB Saunders.

Medical College of Wisconsin International Travel Clinic, Milwaukee, WI, phone (414) 805-3666. http://www.intmed.mcw.edu/travel.html.

U.S. State Department Travel Warning and Consular Information http://www.travel.state.gov/travelfiwarnings.html.

Occupational Health and Safety Tools

Sources for Inspection Checklists
Kornberg, J.P. (1992). *The workplace walk-through.* Boca Raton, FL: Lewis Publishers.

Travers, P.H., & McDougall, C. (1995). *Guidelines for an occupational health and safety service* [AAOHN Publication, Appendix J, Conducting a Safety Walkthrough]. Atlanta: AAOHN Publications.

Sources for Accident Investigation
Travers, P.H. & McDougall, C. (1995). *Guidelines for an occupational health and safety service,* [AAOHN Publication, Appendix K, Sample Corporate Accident Investigation Policy and Procedure, and Appendix L, Sample Supervisor Accident Investigation Form]. Atlanta: AAOHN Publications.

U.S. Department of Labor, Bureau of Labor Statistics, *Evaluating Your Firms Injury and Illness Record,* Reports 813 and 814, available from regional OSHA offices.

Information on Process Safety Reviews
Mullan, R.J. & Murphy, L.I. (1991). Occupational sentinel health events: An updated list for physician recognition and public health surveillance. *American Journal of Industrial Medicine, (19),* 775-799.

OSHA 3133 *Process Safety Management-Guidelines for Compliance,* OSHA Publications Office, 200 Constitution Avenue NW, Washington, DC, phone (202) 219-4667.

Ergonomic Tools and References
ANSI S3.34-1986 (R1997) Hand Arm Vibration Standards—American National Standard Guide for the Measurement and Evaluation of Human Exposure to Vibration Transmitted to the Hand. ANSI S3.34-1986 (R1997). Available for purchase at the ANSI Web site at http://web.ansi.org/default.htm.

Department of Energy ErgoEASER—Ergonomics Education, Awareness, System Evaluation and Recording (ErgoEASER) software package. U.S. Department of Energy, Office of Environment, Safety, and Health (1995). Can be downloaded from the Department of Energy Web site at http://tis.eh.doc.gov/others/ergoeaser/download.htm.

Moore, J.S. & Garg, A. (1995). The Strain Index: A proposed method to analyze jobs for risk of distal upper extremity disorders. *American Industrial Hygiene Association Journal, (56),* 443-458.
http://www.satx.disa.mil/hscoemo/tools/strain.htm.

NOTE: See additional resources in Appendix IV: Web Sites.

Guidelines for Respirator PPE Health Clearance
American National Standards Institute (ANSI) 88.6, *Respirator Use Physical Qualifications for Personnel*, ANSI, 11 West 42nd Street, New York, NY 10036.

Resources for Direct Care Activities

The Agency for Healthcare Research and Quality, in association with the American Association of Health Plans (AAHP) and the American Medical Association (AMA), established a *National Clearinghouse for Guidelines*. http://www.guideline.gov

Centers for Disease Control and Prevention

- Guidelines for occupational infectious disease (ftp://ftp.cdc.gov/pub/Publications/mmwr/rr/rr4618.pdf) or the post exposure prophylaxis

- Recommendations for health care workers exposed to HIV (ftp://ftp.cdc.gov/pub/Publications/mmwr/RR/RR4707.pdf).

- Publications and resources (http://www.cdc.gov/nip/publications/ACIP-list.htm)
  The Adult Immunization Acton Plan can be found at http://www.cdc.gov/od/nvpo/adult.htm.

- Delivery of a vaccine program http://www.cdc.gov/epo/mmwr/preview/mmwrhtml/rr4901a1.htm.

First aid: OSHA Directive CPL 2-2.53—Guidelines for First Aid Programs can be accessed at http://www.osha-slc.gov/OshDoc/Directive_data/CPL_2-2_53.html.

Guidelines for Preventing Workplace Violence for Health Care and Social Service Workers (USDL, OSHA, 1998) can be used to design engineering and administrative controls and for post-incident response and evaluation. Available on-line at http://www.osha-slc.gov/SLTC/workplaceviolence/guideline.html.

The *Guide to Clinical Preventive Services* (2nd ed.) provides research-based screening recommendations for the clinician (U.S. Preventive Services Task Force, 1996).

Healthy People 2010, objectives on immunizations in Chapter 14: Immunizations (http://www.health.gov/healthypeople).

Preplacement resources: federal OSHA standards (http://www.osha.gov), the Americans with Disabilities Act (http://www.usdoj.gov/crt/ada/adahom1.htm), and other mandated programs; for example, the Department of Transportation (http://www.dot.gov) preplacement programs.

Put Prevention into Practice is a program of the Office of Disease Prevention and Health Promotion (http://www.ahrq.gov/ppip/index.html); includes health education materials, *The Clinician's Handbook of Preventive Services,* and other resources (USDHHS, 1998).

Workplace Violence (AAOHN, 2000), AAOHN Advisory: provides an overview of the importance of this issue to occupational health and issues to consider in terms of job safety. Copies can be obtained from AAOHN.

Accident: An undesired event causing harm to people, property or the environment, possibly causing additional losses by interrupting the conduct of business.

Accident investigation: A fact-finding procedure to identify the pertinent factors that allow accidents to occur, with the aim of preventing similar future accidents.

Administrative controls: Supervisory and management practices that promote safe work behaviors to eliminate or limit exposure to hazards.

Air-purifying respirator: A type of personal protective equipment (PPE) that uses filters or adsorbents to remove toxic materials from inhaled air.

Area sample: A sample most commonly collected when doing environmental monitoring to detect where contaminants are most likely to be generated, creating a "map" of levels present.

Assigned protection factor: The minimum anticipated protection provided by a properly functioning respirator or class of respirators to a given percentage of properly fitted and trained users.

Atmosphere-supply respirator: A type of PPE that uses bottled or compressed air via an airline or a tank worn by the worker to protect against inhalation of toxic or oxygen-deficient atmospheres.

Atmospheric monitoring: The testing of air over time to detect the presence and measure the concentration of airborne contaminants to which a worker is being exposed.

Benchmarking: The "process of measuring a company's products, services, and practices against industry-leading competitors" (Collins, 1995) or "against industry's best practices" (Landwehr, 1995).

Budgeting: The process by which programs and activities are quantified into monetary terms for the purpose of planning and managing resources for a given time period.

Case management: A process of coordinating a client's health care services to achieve optimal, quality care delivered in a cost-effective manner (AAOHN, 1994).

Co-employment: A "relationship between two or more employers in which each has actual or potential legal rights and duties with respect to the same employee or group of employees" (Lenz, 1994).

Common law: The legal precedents that have been established as a result of decisions handed down in past cases within a given jurisdiction.

Confidentiality: The implicit promise that information divulged to another will be respected and not released or repeated.

Confined space: An area not designed for human occupancy, with limited entry and egress and often with inadequate ventilation, thus presenting a potential hazard to a worker inside it.

Consensus standard: A standard accepted among professionals and professional organizations and regarded as a guideline, representative of general opinion; it is, however, not legally enforceable unless quoted in a regulation of a legislative body.

Containment: The practice of enclosing a hazardous unit or container inside another container in event of a leak or release of a contaminant or toxin.

Contingent workers: A category of workers also known as floaters, regular part-time, formal intermittents, limited duration hires, informal intermittents, casuals, contract labor services, independent contractors, leased workers, or temporary help services workers.

Dilution ventilation: The circulation of fresh air into the work site to dilute to an acceptable exposure level a contaminant that is emitted into work-site air.

Direct-reading instrument: An instrument that provides immediate data on the contents of the surrounding atmosphere.

Documentation: The written communication of information that is the basis of the legal occupational health record.

Engineering controls: Devices or methods that stop hazards at their source or in the pathway of transmission before they can reach the worker; engineering controls do not depend on the worker to control their effectiveness.

Environmental health: The "freedom from illness or injury related to exposure to toxic agents and other environmental conditions that are potentially detrimental to health" (Institute of Medicine, 1995).

Epidemiology: The study of the distribution and determinants of health-related states or events in specified populations, and the application of this study to the control of health problems. (From *epi*, meaning *upon*; *demos*, meaning *people*; and *logos*, which means *science.*)

Ergonomics: The study of the interaction between humans and their work, ergonomics is concerned with the design of the work site, equipment, physical environment, and organization of work in order to fit them to the worker.

Exposure monitoring: Often done by or with the aid of an industrial hygienist, it is the quantitative assessment of work-site exposures to hazards that are recognized, suspected, or reasonably predictable, based on other preliminary hazard identification methods.

Federal Reserve discount rate: The rate at which the Federal Reserve Bank lends funds to its member banks.

Focused inspections: Periodic inspections of a workplace that target specific processes, equipment, or work areas; investigate an accident; evaluate a reported health or safety hazard; or investigate complaints about such things as a strange odor or loud noise.

Grab sample: An air sample collected over a short period, which may range from a few seconds to less than 2 minutes.

Gross national product (GNP): The total final value of domestic goods and services produced in a national economy over a particular period, usually one year.

Hazard analysis: Procedure performed to identify potential hazards and evaluate data relating to the probability of their occurrence, the severity of their consequences, and the vulnerability of workers to potential exposures.

Hazardous energy control: A device or method that prevents contact between the worker and the sources of hazardous energy.

Hazardous energy source: These can be electrical energy, chemical reactivity, thermal extremes, mechanical energy, and physical energy.

Hazards: Work-site conditions that present the potential for harm or damage to people, property, or the environment. Hazards are classified as physical, chemical, biological, psychological, or mechanical.

Health promotion: The "science and art of helping people change their lifestyles to move towards a state of optimal health" (O'Donnell, 1989).

Incidence rate: An epidemiologic term that describes the "frequency of newly occurring cases in a specified population during a given period of time" (Valanis, 1992).

Incident historical review: The compilation and analysis of accidents and near misses that have occurred over a selected period of time.

Industrial hygiene: That "science and practice devoted to the anticipation, recognition, evaluation, and control of those environmental factors or stresses arising in or from the workplace that may cause injury, illness, impaired health and well-being, or significant discomfort among workers, and may impact the general community" (Harris, 2000).

Informatics: The "specialty that integrates nursing science, computer science, and information science in identifying, collecting, processing, and managing data and information to support nursing practice, administration, education, and research, and to expand nursing knowledge" (ANA, 1994).

Informatics nurse specialists: Nurses who practice in the field of nursing informatics, which "includes the development and evaluation of applications, tools, processes, and structures which assist nurses with the management of data in taking care of patients or in supporting the practice of nursing . . . in all sites and settings of care, whether at the basic or advanced practice level" (ANA, 1994).

Informed consent: A decision made with a complete understanding of a treatment or action, including risks, benefits, and alternative treatments; informed consent must be obtained without coercion or deception.

Integrated disability management: A comprehensive approach to integrating all disability benefits, programs, and services to help control the employer's disability costs and to return the employee to work as soon as possible and maximize the employee's functional capacity.

Integrated, or long-term, sample: A sample that consists of a known volume of air drawn through an appropriate medium for a sampling period of less than 1 hour to a full 8 hours, reflecting the length of time of a worker's overall exposure.

Information management systems: A means to collect, access, and apply large amounts of information from many sources to effectively manage all aspects of the occupational health unit.

Isolation: Interposition of a barrier between a hazard and those who might be affected by that hazard.

Job hazard analysis: The process of carefully studying and recording each step of a job to identify safety and health job hazards and to determine the best way to perform the job to reduce or eliminate those hazards. Also known as *job safety analysis.*

Local exhaust: Removal of contaminated air from the point of origin, away from the worker's breathing zone, through a scrubber or cleaning system to the outside atmosphere.

Machine safeguarding: Eliminating hazards of pinch-, nip-, or shear-points at which it is possible to be caught between the moving parts of a machine or between the materials and the moving parts of a machine.

Malpractice: A type of negligence that involves professional misconduct or unreasonable lack of skill.

Managed care: Any form of health plan that initiates selective contracting between providers, employers, and insurers to channel employees/patients to a specified set of cost-effective providers (a provider network); these providers have procedures in place to ensure that only medically necessary and appropriate use of health care services occurs.

Multiple chemical sensitivity: A condition that has been described as a chemically-induced immune system dysfunction, a low-grade yeast infection, a psychologic response to low-level chemical exposures, antioxidant vitamin deficiencies, and various other causes.

Negligence: The failure to perform one's duties according to acceptable standards.

Net national product: The GNP less capital consumption allowance (allocated costs for depreciation of capital equipment).

Noise exposure assessment: Measurements of sound-pressure levels, expressed in terms of decibels (dB).

Occupational and environmental health nursing: The "specialty practice that provides for and delivers health and safety services to employees, employee populations, and community groups" (AAOHN, 1999).

Occupational health surveillance: The "process of monitoring the health status of worker populations to gather data on the effects of workplace exposures and using data to prevent injury and illness" (AAOHN, 1996).

Occupational illness: Any abnormal condition or disorder, other than one resulting from an occupational injury, caused by exposure to environmental factors associated with employment.

Occupational injury: Any injury, such as a cut, fracture, sprain, or amputation, that results from a single incident in the work environment.

Permissible exposure limits: Standards promulgated by the Occupational Safety and Health Administration that refer to 8-hour, time-weighted averages of airborne exposure to a hazard over 5 working days per week.

Personal protective equipment: Devices, such as respirators, gloves, or special clothing and shoes, that are worn by workers to protect against hazards in the workplace.

Prevalence rate: An epidemiologic term that describes the proportion of the population that has a particular condition at a given time or during a given period.

Primary care: The provision of integrated, accessible health care services by clinicians who are accountable for addressing a large majority of personal health care needs, developing a sustained partnership with patients, and practicing in the context of family and community (Donaldson, Yordy, & Vanselow, 1994).

Primary prevention: Health promotion and health protection measures that prevent the occurrence of disease.

Privatization: A system in which government services are sold or transferred to private businesses and corporations.

Process safety review: A careful evaluation of what could go wrong and what safeguards must be implemented to prevent hazardous chemical releases, explosions, or other process accidents.

Quantity reduction: Reducing the amount of hazardous substances on hand by storing only those amounts that will actually be needed and consumed in a reasonable time, rather than storing large amounts of material over long periods of time.

Reducing the amount stored reduces the potential hazard in the event of a leak, spill, or release.

Risk: The possibility of loss or injury.

Screening: Testing people who are as yet asymptomatic for the purpose of classifying them with respect to their likelihood of having a particular disease.

Secondary prevention: Early detection and treatment of disease so that its progression is slowed or its complications limited; *screening is* a secondary prevention measure.

Self-contained breathing apparatus: Respirable air carried in a tank on the back of the user.

Sentinel health event–occupational: A preventable disease, disability, or untimely death that is occupationally related and whose occurrence may: (1) provide the impetus for epidemiologic or industrial hygiene studies; or (2) serve as a warning signal that materials substitution, engineering control, personal protection, or health care may be required.

Site survey/walk-through: A worksite inspection not related to any particular incident, area, or piece of equipment.

Standard industrial classification: Reference to a four-digit number used by the Bureau of Labor Statistics to classify industries according to type.

Standards of care: Actions that the average, reasonable, and prudent health care provider would perform in similar circumstances; also known as "reasonable and customary care."

Standards of nursing practice: Standards developed by professional nursing associations to guide practice and provide practitioners with a framework for evaluating practice.

Tertiary prevention: The prevention of disability; includes rehabilitative efforts.

Threshold limit values: Guidelines for rating exposure to hazardous substances that are developed by the American Conference of Governmental Industrial Hygienists; they are published annually by that organization and generally refer to 8 hours of time-weighted average exposure in a 5-day week.

Toxic Substances Control Act: A law that requires documentation of worker allegations of previously unrecognized adverse health effects from new chemicals, mixtures, or processes.

Toxicology: The study of adverse effects of chemicals on biologic systems.

Work-conditioning, or work-hardening, program: A "highly structured, goal-oriented, individualized treatment program designed to maximize the person's ability to return to work" (Commission on Accreditation of Rehabilitation Facilities, 1991).

Workers' compensation: A publicly funded insurance system that provides for lost wages, medical costs, and rehabilitation for persons who experience an occupational injury or illness.

Workplace violence: Harassment, threats, and actual physical assaults in the workplace.

References

American Association of Occupational Health Nurses (1994). *Advisory: Case Management.* Atlanta, GA: AAOHN Publications.

American Association of Occupational Health Nurses (1996). *AAOHN position statement: Occupational health surveillance.* Atlanta, GA: AAOHN Publications.

American Association of Occupational Health Nurses (1999). *Standards of occupational and environmental health nursing.* Atlanta, GA: AAOHN Publications.

American Nurses Association (1994). *The scope of practice for nursing informatics.* Washington, DC: American Nurses Publishing.

Collins, M.J. (1995). Benchmarking with simulation: How it can help your production operations. *Production, 107(7),* 51-52.

Commission on Accreditation of Rehabilitation Facilities (1991). *Standards manual for organizations serving people with disabilities.* Tucson, AZ: Commission on Accreditation of Rehabilitation Facilities.

Donaldson, M., Yordy, K., & Vanselow, N. (Eds.) (1994). *Defining primary care: An interim report.* Washington, DC: National Academy Press.

Harris, R.L. (2000). *Patty's industrial hygiene, Vol. 1.* New York: John Wiley & Sons.

Landwehr, W.R. (1995). Focus on benchmarking: Achieving world-class maintenance and superior competitive performance. *Plant Engineering, 49(7),* 120-121.

Lenz, E.A. (1994). Employer liability issues in staffing services arrangements. *Co-employment* (ed. 2). Virginia: National Association of Temporary Services.

Institute of Medicine (1995). *Nursing, health and the environment: Strengthening the relationship to improve the public's health.* Washington, DC: National Academy Press.

O'Donnell, M.D. (1989). Definition of health promotion: Part III: Expanding the definition. *American Journal of Health Promotion, 3(3),* 5.

Valanis, B. (1992). *Epidemiology in nursing and health care.* Norwalk, CN: Appleton & Lange.

APPENDIX

III

Acronyms

AACN: American Association of Colleges of Nursing

AAIN: American Association of Industrial Nurses (AAOHN's name until 1977)

AAOHN: American Association of Occupational Health Nurses, Inc.

ABOHN: American Board of Occupational Health Nurses, Inc.

ACGIH: American Conference of Governmental Industrial Hygienists

ACOEM: American College of Occupational and Environmental Medicine

ADA: Americans with Disabilities Act

AED: automatic external defibrillator

AFL: American Federation of Labor

AIHA: American Industrial Hygiene Association

ANA: American Nurses Association

ANSI: American National Standards Institute

APHA: American Public Health Association

ASSE: American Society of Safety Engineers

ATSDR: Agency for Toxic Substances and Disease Registry

BLS: Bureau of Labor Statistics (USDL)

BPR: Business process reengineering

CAOHC: Council for Accreditation in Occupational Hearing Conservation

CARF: Commission on Accreditation of Rehabilitation Facilities

CCM: Certified Case Manager

CDC: Centers for Disease Control and Prevention

CDL: commercial driver's license

CFR: Code of Federal Regulations

CIO: Council of Industrial Organizations

CISD: critical incident stress debriefing

CO: carbon monoxide

COBRA: Consolidated Omnibus Budget Reconciliation Act

COHC: Certified Occupational Hearing Conservationist

COHN: Certified Occupational Health Nurse

COHN/CM: Certified Occupational Health Nurse/Case Manager

COHN-S: Certified Occupational Health Nurse—Specialist

COHN-S/CM: Certified Occupational Health Nurse—Specialist/Case Manager

CPI: Consumer Price Index

CPR: cardiopulmonary resuscitation

CPWR: Center to Protect Workers' Rights

CQI: continuous quality improvement

CTD: cumulative trauma disorder

dB: decibel

dBA: A sound-pressure measurement derived by using an A-weighted scale that combines frequency with intensity

D-C: demand-control

DFW: Drug-Free Workplace Act

DI: disposable income

DOE: Department of Energy

DOT: Department of Transportation

EAP: employee assistance program

EBD: evidential breathing device

EBRI: Employee Benefit Research Institute

EBT: evidential breath testing

EEOC: Equal Employment Opportunity Commission

EPA: Environmental Protection Agency

ERC: Education and Research Center (funded by NIOSH)

ERISA: Employment Retirement Income Security Act

FAA: Federal Aviation Administration

FDA: Food and Drug Administration

FFDCA: Federal Food, Drug and Cosmetic Act

FHWA: Federal Highway Administration

FIFRA: Federal Insecticide, Fungicide, and Rodenticide Act

FLSA: Fair Labor Standards Act

FMCSA: Federal Motor Carrier Safety Administration

FMEA: failure mode and effect analysis

FMLA: Family and Medical Leave Act

FRA: Federal Railroad Administration

FTA: Federal Transit Administration

FTE: full-time equivalent

GAO: Government Accounting Office

GATT: General Agreement for Trade and Tariffs

GIS: geographic information system

GNP: gross national product

HazCom: hazard communication

HazMat: hazardous materials

HAZOP: hazard and operability

HCFA: Health Care Financing Administration

HCP: hearing conservation program

HCS: Hazard Communication Standard (29 CFR 1910, 1915, 1917, 1918, 1926, 1928)

HCW: health care worker

HEDIS: Health Plan Employer Data Information Set

HEPA: high efficiency particle air

HLPP: hearing-loss prevention program

HMO: health maintenance organization

HPD: hearing protection device

Hz: hertz

ICOH: International Commission on Occupational Health

ILO: International Labour Organization

IMS: information management system

INS: informatics nurse specialist

IPA: independent practice association

ISO: International Organization for Standardization

JCAHO: Joint Commission for Accreditation of Health Care Organizations

JSA: job safety analysis

LC$_{50}$: lethal concentration, 50%

LD$_{50}$: lethal dose, 50%

MCS: multiple chemical sensitivity

MRI: magnetic resonance imaging

MRO: medical review officer

MSDS: material safety data sheet

NAFTA: North American Free Trade Act

NAS: National Academy of Science

NCEH: National Center for Environmental Health

NCQA: National Committee for Quality Assurance

NGO: nongovernmental organization

NHTSA: National Highway Traffic Safety Administration

NIDA: National Institute of Drug Abuse

NIHL: noise-induced hearing loss

NINR: National Institute for Nursing Research

NIOSH: National Institute for Occupational Safety and Health

NRC: National Research Council

NRR: noise reduction rating

NSC: National Safety Council

OHNAC: Occupational Health Nurse in Agricultural Communities

OSH Act: Occupational Safety and Health Act (1970)

OSHA: Occupational Safety and Health Administration

OSHRC: Occupational Safety and Health Review Commission

OTC: over-the-counter

PCP: primary care provider

P-E: person-environment

PEL: permissible exposure limits (OSHA exposure limits)

POS: point-of-service

PPE: personal protective equipment

PPI: Producer Price Index

ppm: parts per million

PPO: preferred provider organization

PT: physical therapy

RCRA: Resource Conservation and Recovery Act

REL: recommended exposure level

RFC: residual functional capacity

RSD: reflex sympathetic dystrophy

RSPA: Research and Special Programs Administration

RTW: return-to-work

SAMHSA: Substance Abuse and Mental Health Services Administration

SARA: Superfund Amendments and Reauthorization Act (1986)

SHE-O: sentinel health event—occupational

SIC: standard industrial classification

SSDI: Social Security Disability Insurance

STD: sexually transmitted disease

STEL: short-term exposure levels

STS: standard threshold shift (also referred to as significant threshold shift)

TCM: telephonic case management

TLD: thermal luminescent dosimeter

TLV: threshold limit value (ACGIH-recommended exposure limit)

TPA: third-party administrator

TQM: total quality management

TSCA: Toxic Substances Control Act

TTS: temporary threshold shift

TWA: time-weighted average

US DOC: United States Department of Census

USDA: United States Department of Agriculture

USDHHS: United States Department of Health and Human Services

USDL: United States Department of Labor

USDL, BLS: United States Department of Labor, Bureau of Labor Statistics

USPHS: United States Public Health Services

UV: ultraviolet

VPP: Voluntary Protection Program (OSHA)

WB: Women's Bureau (USDL)

WBS: work breakdown structure

WHO: World Health Organization

WMSD: work-related musculo-skeletal disorder

WWW: World Wide Web

APPENDIX

IV

Web Sites

Agency for Toxic Substance and Disease Registry: http://www.atsdr.cdc.gov

Airline safety information: http://www.airsafe.com

American Association of Occupational Health Nurses: http://www.aaohn.org

American Board of Independent Medical Examiners: http://www.abime.org

American Board for Occupational Health Nurses: http://www.abohn.org

American College of Occupational and Environmental Medicine:
http://www.acoem.org

American Conference of Governmental Industrial Hygienists:
http://www.acgih.org

American Industrial Hygiene Association: http://www.aiha.org

American National Standards Institute: http://www.ansi.org

American Public Health Association: http://www.apha.org

American Society of Safety Engineers: http://www.asse.org

Association of Occupational and Environmental Clinics: http://www.aoec.org

Association of Occupational Health Professionals: http://www.podi.com/aohp

CCOHS Health & Safety Internet Directory:
http://www.ccohs.ca/resources/occupati.html

Centers for Disease Control and Prevention: http://www.cdc.gov

Children's Environmental Health Network: http://www.cehn.org

CHEMTREC: http://www.cwc-chemical.com

Council for Accreditation on Occupational Hearing loss: http://www.caohc.org

CTD News. Workplace solutions for repetitive stress injuries online:
http://www.ctdnews.com

Department of Defense Ergonomics Working Group:
http://chppmwww.apgea.army.mil/ergowg/index.htm

Drug-Free Workplace Act:
http://www.dol.gov/asp/public/programs/drugs/employer.htm

ErgoWeb—the Place for Ergonomics: http://www.ergoweb.com

Enviro-Net: http://www.enviro-net.com

Human Factors and Ergonomics Society: http://hfes.org/HFES.html

Industrial Hygiene Web site: http://www.industrialhygiene.com

Institute of Medicine (IOM): http://www.iom.edu

National Archives and Records Administration: Federal Register:
http://www.access.gpo.gov/su_docs/aces/aces140.html

National Association of County and City Health Officials:
http://www.naccho.org

National Clearinghouse for Worker Safety and Health training:
http://www.niehs.hih.gov/wetp/clear.htm

National Environmental Education and Training Foundation:
http://www.neetf.org

National Institute for Occupational Safety and Health:
http://www.cdc.gov/niosh

National Institute of Environmental Health Sciences: http://www.niehs.nih.gov

National Library of Medicine: http://www.nlm.nih.gov

National Safety Council: http://www.nsc.org

National Pesticide Telecommunications Network: http://ace.orst.edu/info/nptn

Occupational Safety and Health Administration: http://www.osha.gov

Occupational Health Clinics: http://www.aoec.org

Society of Occupational and Environmental Health: http://www.soeh.org

Travel Health Information: http://www.travelhealth.com

Travel advisory passports visas:
http://www.choosetocruise.com/advisories.html

Travel Tips, Health and Safety: http://www.prevmed.com

University of California Berkeley, Video Display Terminal Health and Safety
Guidelines:
http://www.uhs.berkeley.edu/FacStaff/Ergonomics/ergguide.html

University of Texas at Austin, General Libraries Ergonomics Task Force: http://www.lib.utexas.edu/Pubs/etf/exhibit.html

U.S. Department of Labor: http://www.dol.gov

U.S. Department of Health and Human Services: http://www.hhs.gov

U.S. Department of Travel Warning and Consular Information: http://www.travel.state.gov

U.S. Environmental Protection Agency: http://www.epa.gov

APPENDIX

V

Occupational Safety and Health Administration Act of 1970

To assure so far as possible every working man and woman in the Nation safe and healthful working conditions and to preserve our human resources.

1. By encouraging employers and employees in their efforts to reduce the number of occupational safety and health hazards at their places of employment, and to stimulate employers and employees to institute new and to perfect existing programs for providing safe and healthful working conditions;

2. By providing that employers and employees have separate but dependent responsibilities and rights with respect to achieving safe and healthful working conditions;

3. By authorizing the Secretary of Labor to set mandatory occupational safety and health standards applicable to businesses affecting interstate commerce, and by creating an Occupational Safety and Health Review Commission for carrying out adjudicatory functions under the Act;

4. By building upon advances already made through employer and employee initiative for providing safe and healthful working conditions;

5. By providing for research in the field of occupational safety and health, including the psychological factors involved, and by developing innovative methods, techniques, and approaches for dealing with occupational safety and health problems;

6. By exploring ways to discover latent diseases, establishing causal connections between diseases and work in environmental conditions, and conducting other research relating to health problems, in recognition of the fact that occupational health standards present problems often different from those involved in occupational safety;

7. By providing medical criteria which will assure insofar as practicable that no employee will suffer diminished health, functional capacity, or life expectancy as a result of his work experience;

8. By providing for training programs to increase the number and competence of personnel engaged in the field of occupational safety and health;

9. By providing for the development and promulgation of occupational safety and health standards;

10. By providing an effective enforcement program which shall include a prohibition against giving advance notice of any inspection and sanctions for any individual violating this prohibition;

11. By encouraging the States to assume the fullest responsibility for the administration and enforcement of their occupational safety and health laws by providing grants to the States to assist in identifying their needs and responsibilities in the area of occupational safety and health, to develop plans

in accordance with the provisions of this Act, to improve the administration and enforcement of State occupational safety and health laws, and to conduct experimental and demonstration projects in connection therewith;

12. By providing for appropriate reporting procedures with respect to occupational safety and health procedures which will help achieve the objectives of this Act and accurately describe the nature of the occupational safety and health problem;

13. By encouraging joint labor-management effort to reduce injuries and disease arising out of employment.

APPENDIX

VI

*American Association of Occupational Health Nurses Code of Ethics**

Occupational and environmental health nurses:

- Provide healthcare in the work environment with regard for human dignity and client rights, unrestricted by consideration of social economic status, personal attributes, or the nature of the health status.

- Promote collaboration with other health professionals and community health agencies in order to meet the health needs of the workforce.

- Strive to safeguard employees' rights to privacy by protecting confidential information and releasing information only upon written consent of the employee or as required or permitted by law.

- Strive to provide quality care and to safeguard clients from unethical and illegal actions.

- Licensed to provide health care services, accept obligations to society as professionals and responsible members of the community.

- Maintain individual competence in health nursing practice, based on scientific knowledge, and recognize and accept responsibility for individual judgements and action, while complying with appropriate laws and regulation (local, state, and federal) that impact the delivery of occupational and environmental health services.

- Participate, as appropriate in activities such as research that contribute to the ongoing development of the profession's body of knowledge while protecting the rights of subjects.

*The complete text of AAOHN's Code of Ethics, including the preamble and interpretive statements, can be obtained from AAOHN.

APPENDIX

VII

Occupational and Environmental Health and Safety Legislation

1936	Walsh-Healy Act
1938	Federal Food, Drug and Cosmetic Act (FFDCA)
1947	Federal Insecticide, Fungicide, and Rodenticide Act (FIFRA)
1948	Federal Water Pollution Control Act (later called the Clean Water Act)
1955	Clean Air Act
1965	Shoreline Erosion Protection Act
1966	Solid Waste Disposal Act
1969	Federal Coal Mine and Safety Act
1969	National Environmental Policy Act (NEPA)
1970	Consumer Product Safety Act (CPSC)
1970	Clean Air Act (amended 1977)
1970	Federal Railroad Safety Act (amended 1974, 1975, 1976) (DOT)
1970	Hazardous Materials Transportation Control Act (amended 1975, 1976) (DOT)
1970	Occupational Safety and Health Act (OSH Act)
1970	Pollution Prevention Packaging Act
1970	Resource Recovery Act
1971	Lead-Based Paint Poisoning Prevention Act
1971	Coastal Zone Management Act
1972	Marine Protection, Research, and Sanctuaries Act
1972	Ocean Dumping Act
1972	Noise Control Act
1972	Federal Water Pollution Act (amended and renamed Clean Water Act in 1977)
1972	Federal Insecticide, Fungicide, and Rodenticide Act
1973	Rehabilitation Act (EEOC)
1973	Endangered Species Act
1974	Safe Drinking Water Act (amended 1977)

1974	Shoreline Erosion Control Demonstration Act
1975	Hazardous Materials Transportation Act
1976	Resource Conservation and Recovery Act (RCRA)
1976	Toxic Substances Control Act (TSCA)
1977	Surface Mining Control and Reclamation Act
1978	Lead Standard
1978	Cotton Dust Standard
1978	Uranium Mill-Tailings Radiation Control Act
1980	Asbestos School Hazard Emergency Response Act
1980	Carcinogens Standard
1980	Comprehensive Environmental Response, Compensation, and Liability Act (CERCLA or Superfund)
1982	Nuclear Waste Policy Act
1983	Noise Standard
1984	Asbestos School Hazard Abatement Act
1986	Asbestos Hazard Emergency Response Act
1986	Superfund Amendments and Reauthorization Act (SARA)
1986	Emergency Planning and Community Right-to-Know Act (EPCRA)
1987	Clean Water Act Reauthorization
1988	Indoor Radon Abatement Act
1988	Lead Contamination Control Act
1988	Medical Waste Tracking Act
1988	Ocean Dumping Ban Act
1988	Shore Protection Act
1990	National Environmental Education Act
1990	Clean Air Act Amendment
1990	Oil Prevention Act (OPA)
1990	Pollution Prevention Act (PPA)
1996	Food Quality Protection Act (FQPA)
1999	Chemical Safety Information, Site Security and Fuels Regulatory Act

INDEX

A

AAOHN; *see* American Association of Occupational Health Nurses
AAOHN Journal, 425-426
Absorption from inhalation of toxin, 124-125
Abuse, substance
  lifestyle and, 302
  as stress response, 334
  testing for, 361-367
Accommodation, reasonable, 78
Accreditation, 426
Active surveillance, 381
Activism, social, 9-10
ADA; *see* Americans with Disabilities Act
Adjusted rate, 119
Administration, 147-166
  administrative controls in prevention and, 234-239
  benchmarking and, 164-165
  communication and, 160-161
  critical thinking and, 162-163
  of direct care, 251
  drug testing and, 363
  ethical issues in, 163-164
  fiscal issues of, 154-156, 155t
  human resource issues of, 156-160
  image of nurse and, 163
  leadership in, 147-148
  management process and, 150-152
  organizational culture and, 152-153
  outcome management and, 164
  policies and procedures and, 153-154
  project management by, 161-162
  strategic planning and, 148-150
  time management by, 162
  total quality management and, 165-166
Administration record, 84-85
Administrative control in prevention, 234-239, *238*
Administrative law, 72
Adolescent, in work force, 41-45
Adult education, 307-324; *see also* Education, adult
Advanced practice nursing, 247
Advisory committee on health promotion, 298
Advocacy
  for children in work force, 44
  environmental justice and, 398-399
  responsibility for, 434-435
Age
  children in work force and, 41-45
  implications of, 39-40
  toxicology and, 128
Agency for Toxic Substances and Disease Registry, 401-402
Agricultural worker
  characteristics of, 50-51
  illness and injury in, 51-53, 52t
  young, 43
Air pollution, 406

Airborne contaminant
  sampling of, 135
  standards for, 135-136
Alcohol abuse, 302
Alcohol-related accident, 303-304
Alcohol testing program, 361-367
Alternative worker, changes in use of, 45-48
Altitude sickness, 348t
American Association of Industrial Nurses, 22-24
American Association of Occupational Health Nurses
  behavioral objectives of, 309
  code of ethics of, 427
  competency in nursing and, 427-428
  core curriculum of, 427
  establishment of, 24
  ethics and, 89-90
  journal of, 425-426
  on research, 411
  role of, 425
  standards of, 427
American Nurses Association
  on information systems, 173
  on research, 411
Americans with Disabilities Act
  on alternative worker, 47
  provisions of, 77-78
ANA; *see* American Nurses Association
Analysis
  ergonomic, 218
  hazard, 213-214, 218-219
  incident, 214-215
  job, 272
Analytic study, 121
Anthropometry, 16
Arsenic, 128
Asbestos, 130
Asphyxiant, 123, 133-134
Assault, 329
Assessment
  damage, 374-375
  in direct care, 250-251
  in disability case management, 278-279
  environmental health, 395-396
  of hazard exposure, 20
  of illness exposure, 20
  noise, 351-352
  in program development, 191-193
  of psychosocial factors, 338-339
  risk, 399-400
Associate degree nurse, 411
Atmospheric monitoring, 223
Audiometric testing, 355-357, *356*
Audiovisual aid, 319-320, 321t, 322
Authoritarian management, 149
Automatic protection system, 230

B

Baccalaureate degree nurse, 412
Balance of trade, 96-97
Barrier to health and safety program development, 196

Behavior
  effects of, 142
  stress response, 335
Behavior change theory, 296-298
Behavioral objectives of American Association of Occupational Health Nurses, 309
Benchmarking, 164-165
Benefit
  definition of, 271
  disability, 287-288
  workers' compensation, 88-89
Benzene, 131
Beryllium, 129
Bias in epidemiological study, 121, 122t
Biologic hazard
  environmental health and, 394-395
  to health care worker, 58-59, 58t
  impact of, 15
Biomechanics, 16
Breath testing for alcohol, 366-367
Brownfield, 407
Budgeting; *see also* Financial issues
  as administrative function, 154-156
  project management and, 161
Bureaucratic management, 151
Burnout, 334
Business plan for health and safety program, 205
Business travel, 345-346
Business trend, 102-103

C

Cadmium, 129
CAGE questionnaire, 303
Calculation of incidence rate, 216
Canal cap, ear, 354-355
Cancer awareness, 303
Cap, canal, 354
Capital expenditure budget, 154
Capitalism, 95
Carbamate, 133
Carbon disulfide, 131
Carbon monoxide, 133
Carcinogen, 123
Case-control study design, 120t
Case management
  disability, 271-291; *see also* Disability case management
  in health and safety program, 199-200
  as role expansion, 433
Case management company as practice setting, 27
Case manager role, 28
Cash benefit, 271-272
Centers for Disease Control and Prevention, 402-403
Certification, 426-427
Chain-of-custody procedure in drug testing, 365
Change, planned, 149-150
Characteristic-specific rate, 118
Chart in educational presentation, 322

Page numbers in *italic* indicate figures; those followed by *t* indicate tables.

Chemical hazard
impact of, on workers, 14-15
magnitude of, 393-395
multiple sensitivity and, 227-228
Chemical inventory, 217
Chi square test, 119
Child
environmental health and, 396-398
toxicology and, 128
in work force, 41-45
international, 61
Chromium, 129
Chronic care, 262
Class advocacy, 399
Clean Water Act, 404
Client-centered management system, 172
Climate, organizational, 153
Clinical decision making in direct care, 256-257
Clinician role, 28
Co-employment, 46
Coaching, of staff, 158
Coal dust, 130-131
Coal Mine Health and Safety Act, 9
Code of ethics, 427; *see also* Ethical issues
Coding, 236
Cohort study design, 120t
Cold, monitoring of, 225
Collaboration, 434
Collaborative leadership, 147
Committee
disaster planning, 368
safety, 234-235
Common law, 71
Communicable disease, 346-347
Communication
by administration, 160-161
in emergency response plan, 371
information management and, 171-187; *see also* Information management
risk, 400-401
Communism, 95
Community, environmental risks in, 406-408
Competency
health assessment, 250-251
in occupational and health nursing, 427-428
Competitiveness, 99-100
Comprehensive health history, 252
Compressive force, 137
Confidence interval, 119
Confidentiality
as ethical conflict, 90-92
in health and safety program, 205
in research, 412
Conflict
ethical, 90-92
of interest, 92
Conflict resolution, 160
Confounding in epidemiological study, 121-122
Consent, informed, 72-73
for research, 412-413
Construction worker, 53-55
Consultant
as nursing role, 28
technical, 371

Consultation by Occupational Safety and Health Administration, 76
Consulting company as practice setting, 27
Consumer price index, 95
Container labeling, 361
Contaminant, sampling of, 135
Contamination, noise, 14
Contingent worker, 45-48
Continuing education, 432
Continuous quality improvement, 165
Control
engineering, 383
noise, 351-352
of occupational exposure, 136
in violence prevention, 330
Coordinator
hazard communication, 359
hearing-loss prevention, 350-351
Corporate director, 28
Corrosive, 123
Cost; *see* Financial issues
Cost-benefit analysis, 203-204
Cost effectiveness, of disability case management, 281-282
Cost-effectiveness analysis, 203-204
Cost saving, format for demonstrating, 155t
Council of European Union, 220
Counseling, as nursing role, 29
Countermeasure, 140-141
Crandall, Ella Phillips, 22
Creativity, 163
Credentialing, 426-427
Critical incident stress debriefing, 238-239, 374
Critical thinking, 162-163
Cross-sectional study design, 120t
Crude rate, 118
Culture, organizational, 152-153
as psychosocial factor, 340
Curve, dose-response, 125

D
Damage assessment, 374-375
Data
in direct care, 267-268
in disability case management, 279
on injury and illness, 19-20
research, 416-417
evaluation of, 420-421
Data sheet, material safety, 134-135, 217
hazard communication and, 360
Debriefing, critical incident stress, 238-239, 374
Decision making
in direct care, 256-257
ethical, 163-164
Deconstructionism, 311t-313t
Deductible, 272
Degreaser's flush, 132
Delayed recovery, 277
Delivery models in disability case management, 289-291
Demand-control model, 336
Democratic management, 151
Demographics, workplace
females and, 36
minorities and, 38-39
Department of Energy, 403
Department of Health and Human Services, 402-403

Department of Labor, 7
Department of Transportation, 80-81
Dependence, nicotine, 302t
Depression, 334
Design, study, 120-121, 415-416
Diploma level nurse, 411
Direct care, 247-268
clinical decision making in, 256-257
definition of, 247-248
health history in, 251-253, 254, 255
outcome evaluation in, 267-268
overview of, 248-251
physical examination in, 255-256
practice guidelines for, 257-258
prevention in, 258-262, 267
role expansion in, 433-434
signs of back pain and, 267
of tendinitis, 263-266
Directives, European and non-European, 220
Director, safety, 368-369
Disability case management, 262, 267, 271-291
case study of, 283-284
definition of, 271
delivery models in, 289-291
goal of, 271
historical perspective on, 273-275
integrated programs in, 288-289
practice settings for, 275
program development for, 278-282
assessment, 278-279
data analysis and diagnosis, 279
evaluation, 280-282, 281
implementation, 280
planning, 280
return to work in, 282, 285-288
team roles and responsibilities in, 275-278
terminology in, 271-273
Disabled worker
definition of, 49
demographics of, 49-50
workplace changes for, 50
Disaster plan, 367-376; *see also* Emergency response plan
Disaster planning committee, 368
Disaster response plan, 200
Disposable income, 95
Distraction test, 267
Doctoral degree nurse, research by, 412
Documentation
characteristics of, 81-82, 82t
of emergency response plan, 375
ergonomics and, 385-386
in health and safety program, 200-201
purpose of, 81
records for
access to, 85-87
preservation of, 85
types of, 83-85
Domain, of nursing, 112-113
Dose-response relationship, 125
Dosimeter, noise, 135
Dosimetry, personal, 224
DOT (Department of Transportation), 80-81

Drug abuse
  lifestyle and, 302
  as stress response, 334
Drug Free Workplace Act, 364-365
Drug testing, 361-367
  consequences of abuse and, 367
  Drug Free Workplace Act and,
    364-365
  elements of program, 365-367
  employee assistance program
    and, 363-364
  preliminary considerations in,
    362-363
  program components in, 363
  purpose of, 362
  training and education in, 364
Dust, types of, 130-131
Duty, 72

E

EAP (employee assistance
  program), 304, 306-307,
  363-364
Ear anatomy, 354
Ear muff, 354
Ear plug, 354
Earning capacity, 272
Ecological model, 336-338, 337
Economic indicator, 96
Economics, 95-106
  balance of trade and, 96-97
  economic indicators and, 96
  impact of, on individual, 97-98
  interest rates and, 96
  labor-force statistics and, 96
  occupational injury and illness,
    17-18
  terminology of, 95-96
  in United States, 97
Economy
  business issues and, 103-105
  business trends and, 102-103
  changes in, 99
  global, 99-101
  health care reform and, 106
  managed care and, 106-109
  occupational health nurse and,
    101-102, 105-106, 109
Education
  adult, 307-324
    behavioral objectives in, 309
    characteristics of, 307
    methods and techniques in,
      314, 315t-317t, 318
    motivation in, 310, 314
    philosophies of, 310, 311t-313t
    presentations in, 318-324
    principles of, 307-308
  for children in work force,
    44-45
  continuing, 432
  drug testing and, 364
  on environmental health
    nursing, 409
  ergonomics and, 384
  in hearing loss prevention,
    353-354
  levels of research and, 411-412
  in occupational health
    nursing, 428
  on technology in workplace,
    35-36
Educator role, 28
EEOC (Equal Employment
  Opportunity Commis-
  sion), 78

Electric forklift, focused checklist
  for, 212
Electric shock, 231
Emergency response plan, 367-376
  appendices to include in, 376
  in comprehensive program, 200
  general procedures in, 371-373
  maintenance of, 375-376
  prevention and, 237-238, 238, 262
  purpose of, 367-368
  recovery procedures in, 374-375
  responsibilities for, 368-371
  scope of, 368
  specific procedures in, 373-374
Employee assistance program, 304,
  306-307
  for drug or alcohol abuse,
    363-364
Employee health record, 84
Employee perception survey, 217
Employee recruitment, 156-157
Employer's role in disability case
  management, 276
Employment rate, low, 98
Endogenous host factor, 126-127
Energy source, hazardous, 231
Engineering, human factors, 15
Engineering controls
  ergonomics and, 383
  in prevention, 228-234, 232, 233
Entrapment, nerve, 137
Environment
  of care, 112
  health effects of, 114-115
  work, 4
    of health care workers, 57-59
Environmental assessment, 192
Environmental exposure history,
  253, 254, 255
Environmental health
  access to information on, 403-404
  advocacy for, 398-399
  assessment of, 395-396
  children and, 396-398
  federal regulation of, 401-403
  nurses' roles in, 408-410
  overview of, 393-395
  pharmacology vs. toxicology
    and, 397t
  risk and, 399-401, 404-408
    in community, 406-408
    in home, 404-406
    in school, 406
  role expansion in, 433
Environmental justice, 398-399
Environmental Protection Agency,
  363, 402
Environmental protection manager,
  emergency response plan
  and, 369
Environmental toxicology, 396
EPA (Environmental Protection
  Agency), 363, 402
Epidemic event, 226
Epidemic hysteria, 226-227
Epidemiology
  data sources in, 118
  definition of, 116-117
  environmental, 395-396
  measures of association in,
    117-118
  of occupational injury, 139-140
  rate comparisons in, 118
  types of rates in, 118-119
Equal Employment Opportunity
  Commission, 78

Equipment
  emergency response and, 376
  farm, 51-52
  personal protective, 239-243,
    242, 243
    ergonomics and, 383-384
  program development and,
    193-194
  storage of, 231
Ergonomics
  analysis in, 218
  components of program of,
    379-384
  improvements in, 139
  musculoskeletal disorder
    and, 378
  overview of, 377-378
  purpose of program in, 379
  regulation and, 378-379
  terminology in, 136
Ethical issues, 89-92
  in administration, 163-164
  confidentiality, 90-92
  conflict of interest and, 92
  definitions and principles of, 90
  in direct care, 249
  in health and safety
    program, 205
  professional standards and,
    89-90
  in research, 412-413
Ethylene oxide, 131-132
European Commission, 13
Evacuation procedure, 372
Evaluation
  audiometric, 356
  in disability case management,
    280-282, 281
  ergonomic, 386
  hazard, 218-219
  of hazard communication
    program, 361
  of health and safety program,
    196-197, 202-204
  of research, 419-421
Examination
  Americans with Disabilities Act
    and, 78
  independent medical, 272
Exceptional circumstance, 72
Exclusive remedy, 272
Excretion of toxin, 126
Exogenous host factor, 127
Expatriate worker, 61-62
Experimental study design, 120,
  415-416
Exposure, chemical, 393-395
Exposure history, 253, 254, 255
Exposure monitoring, 221-224
Exposure record, 83-84
Extra-organizational system, 337
Eye protection, 240

F

Face protection, 240
Facility
  for direct care, 251
  emergency response and, 376
  for health and safety
    program, 194
Fagerstrom test for nicotine
  dependence, 302t
Fair Labor Standards Act, on
  children in work force, 42
Family and Medical Leave Act,
  provisions of, 79

Farm worker
   characteristics of, 50-51
   illness and injury in, 51-53, 52t
Fatal injury, 18
Federal Bureau of Labor, 7
Federal law, 71
Federal legislation
   on disability management, 289
   historical perspective on, 7
Federal Motor Carrier Safety
      Administration, 80
Federal regulation of environmen-
      tal health, 401-403
Federal Reserve discount rate,
      disposable, 95
Federalism, 103-105
Female worker
   international, 61-62
   part-time, 46
   temporary, 47
Financial issues
   budgeting
      as administrative function,
         154-156
      in disability case management,
         274-275, 281-282, 288-289
   economics and, 95-106; see also
      Economics
   format for demonstrating cost
      saving, 155t
   in program development, 193
   project management and, 161
   research funding, 421-422,
      421t-422t
Fire brigade, 370
Firs-aid team, 370
First aid, 262
Fiscal issues, administration and,
      154-156, 155t
Floater, changes in use of, 45-48
Flush, degreaser's, 132
Focused inspection, 211-212
Follow-up drug test, 366
Foot protection, 241
Force, compressive, 137
Forklift, focused checklist for, 212
Form, job safety analysis, 214
Formal inspection, 210
Formaldehyde, 132
Functional capacity evaluation, 272
Funding for research, 421-422,
      421t-422t

G

Garment, thermal, 241
Gatekeeper, 272
Gender, in toxicology, 127
Genetic factors in toxicology, 127
Geographic information
      system, 395
Global competitiveness, 99-100
Global marketplace, 101
Goals
   of Healthy People 2010, 11-12
   of occupational health and
      safety, 3-4
Government, economics and,
      97-98
Government agency as practice
      setting, 27
Grid, review, 177t-180t
Gross national product, 96
Guidelines
   competency, 427-428
   for direct care, 257-258
   human capacity, 382

H

Hand protection, 240
Harassment, 329-330
Hazard
   affecting children, 396-398
   to agricultural worker, 52t
   assessment of, 20
   chemical, magnitude of, 393-395
   to construction worker, 55
   ergonomics and, 381-383
   evaluation and analysis of,
      218-219
   to health care worker, 58-59, 58t
   identification of, 210-218,
      212, 214
   impact of, 13-16
   machine, 231, 232, 233
   psychosocial, 328-333
      impact of, 16
      interventions for, 340
      management of, 338-340
      mistreatment and harassment,
         329-330
      shift work as, 331
      stress and, 332-338;
         see also Stress
      unemployment and under-
         employment as, 330-331
      work characteristics and,
         331-332
      workplace violence as,
         328-329
   recognition of, 134-135
   technology changes and, 36
   types of, 380t
Hazard communication program,
      357-361
Hazardous energy source, 231
Hazardous material
   spill of, 373-374
   storage of, 230-231
Hazardous materials response
      team, 370
Health action process
      approach, 298
Health belief model, 295
Health care benefit, 34
Health care management, 385
Health care reform, 106
Health care worker
   demographics for, 56-57
   environment of, 57-59, 58t
   occupational health nursing and,
      59-61
Health center manager, 369-370
Health event, sentinel, 227
Health goal, national, 11-12
Health history, 251-255
Health model, 295
Health promotion, 293-324
   adult education and, 307-324;
      see also Education, adult
   behavior change theories
      and models of, 296
   in direct care, 250
   employee assistance program
      and, 304, 306
   in health and safety program
      development, 199
   health models in, 295
   lifestyle and, 302-304
   national objectives for, 294-295
   nursing science and, 143
   overview of, 293-294
   prevention and, 298
   in prevention program, 237

Health promotion—cont'd
   program development for,
      298-302, 299, 305t
Health promotion model, 295
Health promotion specialist, as
      nursing role, 28
Health record, employee, 84
Health services coordinator, 28
Health surveillance, 260-262
Healthy People 2010
   direct care and, 250
   goals and initiatives of, 11-12
   health promotion and, 294-295
Hearing loss
   in construction workers, 54-55
   in farm workers, 51
   prevention program for, 349-357
      audiometric testing in,
         355-357, 356
      evaluation of, 357
      manager's role in, 350
      prevention coordinator's role
         in, 350-351
      protection devices and,
         354-355
      purpose of, 349-350
      record keeping in, 357
      requirements for, 351
      worker training and education
         in, 352-354, 354
      worker's role in, 351
   toxicity causing, 128t
Hearing protection, 240
Heat, monitoring of, 224-225
High-risk job, 138
Historic review, incidence,
      215, 217
History, health, 251-255
Home, environmental risks in,
      404-406
Home-based telework, 333
Homicide, 328
Horizontal organizational
      structure, 153
Housekeeping, 236
Human capacity guideline, 382
Human factors engineering, 15
Human resource issues, 156-160
Human resources director, 369
Humanism, 311t-313t
Hydrogen cyanide, 133-134
Hygiene, industrial, 134
Hypothesis, 119, 415
Hysteria, epidemic, 226-227

I

Illness
   benefits for, 287-288
   case management of, 287
   of construction worker, 54
   early diagnosis of, 262
   immediate management of, 285
   of international traveler, 346
   mass psychogenic, 226-227
   prevention of; see Prevention
   work-related
      in agricultural workers,
         51-53, 52t
      definitions of, 17
      overview of, 16-20, 19t
      workers' compensation and, 88
Image of occupational health
      nurse, 163
Immunization
   direct care and, 258
   for international travel, 344

Implementation
  in disability case manage-
    ment, 280
  of health and safety program,
    194-196
In-house health and safety
  program, 195-196
Incidence historic review, 215, 217
Incidence rate, 116, 216
Incident
  causes of, 216
  debriefing after, 238-239, 374
Incident analysis, 214-215
Income, disposable, 95
Income benefit of workers'
  compensation, 89
Incremental budget method, 154
Indemnity benefit, 89
Indemnity plan, 272
Independent medical examina-
  tion, 272
Industrial hygiene, 134
Industrial nursing, history of, 21
Industrial revolution, 6
Industry standard in prevention,
  219-221
Infection
  as biologic hazard, 15
  international travel and, 346-347
Informal inspection, 210
Informatics, nursing, 171-187;
    see also Information
    management
Information
  emergency response plan
    and, 372
  on environmental health, 403-404
Information management, 171-187
  Internet in, 181-183
  intranets in, 183-184
  occupational health nursing and,
    185-187
  office management programs
    and, 184
  overview of, 171-172
  selection of system for, 173-174,
    175, 176, 177t-180t, 181
  tools available for, 172-173
Information system,
  geographic, 395
Information technology
  manager, 370
Informed consent, 72-73
  for research, 412-413
Ingestion of toxin, 125
Inhalation of toxin, 124-125
Injury
  benefits for, 287-288
  case management of, 287
  to construction worker, 54
  early diagnosis of, 262
  epidemiology of, 139-140
  fatal, 18
  immediate management of, 285
  prevention of; see Prevention
  work-related
    to adolescent worker, 42
    in agricultural workers,
      51-53, 52t
    overview of, 16-20, 18t
    workers' compensation and, 88
Inspection
  in hazard identification, 210-212
  by Occupational Safety and
    Health Administration,
    75-76

Institute of Medicine, 409-410
Instrumentation, research, 416
Insurance company as practice
  setting, 26-27
Insurer in disability case manage-
  ment, 277
Integrated disability management,
  288-289
Interaction-based theory, 112
Interdisciplinary team, 159
Interest rate, 96
Intermittent worker, 45-48
International Commission on
  Occupational Health, 13
International labor organization,
  12-13
International Labour Organiza-
  tion, 13
International trade status, 100-101
International travel, 343-348
International worker, 61-62
Internet, 181-183
Interpersonal relationship, 341
Interview, employment, 157
Intranet, 183-184
Inventory, chemical, 217
Ionizing radiation monitoring, 224
Irritant, 123

J
Jet lag, 348t
Job analysis, 272
Job description, 156
Job hazard analysis, 213-214
Job safety analysis form, 214
Journal, research, 418
Justice, environmental, 398-399

L
Labeling
  container, 361
  signs for, 236
Labor
  international, 12-13
  organized
    chronology of, 8
    health and safety reforms
      of, 8-9
Labor-Management Relations
  Act, 7
Labor union
  role of, 8-9
  workers in, 48-49
Laboratory, drug testing, 365
Laissez faire management, 152
Law; see also Legislation
  on child labor, 42
  sources of, 71-72
  workers' compensation,
    10-11; see also Workers'
    compensation
Lead
  effects of, 129-130
  in home, 405
Leadership, 147-148
Leave, unpaid, 79
Legal issues
  Americans with Disabilities Act
    and, 77-78
  basic legal concepts of, 72-73
  children in work force as, 42
  Department of Transportation
    and, 80-81
  in direct care, 249
  documentation as, 81-87,
    82t, 86

Legal issues—cont'd
  Family and Medical Leave
    Act, 79
  in health and safety
    program, 205
  Occupational Safety and
    Health Administration and,
    73-77
  responsibility of nurse as, 73
  sources of law, 71-72
  workers' compensation as,
    87-89
Legislation
  Americans with Disabilities Act
    on alternative worker, 47
    provisions of, 77-78
  Clean Water Act, 404
  Coal Mine Health and Safety
    Act, 9
  on disability management, 289
  Drug Free Workplace Act,
    364-365
  Fair Labor Standards Act, 42
  Family and Medical Leave
    Act, 79
  National Labor Relations Act, 7
  Occupational Safety and Health
    Act, 11
  Omnibus Transportation
    Employee Testing Act, 80-81,
    80t, 365
  Safe Drinking Water Act, 404
  Superfund Amendments and
    Reauthorization Act, 404
  workers' compensation, 10-11
    benefits of, 88-89
    controlling cost of, 104-105
    history of, 10-11
    issues related to, 104
    overview of, 87-88
Lethal dose, 125
Lewin's stages of planned
  change, 150
Liberalism, 311t-313t
Licensure, 426
Lifestyle, 302-304
Linear change, 149
Listening, 160
Literature review, 413-414, 420
Lockout, 231-232
Long-range planning, 148-150
Long-term disability, 288

M
Machine hazard, 231, 232, 233
Machinery, farm, 51
Maintenance
  of emergency response plan,
    375-376
  preventive, 232
Maintenance supervisor, 370-371
Malaria, 346-347
Malpractice, 73
Managed care
  definition of, 272
  disability case management
    and, 275
  outcomes in, 108
  overview of, 106-107
  quality control in, 107-108
Management
  emergency response plan and,
    369, 370
  in ergonomics program, 379
  in hazard communication
    program, 358

Management—cont'd
  health promotion program
      and, 298
  in hearing loss prevention, 350
  information, 171-187; see also
      Information management
  outcome, 164
  process of, 150-152
  project, 161-162
  of psychosocial factors, 338-340
  risk, in environmental health,
      399-400
  role expansion in, 433
  time, 162
  total quality, 165-166
  work restriction, 175, 176
Marketplace, global, 101
Mass hysteria, 226-227
Master's degree nurse, 412
Material safety data sheet,
      134-135, 217
  hazard communication
      and, 360
Matrix, risk-analysis, 221
Maximum medical improve-
      ment, 272
Mechanic stress, 137
Mechanical hazard, 15-16
Media tool, 319-320, 321t, 322
Medical examination
  Americans with Disabilities Act
      and, 78
  independent, 272
Medical improvement,
      maximum, 272
Medical removal, 237
Medical review officer, 366
Medical surveillance, 260-262
Megatrend, business, 102-103
Mentoring, 157-158
Mercury, 130
Methylene chloride, 132
Microsystem, 337
Middle Ages, work in, 4-5
Milwaukee Visiting Nurse
      Assocation, 21
Minorities in work force,
      38-39
Mission of occupational health
      and safety, 3
Mistreatment, 329-330
Model
  behavior change, 296-298
  health, 295
  occupational stress, 335-336
  person-environment, 335
Monitoring, exposure, 221-224
  atmospheric, 223
  continuous, 224
  ionizing radiation, 223
  of noise, 222-223
  sampling in, 222
  surface, 224
  temperature, 223-224
Motivation
  in adult education, 310, 314
  of staff, 158
Muff, ear, 354
Multiple chemical sensitivity,
      227-228
Musculoskeletal disorder
  ergonomics and, 377-386;
      see also Ergonomics
  as stress response, 334
  types of, 136-137
Mutagen, 123

N
n-Hexane, 132
National Center for Environmental
      Health, 402
National competitiveness, 99-100
National health goals and
      objectives, 11-12; see also
      Healthy People 2010
National Institute for Occupational
      Health and Safety
  agricultural initiative of, 52
  equation for manual lifting
      of, 218
  establishment of, 7
  function of, 77
  on research priorities, 418-419
  on workplace violence, 329
National Labor Relations Act, 7
Needlestick injury, regulations
      about, 57-58
Needs-based theory, 112
Negligence, definition of, 72
Negotiation, 160
Nerve entrapment, 137
Nervous system, toxic effects on,
      128t
Network, information, 183-184
Networking, 160
Newsletter, safety, 236
Nicotine dependence, test for,
      302t
Nightingale, Florence, 111
NIOSH; see National Institute
      for Occupational Health
      and Safety
Noise assessment, 351-352
Noise contamination, 14
  to farm worker, 51-52
Noise dosimeter, 135
Noise level, 353t
  monitoring of, 222
Noise reduction rating, 355
Nonexperimental study design,
      120-121, 415
Nonfatal injury, number of, 18
Nonoccupational illness benefits,
      287-288
Notification in emergency response
      plan, 372
Nuclear Regulatory Commis-
      sion, 403
Nurse; see Occupational and
      environmental health nurse
Nursing; see Occupational and
      environmental health
      nursing
Nursing Informatics, 171-187;
      see also Information
      management
Nursing organization, 22-24
Nursing practice; see Practice,
      nursing
Nursing science, 111-143; see also
      Science, nursing
Nursing theory, development of,
      111-112

O
Objectives of occupational health
      and safety, 3-4
Observational assessment, 134
Occupational and environmental
      health nurse
  in disability case manage-
      ment, 276
  economics and, 101, 106, 109

Occupational and environmental
      health nurse—cont'd
  environmental health and,
      408-410
  health surveillance by, 261
  in international travel
      program, 344
  worker populations and
      agricultural worker, 53
      children, 44
      construction workers, 55
      contingent workers, 47
      disabled workers, 50
      expatriate worker, 61-62
      females, 37
      health care workers, 60-61
      labor union members, 48-49
      minorities, 37-38
      older workers, 38-39
Occupational and environmental
      health nursing
  advanced practice, 247
  credentialing in, 426-427
  domain of, 112-113
  future challenges and opportuni-
      ties in, 29-30
  history and evolution of, 21-24
  information systems and,
      185-187
  partnerships in, 434-435
  practice of, 24-29
  professional development of,
      428, 429t-431t, 432-433
  professional organizations of,
      22-24, 425-426
  role expansion of, 433-434
Occupational exposure history,
      253, 254, 255
Occupational health and safety
  evolution of, 7-10
  hazards in workplace and,
      13-16
  history of, 4-7
  international, 12-13
  mission and goals of, 3-4
  national health goals and, 11-12
  Occupational Safety and Health
      Act and, 11
  overview of, 3-4
  prevention in, 20-21
  work-related illness and,
      18-20, 19t
  work-related injury and,
      16-18, 18t
  workers' compensation
      and, 10-11
Occupational health and safety
      program, 191-205, 343-386
  assessments needed for, 191-193
  business approach to, 205
  drug and alcohol testing in,
      361-367
  emergency preparedness and,
      367-376; see also Emergency
      response plan
  ergonomics, 377-386; see also
      Ergonomics
  evaluation of, 196-197, 202-204
  hazard communication in,
      357-361
  on hearing loss, 349-357;
      see also Hearing loss
  implementation of, 194-196
  for international travel, 343-348
  outcome of, 201-202
  planning of, 193-194

Occupational health and safety
    program—cont'd
    process of, 199-201, 297t
    structure of, 197-199, 197t
Occupational Health Nurse in
    Agricultural Communities
    program, 52-53
Occupational health nursing
    model of, 4, 5
    temporary workers and, 47-48
Occupational health services
    coordinator, as nursing
    role, 28
Occupational health system review
    grid, 177t-180t
Occupational Safety and Health
    Act, 6-7
    provisions of, 11
Occupational Safety and Health
    Administration
    definitions of, 16-17
    environmental health and, 403
    hazard communication standard
        of, 357-358
    hearing standards of, for
        construction workers, 54-55
    on needlestick injury, 57-58
    records required by, 83
        access to, 85, 86, 87
        preservation of, 85
    responsibilities of, 73-76
    voluntary protection program
        of, 76-77
Occupational Safety and Health
    Review Commission, 77
Office management program, 184
Older worker, 39-40
Omnibus Transportation Employee
    Testing Act, 80-81, 80t, 365
On-site direct care, 248-249
On-site disability case manage-
    ment, 289-290
Operating budget, 154
Organizaed labor
    workers in, 48-49
Organization
    emergency response plan and,
        371-372
    nursing, 22-24
    professional, 425-426
    stress effects on, 335
    of work, as stress factor, 34
Organizational culture, 152-153
    as psychosocial factor, 340
Organizational system, 337
Organized labor
    chronology of, 8
    health and safety reforms of, 8-9
Organochlorine, 133
Organophosphate, 133
OSHA; see Occupational Safety
    and Health Administration
Outcome
    in direct care, 267-268
    in health and safety program,
        201-202
Outcome-based theory, 112
Outcome management, 164
Overreaction, back pain with, 267

P
p-value, 119
Paradigm, of organizational
    culture, 152-153
Paradigm of organizational
    culture, 152

Part-time worker, 45-48
Participatory management, 151
Passive surveillance, 380-381
Performance appraisal, 159
Peri-organizational system, 337
Permissible exposure limit, 135
Permissive management, 152
Permit, work, 235-236
Person-environment model, 335
Personal dosimetry, 224
Personal protective equipment,
    239-243, 242, 243
    ergonomics and, 383-384
Pesticide
    effects of, 133
    in home, 405
Pharmacology vs. toxicology, 397t
Philosophy of adult education, 310,
    311t-313t
Physical examination, 255-256
Physical hazard, 13-14
Physician in disability case
    management, 276
Planned behavior theory, 297
Planning
    in disability case manage-
        ment, 280
    of health and safety program,
        193-194
    of health promotion program,
        298-299
    strategic, 148-150
Plug, ear, 354
Policy
    administration, 153-154
    on drug testing, 363
    health and safety program
        development and, 196
Pollution, air, 406
Population
    research, 416
    worker
        age of workers in, 39-40
        agricultural, 51-53, 52t
        analysis of, in prevention,
            225-228
        changes in, 33
        children, 41-45
        construction, 53-55
        contingent, 45-48
        disabled, 49-50
        expatriate, 61-62
        female, 36-37
        health care, 56-61
        minority, 38-39
        statistics about, 96
Post-accident drug test, 366
Post-incident evaluation, 374
Postindustrial era, 6-7
Postinspection activity, 211
Power of study, 120
PPE; see Personal protective
    equipment
Practice
    nursing
        functional roles in, 27-28
        professionalism and, 432-433
        research and, 112
        science influencing, 114
        scope of, 25-26
        settings of, 26-27
        specialized roles in, 28-29
        standards of, 24-25
    work, controlling of, 234
Practice guidelines for direct care,
    257-258

Practice standard, 427
Predictive value of screening,
    122-123
Preemployment drug test, 366
Preindustrial age, 5-6
Preinspection activity, 210-211
Preplacement examination, 258-259
Presentation, educational, 318-324
    audiovisuals in, 319-320,
        321t, 322
    delivery of, 323-324
    elements of, 318
    evaluation of, 324
    logistics of, 320, 322-323
    preparation of, 318-319
    types of, 318
Prevalence rate, 117
Prevention, 209-243
    assessment of exposure and, 20
    control approaches in,
        228-234, 233
        administrative, 234-239, 238
        engineering, 228-234, 232, 233
        personal protective equipment,
            239-243, 242, 243
    in direct care, 258-262, 267
    in ergonomics program, 382-383
    exposure monitoring in, 221-224
    hazard evaluation and analysis
        in, 218-219
    hazard identification in, 210-218,
        212, 214
    hearing loss; see Hearing loss,
        prevention program for
    industry standards and, 219-221
    levels of, 298
    of lost-time injury, 285
    of malaria, 346
    steps in, 209-210
    surveillance in, 224-225
    of violence, 330
    worker population analysis in,
        225-228
Preventive maintenance, 232
Primary care, definition of;
    see Direct care
Problem solving, 162-163
Problem-specific health history,
    252-253
Process elements in health and
    safety program, 197t,
    199-201
Process safety review, 217-218
Professional issues in direct
    care, 249
Professionalism
    credentialing and, 426-427
    organizations in, 425-426
    partnerships and, 434-435
    professional development and,
        428, 429t-431t
Program
    education and research, 429t-431t
    occupational health and safety,
        191-205, 343-386; see also
        Occupational health and
        safety program
Progressivism, 311t-313t
Project management, 161-162
Promotion, safety, 236-237
Prospective study design, 120t
Protection motivation theory, 298
Protective equipment, 239-243,
    242, 243
    ergonomics and, 383-384
Psychogenic illness, mass, 226-227

Psychologic disorder, 34
Psychology, engineering, 15
Psychosocial hazard, 327-340
  impact of, on workers, 16
  interventions for, 340
  management of, 338-340
  mistreatment and harassment,
    329-330
  overview of, 327-328
  shift work, 331
  stress as, 332-340; *see also* Stress
  unemployment and underem-
    ployment, 330-331
  work characteristics and, 331-332
  workplace violence, 328-329
Public health, 111
Public Health Service, 7

Q

Qualitative data, 417
Quantitative data, 417
Questionnaire
  CAGE, 303
  employee perception, 217

R

Radiation hazard, 394-395
  monitoring of, 224
  protection from, 241
Radicalism, 311t-313t
Random drug test, 366
Rate
  incidence, 116
  prevalence, 117
Rating, noise reduction, 355
Reasonable accommodation, 78
Reasonable suspicion drug
    test, 366
Reasoned action theory, 297
Recommended exposure level, 136
Record
  access to, 85-87
  in hazard identification, 212-213
  in hearing loss prevention
    program, 357
  preservation of, 85
  types of, 83-85
Record keeping
  on drug testing, 363
  in emergency response plan,
    372-373
  ergonomics and, 385-386
  in hazard communication, 361
  in health and safety program,
    200-201
Recovery after emergency, 374
Recruitment, employee, 156-157
Reengineering, 166
Regional strength test, 267
Regulation
  ergonomic, 378-379
  mandatory compliance with, 103
Regulatory agency as practice
    setting, 27
Rehabilitation, 272
Rehabilitation specialist, 277-278
Reliability of research instru-
    ment, 416
...eated trauma disorder, 19
...tion of task, 137
...ing of emergency, 372
..., 411-422
...dren in work force, 45
...onmental health
...ng, 409
...2-413

Research—cont'd
  evaluation of, 419-421
  funding of, 421-422, 421t-422t
  nurses' roles in, 411-412
  as nursing role, 28
  priorities for, 418-419
  procedures in, 413-418
  professional mandates for, 411
  professionalism and, 428,
    429t-431t, 432
  purpose of, 412
  utilization of, 418
Reserves, 272
Residual functional capacity,
    272-273
Resource, in program develop-
    ment, 193-194
Respirable dust, 130-131
Respiratory disorder, 19
Respiratory protection, 241-243,
    242, 243
Respiratory system
  inhalation of toxin and, 124-125
  toxic effects on, 128t
Resume, screening of, 157
Return-to-duty drug test, 366
Return to work
  definition of, 273
  in disability case management,
    282, 285-288
Review
  in hazard identification, 212-213
  historic incidence, 215, 217
  literature, 413-414
  process safety, 217-218
  utilization, 273
Review grid, 177t-180t
Right-to-know statute, 403-404
Rights under Family and Medical
    Leave Act, 79
Risk
  assessment of, 399-400
  calculation of, 221
  environmental, 399-401, 404-408
    in community, 406-408
    in home, 404-406
    in school, 406
  perception of, 401t
  reduction of, 143
Risk-analysis matrix, *221*
Risk appraisal, 300
Risk communication, 400-401
Risk factor
  evaluation of, 138-139
  for musculoskeletal disorder,
    137-138
Risk management
  definition of, 273
  in environmental health,
    399-400
  as nursing role, 28
Role expansion of nurse, 433-434
Role stress, 330-331

S

Safe Drinking Water Act, 404
Safety
  of international traveler, 345
  as nursing role, 28-29
  program development involving,
    191-205; *see also* Occupa-
    tional health and safety
    program
  training in, 235
Safety analysis, 213-214
Safety analysis form, *214*

Safety committee, 234-235
Safety director, 368-369
Safety newsletter, 236
Safety review, process, 217-218
Sampling, 135
  in exposure monitoring, 222
Schedule, work, 235
School environment, 406
Science, nursing, 111-143
  airborne contaminants and,
    135-136
  control countermeasures and,
    140-141
  control strategies in, 136
  domain of nursing and, 113-114
  environmental health and,
    115-116
  epidemiology and, 116-122
    of injury, 139-140
  ergonomics and, 136, 139
  hazard recognition and, 134-135
  health promotion and, 143
  high-risk jobs and, 138
  history of, 111-112
  industrial hygiene and, 134
  inferential statistics in, 119-120
  musculoskeletal disorders and,
    136-138
  nursing practice and, 115
  nursing theory and, 114-115
  occupational health nursing
    and, 141
  research-theory-practice linkages,
    112-113
  risk factor evaluation in,
    138-139
  sampling methods in, 135
  screening and, 122-123
  social conditions and behavior
    and, 142
  toxicology and, 123-134;
    see also Toxicology
Screening
  characteristics of, 122-123
  in direct care, 259-260
  employment, 157
Secret, trade, 360-361
Security, workplace, 34-35
Security personnel in emergency
    response, 370
Self-directed learning, 308
Sensitizer, 123
Sentinel health event, 227
Servant leadership, 147
Service effectiveness, 281
Service efficiency, 281
Service sector job, 35
Sexual harassment, 329-330
Sexually transmitted disease, 347
Shift work, 331
Shock, electric, 231
Sign, warning, 236
Silica, 131
Simulation test, 267
Site-centered management
    system, 173
Skin disorder
  number of, 19
  toxin causing, 125, 128t
Skin protection, 240
Skin wipe, 135
Sleep disorder, 334
SOAP formula for documenta-
    tion, 82t
Social activism, 9-10
Social behavior theory, 298

Social factor
  children in work force as, 43-44
  effects of, 142
  females in workplace and, 37
Social learning theory, 296-297
Solvent, 131-132
Specialist, rehabilitation, 277-278
Spill, hazardous material, 373-374
Staff development, 157-158
Stages of change model, 296, 297t
Standard
  of care, 72
  ethical, 89-90
  hazard communication, 357-358
  industry, 219-221
  practice, 427
Standardized rate, 119
State law, 71
State legislation, 7
Statute
  definition of, 71
  of limitations, 73
  right-to-know, 403-404
Storage
  of equipment, 231
  of hazardous material, 230-231
Strategic planning, 148-150
Strategy, control, 136
Stress, 332-338
  of business travel, 345-346
  causes of, 332-333
  as common problem, 34
  critical-incident stress debriefing
    and, 238-239, 374
  epidemic, 227
  mechanical, 15, 137
  occupational, 333-340
    conditions leading to,
      333-334
    definition of, 333
    ecological approach to,
      336-338
    effect of, 334-335
    facts about, 333
    management of, 338-340
    models of, 335-336
  psychosocial, 16
  thermal, 14
  monitoring of, 223-224
Study design, 120-121, 415-416
Substance abuse
  lifestyle and, 302
  as stress response, 334
  testing for, 361-367
Superficial tenderness with back
    pain, 267
Superfund Amendments and
    Reauthorization Act, 404
Superfund site, 407
Supervisor
  emergency response plan
    and, 369
  maintenance, 370-371
Surveillance
  ergonomics program and,
    380-381
  medical, 260-262
  in prevention, 224-225
Survey, employee perception, 217
Switchboard operator in
    emergency response, 370
Systems model, 336

T

Tactical leadership, 147
Tagout, 231-232

Teaching; *see also* Education
  effective, 308
  methods and techniques of, 314,
    315t-317t, 318
Team
  disability case management,
    275-278
  information systems, 173-174
  interdisciplinary, 159
Team building, 158-159
Technical consultant, 371
Technician, audiometric, 356
Technology, trends in, 35-36
Telecommuting, 34
Telephonic disability case
    management, 290-291
Telework, 333
Temperature-related stress, 14
Temporary worker, 45-48
Tendinitis, 263-266
Teratogen, 123
Terminology
  of economics, 95-96
  in ergonomics, 136
  surveillance, 224
Testing
  audiometric, 355-357, *356*
  drug, 361-367
  under Omnibus Transportation
    Employee Testing Act,
    80-81, 80t
Theory
  behavior change, 296-298
  nursing
    development of, 111-112
    early, 112
    middle-range, 113-114
    research and, 112
Therapeutics, nursing, 113
Thermal garment, 241
Thermal stress, 14
Third-party administrator, 273
  as practice setting, 26-27
Threshold limit value, 135-136
Time management, 162
Tobacco use, 302
Toluene, 132
Tool
  information management,
    172-173
  media, 319-320, 321t, 322
Tornado, 373
Torso protection, 241
Tort, 72
Total quality management,
    165-166
Toxic chemical, 14-15
Toxicology, 123-132
  definitions in, 123-124
  dose-response relationship
    in, 125
  effects of toxin and, 125-126
  environmental, 396
  excretion of toxin and, 126
  exposure in, 124-125
  host factors in, 126-127
  pharmacology *vs.*, 397t
  work-related exposure and,
    128-134
    asphyxiant, 133-134
    dust, 130-131
    metals, 128-129, 128-130
    pesticide, 133
    solvent, 131-132
Trade secret, 360-361
Trade status, 100-101

Training
  in drug testing, 364
  in emergency response, 375-376
  ergonomics and, 384
  in hazard communication,
    359-360
  in hearing loss prevention,
    353-354
  for older workers, 40
  safety, 235
  staff, 158
Transactional leadership, 147
Transformation of toxin, 126
Transformational leadership, 147
Transitional work in disability case
    management, 273, 286-287
Transtheoretical theory, 296, 297t
Travel, international, 343-348
Trend, business, 102-103
Trichloroethylene, 132

U

Underemployment, 330-331
Unemployment, 330-331
United States Department
    of Agriculture, 403
United States Department
    of Labor, 7
United States Public Health
    Service, 7
Urgent care, 262
Utilization review, 273
Utilization review company,
    as practice setting, 27

V

Validity of research instrument, 416
Variable in study, 415
Vendor-contracted health
    and safety program, 196
Ventilation, in prevention
    system, 230
Vertical organizational
    structure, 153
Vibration, 137-138
Videotaping in risk evaluation,
    138-139
Violence, work-site, 228, 328-329
  increase in, 34-35
Virtual office, 34
Vision, toxic effects on, 128t
Voluntary protection program,
    76-77

W

Waddell's signs for low back
    pain, 267
Warning labeling, container, 361
Warning sign, 236
Water, federal regulation of, 404
Wellness program, establishment
    of, 10
Work
  organization of, as stress
    factor, 34
  shift, 331
  transitional, 273, 286-287
Work environment of health care
    worker, 57-59
Work force
  age of workers in, 39-40
  agricultural workers in,
    51-53, 52t
  changes in, 33
  children in, 41-45
  construction, 53-55

Work force—cont'd
   contingent workers in, 45-48
   disabled workers in, 49-50
   expatriate, 61-62
   females in, 36-37
   health care, 56-61
   minorities in, 38-39
   statistics about, 96
Work permit, 235-236
Work physiology, 15
Work-related exposure, 128-134
Work-related injury, 16
Work-related musculoskeletal
      disorder, 377-386
Work restriction management,
      175, 176
Work schedule, exposure control
      by, 235
Work-site analysis, 379-380

Work-site violence, 228, 328-329
   increase in, 34-35
Worker; *see also* Work force
   characteristics of, 341
   emergency response plan
      and, 370
   in ergonomics program, 379
   hazard communication and,
      359-360
   in hearing loss prevention, 351
   in labor union, 48-49
Worker population; *see* Population,
      worker
Worker-related assessment,
      191-192
Workers' compensation
   benefits of, 88-89
   controlling cost of, 104-105
   history of, 10-11

Workers' compensation—cont'd
   issues related to, 104
   overview of, 87-88
Workload, 330
Workplace
   assessment of, 192
   environments of, 4
   historical perspective on, 6-7
   international, 61-62
   technologic trends in,
      35-36
   violence in, 34-36
Worksite engineering design,
      229-230
World Health Organization, 13
Wright, Florence, 21

Z
Zero-based budget method, 155